The Humanistic Nursing Process

The Humanistic Nursing Process

Elaine Lynne La Monica, Ed.D., F.A.A.N.
Teachers College, Columbia University

 Wadsworth Health Sciences Division
Monterey, California

Wadsworth Health Sciences Division
A Division of Wadsworth, Inc.

Printed in the United States of America

10 9 8 7 6 5 4 3 2 1

Library of Congress Cataloging in Publication Data

Main entry under title:

The Humanistic nursing process.

　　Includes some articles reprinted from various
sources.
　　Bibliography: p.
　　Includes indexes.
　　1. Nursing—Philosophy. 2. Nursing—Problems,
exercises, etc. 3. Medicine and the humanities.
I. La Monica, Elaine Lynne, [date]　　. [DNLM:
1. Humanism. 2. Nursing Process. WY 100 H9183]
RT84.5.H85　　1985　　610.73'01　　　　84-23694
ISBN 0-534-04428-X

Sponsoring Editor: Aline Faben
Editorial Assistant: Mary Beth McDavid
Production Editor: C. Diane Brown
Manuscript Editor: Marilu Uland
Permissions Editor: Mary Kay Hancharick
Interior Design: Richard Kharibian
Cover Design: John Edeen
Interior Illustration: Brenda Booth
Typesetting: Omegatype Typography, Inc.,
　　Champaign, Illinois
Printing and Binding: Malloy Lithographing, Inc.,
　　Ann Arbor, Michigan

A Spirit grows...
           It brings Life.

Life grows...
           Love follows.

In the fullness of love
Is a flower.
Each delicate petal grows bigger

      And cares more...

To this process
      This book is dedicated.

           Elaine Lynne La Monica

27 January 1984

Preface

The wet, cold snow squeezed under my fleece-lined boots; wind tore through the trees; yet, snowflakes melting on my nose felt like a pleasant sting embraced in warmth. I was alone and the night was dark, but out of this frosty, angry night fell pure white, delicate sculptures. I could never fully describe or share what I saw and what I felt that night. For a person to know the beauty of anger and happiness, cold and hot, pain and health, crystal and wood, darkness and sunshine, one must either experience by seeing, touching, listening, smelling, or tasting, or one must fantasize on the basis of a shared experience.

That night I was relieved at 11 P.M. from my work as a nurse in the intensive-care unit of a large city hospital. The expressions of anguish and peacefulness in a dying patient, the joy and sorrow of a new mother, the pain and serenity of a human being disfigured . . . . "A paradox," I thought, "a complete, utter paradox. What if it were me? I would be angry with the disfigurement, I would hate, I would toss with the pain, and I would cry out, seeking an answer to 'Why me? I have not finished yet.'"

Later I sat at my dining room table thinking: If they can know and understand, why is it so difficult for me to know and understand? I should be helping them. I should bring them relief, hope, and comfort. I should understand, but, in fact, they knew and I did not.

The parted curtains allowed the whiteness of the snow to shine in like a warm, protective beacon. I opened my window and felt the bite of the air; I put a handful of snow to my lips and felt the numbness slowly replaced by a glowing, spreading warmth. Reflecting on myself, my form took a new shape and my mind a new form: I am a person with experience first, a teacher second. I know in each of these facets the only absolute is me as an individual.

My communion with nursing seemed a separate turmoil, but it was actually one with my experience of the night since I believe that the strongest contribution I can offer is to be present and share me—my thoughts, my experiences, and my feelings. I also believe that, as a teacher, I should share myself and enable others to develop inner experiences and awarenesses that will be uniquely their own.*

This book grows from my experience in trying to develop effective ways to teach both prospective and practicing nurses the importance and meaning of the nursing process in the implementation of professional nursing care. Regrettably, my experience with students and colleagues makes it all too clear that cognitive knowledge frequently does not get carried into behavior. Information confined to printed words and case studies essentially restricts students to "head trips" and fails to build the necessary bridges among formalized learning, attitudinal development, and resulting professional practice.

In my search for ways to provide learners with an opportunity to observe, experience, and carry out actual behavior, I have used humanistic approaches in learning with human-relations techniques. The humanistic teaching process involves cognitive and affective components of learning, including formalized classroom teaching, personalization of vicarious experience, and actual professional practice. Learners are able thereby to study and consider theory, to employ individual resources in the educative process, and, ultimately, to enter into practice with learned, new behaviors that are truly integrated components of the learners' beliefs.

The humanistic approach corresponds with our current trend in nursing to administer individualized care. Since the student is the focus in academic settings, it follows that the learning process must be individualized. Theory must be presented in a way that provides students with the opportunity to bring these ideas into step with their own personal learning processes, to adapt these ideas into their own individual frameworks and definitions of nursing, and then, to practice accordingly. The result is *knowing* the nursing process as opposed to *knowing about* it. Several years of experimenting with this teaching approach has convinced me that it is far superior to any other method with which I am familiar. The results have been learners with increased empathy for clients and colleagues; heightened sensitivity to the needs of others, as well as ways in which to meet them; and most importantly, increasing behavioral consistency between classroom and service environments.

This book follows a course that covers the entire nursing process by examining the individual components that make up the whole. The book contains humanistic, multimedia approaches to integrating theory with practice and beliefs. It is suggested that study be weighted so that greater time is devoted to the experiential elements, since enriched learning can be derived from actual and vicarious experience. Pertinent articles relating to chapter topics are included to increase the learner's perceptions of a particular area. The reader should conceptualize the material, using knowledge from all of life's resources, and should subsequently form individual attitudinal bases

---

The above was a personal experience of E. L. La Monica. From "A Creative Approach to Individualized Nursing Care," by S. M. Brainerd and E. L. La Monica, *Nursing Forum*, 1975, 14, 188–193. Reprinted by permission.

for practice. The text provides the groundwork in nursing-process theory. Humanistic exercises at the end of each Part provide the learner with an experiential base. Careful explanations of the purpose of each exercise are included. The text and exercises are designed for use both in self-learning and classroom environments and for use in both individual and group learning experiences.

The primary thrust of this book is the study of the nursing process, our foundation of professional nursing practice. It is intended to be used in nursing process and practice courses at all levels of nursing education and as nursing inservice or continuing-education experiences.

ACKNOWLEDGMENTS

The theory, exercises, and philosophy in this book have been derived from many personal and professional resources. Some are original, and some are from established sources to whom credit is most gratefully given; others have evolved from a constant interchange with professionals whose commitment has been to professional quality. I would like to particularly thank Maxine Greene, colleague and friend, for her eloquent and sensitive chapter on ethics; Eunice M. Parisi-Carew, Sister Kathleen Black, and Virginia Earles, whose knowledge and experience are woven into the content of this entire book; Beryl Skog for her clinical expertise; Aline Faben and James Keating for their unending assistance; and Mary Conlon for her help in preparing the final manuscript of this book.

To all who have molded my beliefs, to all from whom I have received, I express my sincere gratitude.

Elaine Lynne La Monica

Contents

HUMANISTIC EXERCISES
Implementing: Initiating and
Completing Actions   239

PART V
Evaluating: Determining Extent
of Goal Attainment   245

HUMANISTIC EXERCISES
Evaluating: Determining Extent
of Goal Attainment   287

PART VI
Nursing: A Helping
Profession   305

The Humanistic
Nursing Process

Introduction: The Nursing Process and Its Presentation

The nursing process is the scientific method of the nursing profession. It is the approach used to increase the effectiveness of nursing care based on the client's individual system. Grounded on scientific rather than intuitive bases, it can be used developmentally; continuity of care is therefore implicit. As a system within itself, it is dynamic, since it moves and changes in response to the system within which it is applied. Moreover, the nursing process provides the framework upon which education of the future nurse is built.

Maintaining step with all variations of the scientific method of problem-solving processes, the nursing process is respectful of and applicable in any setting or system with any client regardless of the client's place on the health-illness continuum. Furthermore, the process can be interpreted within the construct of any theoretic framework of phenomenologic experience. The nursing process, along with effective actualization of the process, frames the entire profession of nursing—practice and education. It provides a strategy for individualized nursing care and is the foundation for nursing education.

The term *nursing process* was initially coined by Hall (1955). Describing care on a scale of bad to good, Hall designated four prepositions in the nurse/client relationship. Moving from poor to very good, they were: nursing *at* the client, *to* the client, *for* the client, and *with* the client. Thus, the preposition *with* denotes higher processes than those prepositions preceding it; *with* implies being a part of the client's system and moving toward effective nurse/client outcomes. The client is the leader of his or her system, and, hence, also the leader in care.

Later in the fifties, Kreuter (1957) discussed the steps of the nursing process as we know them today but did not label them as such. Coordinating, planning, and evaluating nursing care were seen as promoting quality and professional practice. Johnson (1959) later included the need to assess, make decisions, and delineate actions.

Many subsequent authors have used variations on the theme in describing the nursing process, but the intent remains similar. Orlando (1961) identified three factors as the process: (1) client behavior, (2) nurse reaction, and (3) nursing actions. Knowles (1967) described nurse activity with five verbs: discover, delve, decide, do, and discriminate. Three steps of nursing care are explicated by Orem (1980): (1) secure information from the client and make decisions regarding the need for nursing care, (2) design nursing actions and plan for delivery, and (3) control and evaluate care. Yura and Walsh (1983) delineated the steps of the nursing process as assessment, planning, implementation, and evaluating nursing care.

This author uses the steps of the nursing process as defined and described by the National Council of State Boards of Nursing (1982). These steps are assessing, analyzing, planning, implementing, and evaluating. The Council viewed these steps as nursing behaviors. Then, there are three decision styles: what the nurse does in a system (1) when the locus of decision lies with the nurse, (2) when the locus of decision is shared by the nurse and the client, and (3) when the locus of decision is centered in the client's control. The test plan for the current national licensure examination of registered nurses defines the health requirements of clients within systems that relate to the three decision styles; each decision style then focuses on each of the five steps of the nursing process.

Nursing is a human service. Yet, too often one hears of "dehumanization" in health care brought on by technologic advances in medicine as well as by practitioners who function in an automatic, mechanical manner. It is hoped that dehumanization is the exception, not the rule, in health care today. Nursing, because of its unique position in the health team of being most closely and directly involved with clients, certainly has a primary goal that is vital to total client well-being: to provide humanistic care adapted to individual needs, thereby enabling the client to reach fullest health potential.

This author sees the humanistic approach to the nursing process as being essential to quality care, as well as to the future of health care. The humanistic approach takes into consideration all that is known about an individual, such as thoughts, feelings, values, experiences, likes, desires, behavior, and body. The humanistic approach involves a continual learning process in which the student is an active participant. Each facet of the learner—thoughts, feelings, body, and all others—is integrated into a learning modality that is based on content and experience. Learning then becomes an individualized experience, parallel to nursing's goal of giving individualized nursing care.

The learner need not be only the student of nursing. Rather, the student is also the practicing nurse, the client, the client's entire system, and other members of the health team. The humanistic use of the nursing process yields a continuous learning experience in giving and receiving care. New data are continuously accumulated, learned, and used; new experiences are constantly occurring; and new behaviors are continuously being exchanged for old, unworkable, unhealthy ones. The client is as involved in the nursing process as is the nurse. The intent of humanism, therefore, is to enable a self-aware nurse to provide care for and with an individual, whole client—that is, a client with feelings, thoughts, values, and experiences, as well as a body. (See Part VI for a further discussion of humanism.)

To set the humanistic approach to the nursing process into motion, a systems approach is recommended. The systems approach involves taking into consideration all interrelated aspects of a person, a situation, a group, or an environment. A client's system, for example, could include the client's family, employer, fellow workers, and members of the health team; each of these "components" of the client's system interact. In addition, environmental factors influence the client's system. By taking a systems approach, all persons and things affecting the client are considered as well as the interactions among the parts of the system.

It is important to note that each system is unique, is composed of parts that may change, and has a definite purpose. Often, identifying the purpose of a system makes it easier to study the system and to determine the problems and assets of the system.

Nursing itself is a dynamic, open system. *Dynamic* means it is everchanging; *open* means that people and environmental factors move in and out in response to the system's purposes or goals. The client, of course, is also an open, dynamic system, as are almost all systems involved in health caregiving. (For a theoretic discussion of the systems approach as it relates to nursing, refer to Part VI.)

In this book, the systems approach forms a basic organizational structure that enables the nursing student or practitioner to integrate elements of humanism with knowledge and skills. The book moves from simple to complex, beginning with simple concepts and methods and building on these to form a spiraling network of interrelated elements comprising the entire nursing process. Each chapter presents information and experiences that build upon each other. As the book progresses, the importance and interrelatedness of each method, skill, and concept emerge with more clarity. It is the intent of this book that the nursing student and practitioner ultimately *know the nursing process, rather than know about it.*

The book is organized into Parts by the steps of the nursing process: assessing, analyzing, planning, implementing, and evaluating. Each step provides the basis for the methods and concepts that follow. In addition, the skills and competencies that are essential in order to carry out the specific step of the process are presented in the same Part. The last Part, entitled "Nursing: A Helping Profession," takes a closer look at nursing as a helping profession in addition to providing a conceptual framework for the nursing process itself and the ideals of humanism. Nursing definitions are also provided. The goals of the nursing process are amplified using the expanse of knowledge that has accumulated throughout the book. These concepts of the humanistic nursing process are both the beginning and the end of the nursing process. Therefore, you may wish to refer to Part VI throughout the course of study.

In fulfillment of the objectives of this book, content, theory, and applications all are presented in each chapter. These discussions are often followed by classic selected readings by other authors to amplify and extend the material presented by this author. The appendix contains a key to abbreviations used in the book.

Learning exercises are provided following each Part of the book. Many can actually be done in the book and used as assignments or be done in discussion groups at home, in the learning laboratory, or in the classroom. It is the purpose of these exercises to provide practice experiences that illustrate the content of the chapters, as well as to expand your own range of experience. This book is intended as a learning tool that can be used in any stage of your professional development.

The purposes of the exercises following Part VI are to help you explore the professional portion of your life and to help you build a personal philosophy of nursing. This process facilitates an individual definition of nursing and illuminates the unique experiences of each learner. The exercises commence with ice-breaking and getting-acquainted activities; these are designed to help in the formation of effective groups and may be used at the beginning of studying the nursing process in formal settings.

Throughout the book, emphasis is always placed on the person—whether client or nurse—as a unique individual with unique needs, desires, and feelings. By integrating the ideals of humanism within the structure of a systems approach, the nursing process should become a workable, applicable, dynamic human process.

The ultimate goal of this book is identical to the ultimate goal of nursing: to assist the client to fullest health potential. This book provides a careful method for that assistance.

In order to set the stage for learning, let us review the phases of the nursing process as delineated by the National Council of State Boards of Nursing (1982), which are followed in this book.

Assessing. This is the beginning of the nursing process. The nurse must be aware of the overall purposes of nursing care and must establish a data base about a client. Involved in this phase are all known (surface) and surmised (underlying) facts and suppositions about the client. The health assessment, nursing history, medical history, and system analysis are included in data collection. Skills of observation, listening, communication, and interviewing are vitally important.

Analyzing. After the collection of data, client needs must be identified with the goals of care. Data processing provides the procedure for coordinating the pre-established responsibilities of professional nursing with the individual pieces of information from the client. It is this coordination that facilitates individualization in client care.

In response to the client's system, the areas of nursing responsibility, and data processing, the following question is posed: "What are the actual or potential health problems for which the client needs nursing assistance?" Your response develops the nursing diagnoses. The diagnoses are then ranked in terms of their importance in a specific time and place.

Planning. This involves designing the strategy to meet the goals of nursing care, cooperating with appropriate health personnel, and recording information. Priority diagnoses are put into operation in terms of what must be done by the nurse with the client and the client's system to accomplish the designated goals and objectives of care. Specific steps are delineated for each diagnosis.

Implementing. This component involves either directly carrying out nursing orders, delegating them to other professionals or technicians, and/or establishing collaborative actions with associates. The teaching skill is emphasized in this Part.

Evaluating. In this step the nurse determines the extent to which the goals of care have been achieved. This Part also contains chapters on nursing audit, client rights, and ethics.

Even though the steps of the nursing process seem sequential, they are circular. Evaluation of each nursing action by the nurse and client provides more data, and the process flows with the additions, deletions, or alterations indicated; constantly, feedback is received and given between all parts of the client's system. This is consistently evaluated and provides additional data. Hence, the nursing process is a dynamic process that can be shaped and applied to unique, open, and changing human systems.

The purpose of the nursing process is to use a definitive, scientific method in the delivery of quality, individualized nursing care.

REFERENCES

Hall, L. (1955). Quality of nursing care. *Public Health News*. Newark, NJ: State Department of Health, June.

Johnson, D. (1959). A philosophy of nursing. *Nursing Outlook, 7,* 198–200.

Knowles, L. (1967). *Decision-making in nursing: A necessity for doing.* New York: Appleton-Century-Crofts.

Kreuter, F. (1957). What is good nursing care? *Nursing Outlook, 57,* 302–304.

National Council of State Boards of Nursing. (1982). *Test plan for the National Council licensure examination for registered nurses.* Chicago: Author.

Orem, D. (1980). *Nursing: Concepts of practice* (2nd ed.). New York: McGraw-Hill.

Orlando, I. (1961). *The dynamic nurse-patient relationship.* New York: G. P. Putnam's.

Yura, H., & Walsh, M. (1983). *The nursing process: Assessing, planning, implementing, evaluating* (4th ed.). Norwalk, CT: Appleton-Century-Crofts.

Part I

Assessing: Establishing a Data Base

Chapter 1

Data Collection

To work toward a whole process of individualized, comprehensive client care, it is necessary to proceed through specific steps. Assessment is the initial phase in the nursing process, and data collection is a primary tool in this assessment. Although authors differ in their definitions of nursing assessment (Bower, 1982; Kozier & Erb, 1979; Sundeen, Stuart, Rankin, & Cohen, 1981), all discussions converge on the fact that assessment means critically evaluating the various conditions and situations involved in a client's system. The nurse assesses the status of the client's health, mood, family situation, response to illness or hospitalization, and any other elements necessary to assist the health team in providing treatment and care.

The assessment phase begins with the collection of data. *Data collection* is the continuous process of obtaining information needed in providing care. It is a dynamic process with changes occurring as more data are collected and as the patient's condition alters. Data collection is done both formally and informally by such means as observation, interviewing, physical examination, research into the client's medical history, and communication, among others. Many sources are available for data collection, ranging from information provided by the client personally to such things as physician's orders or results of laboratory tests.

As the member of the health team who is responsible for total care of the client, the nurse must view and validate all data pertaining to a client's system. In addition to studying the client data that are already available, the nurse also takes action personally to obtain certain information needed to provide total client care. Among these actions is included the obtaining of a nursing history, which will be discussed later.

Sources of data collection can be grouped into primary and secondary sources. McCain (1965) cited the client as the *primary source* of data; in other words, the client provided basic, firsthand information that has not been interpreted or recounted by someone else. All other components of the evolving client system are *secondary sources* of data—that is, sources of data that are derived from the primary source. Thus, secondary sources are indirect, whereas primary sources are direct. These secondary sources may include the physician, family members, colleagues, social worker, developmental records, information from computer systems, nursing notes, nursing rounds, books, journals, experts, and others (Marriner, 1983). Secondary sources also include such information as previous health records or charts, medical histories, reports of previous physical examinations, reports of x-rays and laboratory tests, and all subjective data informally and formally noted. This brief list is not all-encompassing; the nurse searches for all data available about the client from any source believed to be useful in nursing care. Of course, this should all be relative to the evolving goals of care for the client and should be reflective of priorities. Data known to be unnecessary for planning care should never be collected. To do so is to exploit the client.

THE SYSTEMS APPROACH

Just as this book's study of the whole nursing process involves a systems approach, the study of the various steps of the process involves a

systems approach as well. The systems approach requires that the client be studied concomitant with all the environmental elements (people and things) that have an effect on the client's present existence. Since the environment exerts effects and forces on an individual, all elements become both part of the problem and part of the solution. (See Chapter 16 for further study of General System Theory.)

Data collection, therefore, covers the entire expanse of a client's system. Yet, it is merely the initial phase of the nursing process. This should illustrate the broad scope of the nursing process itself.

The following equation will help you visualize the initial steps of the nursing process as discussed in Parts I, II, and III of this book:

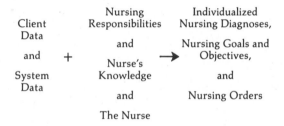

This chapter is concerned with the first elements of this equation: client data (primary data source) and system data (secondary data sources). These data provide the foundation upon which the second part of the equation acts. The combination of the first two parts results in the third part of the equation: the nursing-care plan consisting of individualized nursing diagnoses, nursing goals and objectives, and nursing orders.

To study client data and system data using the systems approach, it is important to visualize the relationship of these components to the whole (see Figure 1–1), but it is equally important that a purpose is ascribed to the whole nursing process and, indeed, also to the specific components of the process. Banathy (1968) described determining a system's purpose as a

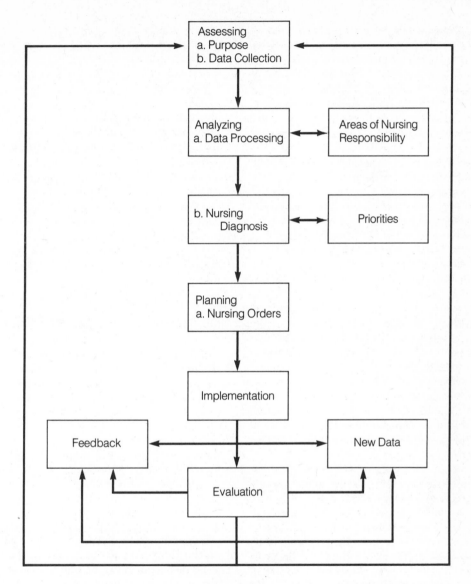

Figure 1–1

Schematic Diagram of the Nursing Process

means of classifying and clarifying the system. By determining a system's purpose, study of the system is facilitated.

Several systems are at work in the context of the nursing process. The primary system is the nursing process itself. Subsystems include the client, the nurse, and the various components of the process, such as data collection. Each system and subsystem has a definite purpose with definite goals.

The generalized, overall purpose of nursing care is to facilitate the client's growth toward maximum health potential for the unique person. The nursing process provides the systematic means to fulfill this goal. Investigation of the purpose of the nursing process demands a response to two specific questions: (1) Why does the client need care and (2) how can and why does the nurse give care?

To respond to why the client needs care, it is necessary for the nurse to collect data. At times, the nurse collects data even before meeting the client; for example, the nurse may study a medical history provided by a physician for a patient who is scheduled to be admitted to the hospital for surgery. Despite the time or source of data collection, however, the overall purpose is to determine general reasons and goals for care.

To answer the second question—how can and why does the nurse give care?—it is again necessary for the nurse to collect data. By obtaining and studying information, the nurse uses knowledge and experience to determine how to provide care for a particular client, as well as why a particular type of care is provided.

These questions obviously are interrelated and point to the ultimate purpose of data collection by the nurse: to provide care suited to the individual.

Before proceeding to methods of data collection, however, there is one more important point connected with the "how" and "why" of providing nursing care: the nurse's personal philosophy. This combination of the nurse's knowledge, experience, beliefs, and values is vital. Henderson (1966) eloquently called for nurses to develop and be aware of a personal philosophy of nursing practice, and it is this author's belief that the development of a personal philosophy is an absolute for the nurse as a caring individual. Since behavior is a result of our attitudes (Campbell, 1947; Hersey & Blanchard, 1982; Katz & Stotland, 1959; Lott, 1973), awareness of one's philosophy is pursued so that the basis of all actions is conscious and controllable. It is assumed that all nurses believe

clients to be individuals and that individualized nursing care is the ultimate desire of practitioners. Working from this basic assumption, it follows that the human aspect of all individuals must be respected. Although the nurse and the client may be categorized as systems to provide an organized, convenient means for study and for giving care, it is important to remember a basic fundamental of the nursing process: nurses and clients are people. Each is an individual person with wants, needs, and capabilities.

A nurse's personal philosophy should also include a fundamental belief in one or more nursing theories. Nursing theory can guide what nursing practice involves as well as indicate how to carry out nursing responsibilities.

METHODS OF COLLECTING DATA

Even though formally discussed only in this chapter, data collection occurs throughout the nursing process since data are always changing and, therefore, always incomplete. Each passing minute for each human being results in a change in the person. Decisions, therefore, are made on limited and incomplete data. Nevertheless, each decision should be explored to the fullest degree possible as dictated by time.

All sources of data—primary and secondary—that involve the client and the client's system should be considered when making nursing decisions. The methods used to collect data with the aim of providing total care will depend on the skills necessary to carry out the task; as the practitioner gains more knowledge and more experience, more methods of data collection become available. For example, some methods of data collection, such as physical examination, require much technical skill and practice. Each Part of this book is devoted to a discussion of major skills necessary for each specific step of the process; in addition, the humanistic exercises provide simulated learning experiences for practice. Other methods of data collection require fewer technical skills and are an excellent means of becoming familiar with principles of obtaining information. An example of one such method is obtaining a nursing history; interpersonal skills are most important in this method.

Methods of data collection include communication with physicians, family members, colleagues, social workers, technicians, teachers, and others. Information may also be obtained from previous health records, patient charts, medical histories, reports of physical examinations, results of x-rays and laboratory tests, admitting records, and informal observation. These methods all involve secondary sources.

Methods of collecting data from the primary source—the client—include informal conversation, formal interviews, nursing histories, and actual physical examination. Because the nursing history involves information from the primary source and because obtaining it involves fewer technical skills than certain other methods of data collection, the next section will discuss in detail the obtaining of a nursing history.

THE NURSING HISTORY

The nursing history is the foremost method of collecting data. The procedure usually involves purposeful observation and an interview or oral history, but occasionally the nursing history is first written by the client from a list of questions and then elaborated upon by the nurse.

The nursing history is viewed by McPhetridge (1968) as a primary means of personalizing nursing care. It provides a skeleton of pertinent information from which problems can be identified initially and then pursued. This knowledge about the client is used in planning individualized nursing care as well as in attempting to prevent misunderstandings or problems from arising.

The nursing history differs from the medical history. The medical history is a record of the client's previous illnesses, medical problems, hospitalizations, physical traits, and familial medical patterns. By contrast, the nursing history is a record of the client's habits, emotional status, expectations, and other such factors. Though both the medical history and the nursing history have the same overall purpose—to provide a basis for optimum treatment and care—they differ in specifics.

Erikson (1964) described data collection as the responsibility of the clinician for obtaining evidence relative to clinical problems, evaluation, and diagnostic inferences. McManus (1951) referred to the data-collecting process as clinical thinking. The nursing history, then, is that part of the clinical data-collection process that is concerned most directly with the client as a person. Smith (1968) viewed the nursing history as a pathway by which the nurse can get to know a client, and vice versa.

A nursing history, however, is not an end in and of itself; rather, it is a tool to obtain what the nurse needs to provide comprehensive care. The nurse's responsibility is to assist the client *when the client is in need of help*. It follows that the nurse will not delve into areas of the client's life where intervention is not needed. Only data that are usable and that the client feels ease in providing should be obtained. Furthermore, the data should be collected in a way that respects the nurse's philosophy, beliefs, and expertise, as well as the environmental elements of the particular system. In other words, consider the persons, things, and situations surrounding yourself and the client.

Smith (1968) earmarked the need for a conceptual and procedural frame of reference in obtaining a nursing history. The following nursing-history guide is a structured interview format that is intended to be a compilation of areas and questions that can be pursued by the nurse interviewer. The depth to which each area is investigated depends on the individual client and the individual nurse. The following nursing history is only a guide and is to be used according to the purposes of care with respect to the skills and techniques of the nurse. How you interview (structured or unstructured), the order of questions asked, and the depth of exploration should be flexible and should be determined by the reactions and responses of the client. Information already known should not be reintroduced; areas requiring further information can be amplified; possible problems can be noted for future study. After becoming familiar with this nursing-history guide, you may wish to develop your own. Or, you may find it best to use different formats of nursing histories with different clients. The key to obtaining the nursing history is personalizing the format to the unique client and to the unique nurse and listening.

NURSING HISTORY GUIDE

A. General Information

   1. Date of Interview:

   2. Date of Admission:

   3. Hours of Time Elapsed from Admission to First Interview:

   4. Patient's Name:

   5. Patient's Age:

   6. Diagnosis (Medical):

   7. Profession/Occupation

     a. Patient's:

     b. Spouse's:

   8. Religion:

   9. Educational Level:

   10. Residence (City and State):

   11. Marital Status:

B. Guide Questions

   1. Family Situation

     a. With whom do you live?

     b. How many children do you have, if any?

     c. Who is caring for them while you are here?

     d. How many brothers and sisters do you have?

     e. Do your parents live nearby?

     f. Was there anything that happened to you or your family in the past year, other than this illness, that was upsetting to you?

   2. Work Situation (including financial aspects)

     a. What type of work do you do?

     b. How long have you done this type of work?

     c. Are you on sick leave from work?

     d. Do you think your illness will interfere with your work?

     e. Do you have health insurance?

   3. Patient's Activities

     a. What kind of environment and pace are you used to?

     b. What are your feelings concerning your activity schedule in the hospital?

     c. Do you have any special interests or hobbies that you would like to pursue, if feasible, while you are here?

     d. What habits have you had to change here?

   4. Eating Habits

     a. Are you on a restricted diet?

     b. Are you allergic to any foods?

     c. Are there any particular foods you like or dislike?

     d. Do you eat breakfast?

     e. Do you need an early morning cup of coffee or the like?

     f. How many times do you eat each day?

     g. When do you usually eat your meals?

     h. Has being sick affected your eating habits? How?

     i. Do you foresee any difficulty with hospital food?

     j. Do you prefer plain or ice water?

     k. Are you accustomed to eating snacks? At regular times?

5. Sleeping Habits

    a. How long do you usually sleep? Between what hours?

    b. Do you sleep well at home?

    c. Do you nap? Occasionally? Regularly? Rarely?

    d. Are you an early riser?

    e. Do you need medication to sleep?

    f. Do you get up at intervals?

    g. Does light or noise disturb you?

    h. If you are awakened at night, can you go back to sleep?

    i. Do you sleep with a night light on?

    j. Do you like an extra blanket at night?

    k. Do you usually sleep with a window closed or open?

    l. Have you found that strange surroundings decrease your ability to sleep soundly?

    m. How many pillows do you use?

6. Elimination Habits

    a. What are your elimination habits at home?

    b. Do you have any difficulty with elimination?

    c. Do you take laxatives? If so, how often? What kind?

    d. Do you take any special foods to aid in elimination?

7. Allergies

    a. Do you have any special allergies to drugs, food, adhesive tape, and so forth?

8. Drugs or Special Diets

    a. Were you on any medications before you came to the hospital?

    b. Do you routinely take any "over-the-counter" medicines?

    c. Did you bring any of these medications with you?

9. Previous Illnesses or Hospitalizations

    a. Have you had other experiences when you or members of your family were ill?

        (1) What kind of experience was it—good, bad, indifferent?

        (2) What problems, if any, did you or they encounter?

    b. Have you ever been sick before?

        (1) What was wrong?

        (2) Were you in the hospital?

        (3) How long were you sick?

        (4) What do you remember most about being hospitalized?

        (5) What did you like most about the hospital care, routines, and so forth?

        (6) What did you like least?

    c. Do you have any disability other than your present illness that may restrict your normal activity?

    d. Who cares for you when you are sick at home?

    e. What can you do when you are sick at home that makes you feel better?

10. Current Illness

    a. Why are you in the hospital?

    b. What do you think made you ill?

    c. How long have you been ill?

    d. Can you tell me what you feel concerning your illness?

    e. What kinds of things usually make you feel better when you are sick?

    f. Were there other things that happened when you first became ill?

    g. What do you feel concerning the outcome of your illness?

    h. What is causing you the most discomfort at this time?

11. Current Hospitalization

    a. What do you think you need done for you while you are here?

b. What do you feel about being here in the hospital?

c. What do you miss most by being in the hospital?

d. Are there some things at home that you would like to have here with you? If so, what?

e. Are there things at home that might bother or worry you while you are here?

12. Personal Preferences Regarding Visitors: Family and Friends

   a. If feasible, would you prefer to be with other patients during the day, or would you rather be alone?

   b. Would you like to have visitors?

      (1) Just family?

      (2) Just friends?

      (3) Both family and friends?

      (4) Just certain individuals? Who?

   c. How many visitors would you like at one time and how frequently?

   d. Is it possible for your family and friends to visit you if you so desire?

   e. Has anyone visited with you yet or did anyone come with you when you were admitted?

   f. (For persons with serious illness, or as hospital policy allows): Would you feel better if it were possible for some of your family to stay here with you overnight?

13. Patient's Expectations of Hospital Personnel and Physician

   a. Would you like your doctor and nurses to explain everything that is going on with you?

   b. Would you be comfortable enough to ask them questions if they do not explain?

   c. Would you like someone to come in frequently during the day just to talk or be with you?

d. Is there anything special you expect or would like me to do for you or see that gets done, if feasible, while you are here?

e. What do you expect from nurses?

f. What do you expect from other personnel?

g. What has your doctor told you about your illness and what to expect while you are in the hospital?

h. What do you expect from your doctor?

i. What do you expect from the hospital?

j. What do you expect from hospital policy or routine?

k. Would you like a minister to visit you?

l. How best can I help you while you are in the hospital?

C. Visual Observation on General Appearance

   1. Immediate General Impression of Appearance:

   2. Overall Physical Appearance:

   3. Motor Activity/Posture:

   4. Build and Weight:

   5. Prosthesis/Limitations/Debilitations:

   6. Complexion and Appearance of Skin

      a. Color:

      b. Lesions:

      c. Abrasions:

      d. Rash:

   7. Subjective Symptoms

      a. Watery eyes:

      b. Running nose:

      c. Cough:

   8. Mouth

      a. Oral hygiene:

      b. Dentures:

9. Eyes
   a. Eye glasses:
   b. Contact lenses (soft or hard, extended wear or regular):
10. Age Group:
11. Clothing:
12. Belongings and Objects in Environment:
13. Speech:
14. Apparent Cultural, Educational, and Intellectual Levels:
15. Other Pertinent Factors:

D. Nonverbal Behavior Observations
   1. Emotional Tone, Facial Expression, Attitude:
   2. Gestures, Movements, or Activities During Interview:
   3. Main Theme of Patient's Conversation and Behavior:
   4. Topics the Patient Seemed to Avoid:
   5. Patient's Response to Interviewer:
   6. Interviewer's Response to Patient:
   7. Other Pertinent Factors:

E. Summary

NURSING CARE: AN ENCOUNTER

Nursing care can be viewed as an encounter between persons—the nurse and the client. Carkhuff (1969) noted that the growth or deterioration of all people in a relationship depends on the interaction of all. The first person (or leader, for example) has the most critical effect on the interaction. Since the nurse is the leader in the client/nurse situation, the nurse naturally assumes added responsibility in the encounter. Moreover, since no interaction remains in neutrality, each encounter will be either harmful or helpful to all involved participants. Therefore, even though the professional is not the primary focus, the benefits and/or detriments of nursing care are experienced by all involved members of the system.

To make Carkhuff's statements meaningful in nursing, let us consider the following example. Picture yourself as a 19-year-old student who is assigned by an instructor to obtain a nursing history from Mr. Blanche. Mr. Blanche is 46 years old and has just been admitted to the hospital with a medical diagnosis of angina with a possible myocardial infarction. This is your first encounter in interviewing and the client's first admission to a hospital. You have a written history form to follow and, being an enthusiastic learner, you have studied the disease process. Entering the room, you quickly observe that Mr. Blanche is sitting in bed watching television. His color is pink, and he seems to be comfortable. You introduce yourself and tell him you would like to ask some questions to make it possible for you and your colleagues to plan nursing care reflecting his individual needs. You begin. All goes smoothly until you ask when he first noticed the pain. You ask the question, and he hesitates, blushes, and hurriedly states that it was when he was having intercourse with his wife. Is this area important to pursue? Do you believe further information is necessary to help him? What questions does your education lead you to ask? Are you comfortable? Can you handle this with ease? Can you decrease the client's anxiety while interviewing? These are important questions to ask yourself. If both you and the client cannot proceed comfortably with this line of assessment, the interviewing experience will be negative. Furthermore, you will probably not be able to obtain the information needed to plan individualized care.

Preplanning is the key in situations such as this. Since the nurse is as much a part of the data-collection process (and of all nursing) as the client, it becomes crucial to look at yourself in these initial stages so that a negative encounter with a client can be avoided.

Follow these steps in preplanning your first interaction with the client. Begin by determining the purpose of nursing care. Next, specify the goals of care from the existing data, and earmark those areas that need further exploration. Then, ask yourself the question, "Do I have the knowledge, experience, and ease necessary to pursue these areas with the client?" If you answer "yes," then carry on. Should your response be "no" or any combination of "yes/no," you should then get the experience needed by practicing the required skills in a safe, low-risk way. For example, you might share your feelings with your instructor. You might request that the instructor interview the client with you, giving the instructor the areas to pursue in which you are unsure or unclear. Learn by observation. Or, you may role-play the situation in a nursing laboratory or conference room with peers. The point is to learn to handle a situation positively and effectively. The myth that the best way to teach a child the effects of fire is to burn the child maintains its mythic status in nursing and in most other situations. It is not necessary to experience pain or discomfort to learn about it. By placing the learning situation in the proper perspective, you assume responsibility for both yourself and the one looking to you for help. Thus, you can ensure a positive first encounter.

In short, build yourself a foundation of comfort with respect to your needs, feelings, knowledge, and experience prior to encountering the client. Do whatever you must, request the help you desire, and delegate those aspects you cannot handle. As long as total care of a client is carried out by one nurse or a combination of nurses, professional responsibility is maintained. A supragoal of nursing care, as well as of learning and teaching, is that the experience be positive. Even though negative learning on the part of the nurse and/or client may occur, all attempts should be made to diminish negativity as much as possible for all concerned.

SUMMARY

Chapter 1 discussed the beginning of the nursing process—assessing by collecting data. Data collection is viewed as necessary at the onset of care for the purpose of planning individualized care, but data collection is continuous throughout the nurse/patient relationship. The nursing history was earmarked as an important means of collecting information that is responsive to the goals and purposes of nursing care and that is reflective of priorities. The skills used by the nurse in the process of data collection should be those with which the interviewer is most comfortable.

Chapters 2, 3, and 4 discuss the major skills and competencies needed to carry out the assessment phase of the nursing process. The chapter topics are not meant to be all-inclusive but, rather, should reflect basic skill areas that the practitioner can expand through experience and continued education. Chapter 2 focuses on observation and listening.

REFERENCES

Banathy, B. (1968). *Instructional systems.* Palo Alto, CA: Fearon.

Bower, F. (1982). *The process of planning nursing care: Nursing practice models* (3rd ed.). St. Louis: Mosby.

Campbell, D. (1947). *The generality of social attitudes.* Doctoral dissertation, University of California, Berkeley.

Carkhuff, R. (1969). *Helping and human relations: A primer for lay and professional helpers* (Vol. 1). New York: Holt, Rinehart and Winston.

Erikson, E. (1964). *Insight and responsibility.* New York: Norton.

Henderson, V. (1966). *The nature of nursing.* New York: Macmillan.

Hersey, P., & Blanchard, K. (1982). *Management of organizational behavior: Utilizing human resources* (4th ed.). Englewood Cliffs, NJ: Prentice-Hall.

Katz, D., & Stotland, E. (1959). A preliminary statement to a theory of attitude structure and change. In S. Koch (Ed.), *Psychology: A study of a science* (Vol. 3). New York: McGraw-Hill.

Kozier, B., & Erb, G. (1979). *Fundamentals of nursing: Concepts and procedures.* Menlo Park, CA: Addison-Wesley.

Lott, A. (1973). Social psychology. In B. Wolman (Ed.), *Handbook of general psychology.* Englewood Cliffs, NJ: Prentice-Hall.

Marriner, A. (1983). *The nursing process: A scientific approach to nursing care* (3rd ed.). St. Louis: Mosby.

McCain, R. F. (1965). Nursing by assessment—not intuition. *American Journal of Nursing, 65,* 82–84.

McManus, R. (1951). Assumptions of functions of nursing. In *Regional planning for nursing and nursing education* (p. 54). Report of a work conference at Plymouth, New Hampshire, June 12–23, 1950. New York: Bureau of Publications, Teachers College, Columbia University.

McPhetridge, L. M. (1968). Nursing history: One means to personalize care. *American Journal of Nursing, 68,* 68–75.

Smith, D. (1968). A clinical nursing tool. *American Journal of Nursing, 68,* 2384–2388.

Sundeen, S., Stuart, G., Rankin, E., & Cohen, S. (1981). *Nurse-client interaction: Implementing the nursing process* (2nd ed.). St. Louis: Mosby.

SELECTED READINGS

Two articles are recommended for further reading. In the first, McCain (1965) provided a rationale for assessment, underscoring that it should be a concrete and deliberative process. She introduced an assessment tool that delineated topic areas for client inquiry. In the second article, McPhetridge (1968) used the nursing home as a means for providing individualized care and suggested a nursing-history format.

Nursing by Assessment—Not Intuition

R. Faye McCain

To practice effectively, a nurse must assess. She must—consciously or unconsciously—determine the patient's nursing needs on the basis of his diagnosis, symptoms, medical orders, laboratory data, and so forth. But no precise method of such assessment has, as yet, been widely accepted. In this article, the author describes an approach to assessment which is being developed with graduate students in medical-surgical nursing.

Nursing, as it is taught and practiced today, is primarily intuitive. Unlike the professions of law, engineering, and medicine, nursing has not developed a precise method of determining when nursing intervention is needed. However, the need for a precise method has been recognized. Several years ago, Abdellah and associates described an approach to planning care, using as a guide "the twenty-one nursing problems" (1). More recently Bonney and Rothberg suggested a method of identifying the needs for nursing services of the chronically disabled person (2). But, as yet, neither of these approaches have been widely accepted by nursing educators and practitioners.

For the past three years graduate students in medical-surgical nursing at the University of Michigan have been evolving a method of systematically assessing functional abilities of patients. These assessments serve as the basis for making nursing diagnoses, for planning and evaluating the nursing therapy, and for writing the various nursing orders.

This method is far from precise and complete at this stage of its evolution. Some aspects

of the method are developed to a higher degree than others; none have yet been developed in complete detail. We recognize that further experiential evidence is needed and that, ultimately, a controlled study should be done to validate the method. So far, we believe that it does have merit and does deserve further consideration by members of the nursing profession.

FUNCTIONAL ABILITIES APPROACH

The functional abilities of the patient were selected as the basis for assessment because such an approach agreed with our concept of nursing care. This concept incorporates the belief that the primary goal of nursing care is to assist a patient to attain and maintain a state of equilibrium as he reacts to internal and external stimuli. Equilibrium, as advanced by Johnson, represents a momentary balancing of opposing forces and does not imply a state of health or well-being (3). To carry this concept further, the extent to which a patient does or does not achieve equilibrium is reflected in his physiological, psychological, and social behavior. Functional abilities, then, become another way of expressing behavior.

A patient, today, is expected to do for himself whatever he is capable of doing; in other words, he is expected to participate in his therapeutic regimen. But in order to help him be a participant, the nurse must know his functional abilities as well as his disabilities. When she plans nursing care and writes nursing orders, the nurse will capitalize on the patient's abilities but, at the same time, she will endeavor to assist him to live with his disabilities, whether they are temporary or permanent.

Before describing the proposed method of patient assessment, it is appropriate to consider some of the basic factors underlying the process. The systematic assessment of a patient's functional abilities is an orderly and precise method of collecting information about the physiological, psychological, and social behavior of a patient. The data collected from such an assessment provide a rationale for determining the patient's nursing needs and serve as a basis for planning and evaluating nursing therapy, writing nursing orders, and guiding and directing nursing activities. It is our working hypothesis that the nursing diagnosis, per se, is the identification of the patient's functional disabilities, or symptoms, as well as identification of his most important functional abilities. One can speculate, however, that with time, creativity, and sufficient precise data, symptoms that have a meaningful relationship in the nursing process can be grouped together, given a descriptive name, and be considered a nursing syndrome.

THE ASSESSMENT

Four resources are available for making an assessment: the patient, his family, health team members, and records. The primary resource, in most instances, is the patient; the other resources enlarge, clarify, and substantiate the information obtained from him. Interview and direct observation or inspection are the tools used by the nurse. Although these tools have long been recognized as essential to nursing care, in the patient assessment process they are used with direction and precision. Here again, one can speculate that with time, creativity, and sufficient precise data, specific nursing diagnostic tests could be evolved.

In assessing the patient's functional abilities, both objective and subjective data are collected and recorded. The time is long since past when the collection of only objective data

should be advocated. Professional nurses can, do, and should make judgments. When professional nurses are more knowledgeable in the contributing sciences and become more competent in analytical thinking, some of these judgments probably will be independent judgments upon which nurses will make decisions without waiting for medical direction.

Patient assessment is the responsibility of the professional nurse. She initiates the assessment as soon as possible after the patient is admitted and continues to assess and evaluate, modifying the plan of care as the patient's behavior or functional abilities change.

In developing the method for systematic assessment of a patient's functional abilities, it was necessary to classify body functions. To date we have identified and used 13 functional areas: The patient's social, mental, emotional, body temperature, respiratory, circulatory, nutritional, elimination, and reproductive status; state of rest and comfort; state of skin and appendages; sensory perception; and motor ability. Although these functions are not mutually exclusive, for purposes of assessment we consider them separately. Social status may be questioned as a functional area, but after considerable thought and discussion, we decided it should be included. Our aim is to determine the patient's position in his family and community and discover, if possible, what social stimuli may be contributing to or detracting from his ability to function at an optimum level. In some instances, we decided to include a specific function under a category where the relationship cannot be validated by authorities, for example, placing the function of speech under sensory perception, and including intake and output in circulatory status.

SUGGESTIONS FOR USE OF GUIDE

Factors included in the guide we have developed are suggestive only. In a given patient, some factors will not be pertinent. The professional nurse in making the assessment, however, must consider all functional aspects and judge which ones do or do not apply.

We have included only those functional elements whose data can be collected by the professional nurse, using, primarily, the techniques of interview, direct observation, or inspection. It is well recognized, however, that more information will be needed before the nursing therapeutic regime for a specific patient can be planned and evaluated; for instance, findings from the medical history and physical examination, results of x-ray and laboratory tests, medical diagnosis, plan of medical management, medical prognosis, and data from hospitalizations will be needed. This information can be obtained from the patient's record or from his physician and should not be duplicated in the assessment done by the nurse.

The graduate student using the guide approaches each patient much as a physician might in taking the patient's history and doing the physical examination—with a definite plan in mind of data to be collected. After the data are collected, she proceeds to analyze the data, make the nursing diagnosis, and decide upon a plan of care. This plan then is discussed with those who will be a part of the nursing team before it is implemented. Naturally, there will be instances when collecting data and carrying out care will be simultaneous, particularly when the patient is in acute need. At these times when symptoms are acute and may be changing rapidly, filling in the data collection forms comes after the emergency moment. However, nurses must, with the majority of patients, reach a point where their plans for care are not based on hunch alone.

Reactions to this method of patient assessment have been favorable, and there is general agreement on the wards that the nursing care plans based on the assessments take all of the nursing needs of the patients into consideration. Increased knowledge about patients and increased awareness of them have given graduate students greater satisfaction in carrying out their responsibilities. Further, we have noticed that whenever baseline data are available, evaluation of the effectiveness of nursing therapy has improved.

In the beginning, we wondered how patients and physicians would react to this process. Our experiences so far indicate that patients are pleased that nurses take time to listen to their problems, demonstrate an interest in them, and obviously base nursing care on their expressed needs. Physicians' responses have been more general than those of patients, but they, too, have seen the value of the assessment process.

Mental Status

State of consciousness
- Alert and quick to respond to surroundings
- Drowsy and slow to respond
- Semiconscious and difficult to arouse
- Comatose and unable to arouse
- State of automatism

Orientation
- To time
- To place
- To person

Intellectual capacity
- Level of education
- Ability to recall events: recent; past

Attention span

Vocabulary level
- Use of simple, nontechnical words
- Use of complex, technical words

Ability to understand ideas
- Slow to learn meaning and make relationships
- Quick to gain meaning and make relationships
- Insight into health problems

Emotional Status

Emotional reactions
- Mood
- Presence or absence of anxiety
- Defenses against anxiety: such as, aggression; depression; fantasies; identification; rationalization; regression; repression; sublimation

Body image
- Effect of illness on self-concept
- Adaptation of self-concept to reality demands

Ability to relate to others
- To family
- To other patients
- To health team members

Sensory Perception

Hearing
- Sensitivity to sound
  - Voice tone that distinguishes sounds: low; moderate; loud
  - Distance that sounds distinguished
  - Need to see speaker to distinguish sounds
- Presence of impairment
  - Partial or complete
  - Unilateral or bilateral
  - Ability to lip read
  - Use and effectiveness of supportive aid

Vision
- Acuity
- Presence of impairment
  - Partial or complete
  - Unilateral or bilateral
  - Type: hyperopia; myopia; astigmatism; color-blindness; diplopia; photophobia; nyctalopia; other
  - Use and effectiveness of supportive aid
- Enunciation
  - Unilateral or bilateral
  - Use of prosthesis

Speech
- Has auditory expression
- Aphasia
  - Verbal defect
  - Syntactical defect
  - Nominal defect
  - Semantic defect
- Anarthria
- Mute
- Laryngectomy
  - Use and effectiveness of esophageal speech
  - Unusual speech patterns: such as, lisping; repetitive; staccato; stammer; stutter

Touch
- Hyperesthesia
- Anesthesia
- Paresthesia
- Paralgesia

Smell
- Anosmia
- Hyperosmia
- Kakosmia
- Parosmia

Taste
- Distinguishes: sweet; salt; sour; bitter
- Aftertaste present

Motor Ability

Mobility
- Complete bed rest
- Bed rest with bathroom privileges
- Sit in chair
- Ambulatory
  - Without assistance
  - With supportive aids: person; crutches; walker
  - Use of wheel chair
  - Use of stretcher
- Posture
  - In bed
  - Upright

Range of motion
- Passive
- Active

Gait

Equilibrium

Abnormal movement
- Clonic
- Tonic
- Spastic
- Flaccid
- Tic
- Ataxia

Muscle tone
- Spasm
- Contractures
- Weakness

Paralysis
- Hemiplegia
- Paraplegia
- Quadriplegia

Loss of extremity
- Location
- Extent
- Use and effectiveness of prosthetic

———————————

Many factors, of which those listed above are only a small sample, are taken into consideration when the graduate student first sees, talks with, and examines the patient.

REFERENCES

1. Abdellah, Fay G., et al. *Patient-Centered Approaches to Nursing.* New York, Macmillan Co., 1960.

2. Bonney, Virginia, and Rothberg, June. *Nursing Diagnosis and Therapy—An Instrument for Evaluation and Measurement.* (League Exchange) New York, National League for Nursing, 1963.

3. Johnson, Dorothy E. The significance of nursing care. *American Journal of Nursing* 61: 63–66.

Nursing History: One Means to Personalize Care

L. Mae McPhetridge

Early, full knowledge of what the patient perceives about his illness and hospitalization and what he prefers about his care enables the nurse, says this author, to personalize his nursing during his stay and to prepare more successfully for his departure from the hospital. Completing the history form which records this enabling information is claimed to take far less time than to gather the same facts over a period of several days' nursing care.

Personalized nursing care is increasingly difficult to achieve despite the fact that it remains a consistent goal of nurse practitioners and nurse educators. Growing numbers of patients, greater nurse participation in more and more complex plans of medical care, and responsibility for larger numbers of auxiliary personnel are all cited as reasons for failure to give patient-centered nursing care.

Legitimate deterrents though these are, nurses must find a way to individualize nursing care. One means, a nursing history form, has been developed to help the nurse make maximum use of her limited time with the patient by obtaining systematically the information needed to plan his nursing care.

Any usable nursing history should identify the patient's perception and expectations related to his illness, hospitalization, and care. The history also should furnish clues to the patient's ability to meet his personal needs and to cope with problems he faces. From such data, the nurse can deduce the amount and kind of nursing assistance he requires.

A nursing history differs from a medical history in that it focuses on the meaning of illness and hospitalization to the patient and his family as a basis for planning nursing care. The medical history is taken to determine whether pathology is present as a basis for planning medical care.

One patient expressed this difference succinctly when he said during a nursing interview, "I'm glad to know someone's interested in me as well as my illness." Of course, physicians, too, are interested in patients' perceptions and ways of coping just as nurses are interested in patients' pathologies. But a history that is quite adequate for developing a medical regimen may be just as unsatisfactory for planning nursing care as a nursing history would be for planning medical care. Since information taken in a nursing history may be useful to the physician, the two histories are complementary, valuable to both nurse and physician.

NURSING HISTORY FORMAT

Our nursing history format, developed as an interview guide, consists of questions directed to the patient and space for his answers. The recording of direct quotes and key phrases captures the patient's meaning with a minimum of writing. His identifying data on the face sheet should be obtained from his record to avoid repetitive questioning. The history format is organized in four parts.

Patient perceptions and expectations about the meaning of illness and hospitalization to him and his family are elicited in the first section. Asking why the patient sought medical care, what he thinks caused him to get sick, and how his illness has affected his usual way of life all tend to reveal his understanding of his condition and how it has affected him. What hospitalization means to him is learned by asking what he expects will happen to him, what it is like to be in the hospital, and how long he expects to stay.

The patient's view of the effects of his illness and hospitalization on his family or other significant persons is obtained by asking with whom he lives, who is the most important person(s) to him, what effect his entering the hospital has had on his family or the person closest to him, and whether the significant person(s) is able to visit him. Inquiring what the patient does for recreation provides some guidance for considering this aspect of care. Asking how he expects to manage after leaving the hospital gives further indication of his understanding and feelings about his illness. This question also lays the foundation for early planning of care after discharge.

Basic needs are explored in the second section which investigates the patient's ability to care for himself and serves as a basis for determining whether nursing intervention will be necessary to insure comfort, rest, and sleep. Questions about these basic needs also embrace pain and personal hygiene; safety, including items related to locomotion, vision, and hearing; fluids and nutrition; elimination; oxygen; and sexuality.

Each need is considered from the patient's standpoint, from his perception of problems he is encountering at present, whether he has experienced similar problems in the past and how he coped with them, and with what success. What nursing assistance does he expect with each need at this time? The help he wants and that which the nurse thinks he should have may differ widely. This incongruity must be reconciled or it may give rise to conflict that will hinder the nurse's therapeutic effectiveness. Data concerning anticipated problems and how he expects to manage suggest the nursing assistance needed to provide continuity of care.

Additional information is secured in the third section, labeled "Other," which asks questions that do not fit logically into the first two sections. Does the patient have a history of allergy? This is important information with the widespread use of pharmaceuticals. A question asking how far the patient went in school is placed in this section rather than earlier in the interview so that he will not think the nurse measures his worth in terms of his education. This question aids in assessing the patient's intellectual capacity, a prerequisite for successful communication and future planning. A final, open-ended question lets the patient tell anything else he thinks would help the nurse with his care. For instance, knowing whether he is being assisted by other health or social agencies is useful for continuity of care.

Nurse's impressions and suggestions, the last section, is completed after the interview. From the data, the nurse summarizes the significant findings and from this summary develops a plan for this person's nursing care. All sections except the last may be completed during the interview or the nurse may jot down a word or two as a reminder and fill in more detail out of the patient's presence.

The form is not intended to limit nurse-patient communication. Using the form only as a guide, the interviewer is free to rephrase questions and explore more deeply any areas of concern that need probing. The questions about patient's perception simply suggest material that may be significant to his nursing care and may require further discussion, depending on his response or lack of response to a given question.

After initial testing by the author with eight patients, the form was tested by junior and senior baccalaureate students during an entire school year. Students' and patients' overall reactions were positive. Questions were generally understood by patients and elicited in minimum time the information necessary to plan individualized care. Interview time ranged from 20 to 60 minutes with an average of 25 minutes. Like any nursing activity, the time varied according to the patient's response and the nurse's skill.

NURSING IMPLICATIONS

Asked why he was in the hospital and what he thought caused him to get sick, one patient with cancer of the neck responded, "I have cancer of the neck." Here, the nurse immediately learned that the patient knew his diagnosis. Accordingly she could approach him appropriately concerning his illness and thus avoid a nonverbal guessing game that is potentially destructive to a therapeutic relationship. Another person, with diagnosed lung cancer, answered these questions by saying he had had pneumonia and his lung had "closed up" so that it was hard for him to breathe. This response guided the nurse in further communication, particularly in choosing words to help the patient talk about concerns relating to his illness. A third patient, who had had a node resection for cancer of the groin, attributed this "lump" to heavy lifting. Obviously, this patient's understanding and acceptance of follow-up care was quite different from that of the man who said he had a cancer on his neck. Hence the nurse's approach must differ.

Statements about effects of illness on patients' usual ways of life demonstrated the great variation in meaning that illness holds for different persons. To one man, it meant economic disaster. To another, illness meant dependence on other people to an extent he found repugnant. To still another patient, the most significant effect had been his sexual impotence for several months. If the nurse is to assist these patients in coping with these problems, it is apparent that she must offer very different kinds of help. For the first patient, the proper assistance might be referral to social service. For the second, the nurse might plan with the patient so that he could make as many decisions as possible and thereby strengthen his feelings of independence. Perhaps the help needed by

the third patient is merely to know that those caring for him appreciate his feelings.

Patients' reactions to hospitalization were equally varied. One man expressed immense relief at being in the hospital and receiving medical care from highly qualified staff. But being in the hospital meant overwhelming loneliness to one woman because of separation from her family, who were unable to visit. The man apparently did not need nursing assistance related specifically to his hospitalization, but the woman required considerable help from the nursing staff to deal with her loneliness and thus conserve the psychic energy she sorely needed to combat her illness.

Assuming that people cope better with the known than the unknown, their needs for nursing assistance will vary in proportion to their understanding and expectations during hospitalization. One patient, for instance, arrived with detailed knowledge of her proposed care, which included a proctoscopic examination and bowel x-ray. Another person had no idea what was to be done during his hospital stay or, for that matter, how long he was to stay. Some patients replied, "I don't know," to all questions related to perception of illness and expectations.

While such responses give no immediate clue to nursing needs, they do suggest questions worth further exploration. Was any information given to the patient? If so, did he comprehend it? Was he too anxious to hear? Does his pattern of response represent denial of illness? If such an explanation can be verified with the patient, the nurse can begin appropriate action. For example, assistance for a patient who does not know what to expect because he does not understand the terminology used in explanation would be very different from that for a patient whose responses stem from denial.

Asking the patient how he expects to get along after leaving the hospital also helped determine nursing needs. Some patients had specific, firm arrangements for their continued care. Others had not looked that far ahead. By asking the question early, nurses could begin discharge planning much sooner.

This question also gave a clue as to whether the patient's understanding of his illness was realistic. One woman, for example, who had a hysterectomy for a benign condition and presumably would be considered cured upon discharge, said she expected to go to bed indefinitely after leaving the hospital and be unable to do anything for herself. To help this patient plan realistically, the nurse must know not only what the patient thinks but why. If her response is based on fear of cancer, one kind of nursing action is indicated. If her answer reflects an exaggerated dependency need, an entirely different nursing measure is required.

The section dealing with the patient's basic needs yielded much useful information for planning nursing care. For example, if the patient had pain, a major nursing aim would be to relieve it. To do so, the nurse needs more information. Besides her own observations, she must consider the patient's description of his pain, whether he has had it previously, what he did to relieve it, and whether he succeeded. One patient said he gained partial relief by walking about, while another man's pain was lessened by remaining very quiet. In addition to administering their prescribed medications, some patients wanted the nurse to talk with them or help them find comfortable positions. A 28-year-old man with peptic ulcer responded that he had little faith in medications and what he wanted most was that the nurse allow him to tell her how much it hurt.

The vast majority of patients interviewed had distinct preferences about the frequency and time for bathing as well as the type of bath. There were no consistent patterns. Some patients preferred a daily bath; a few wanted to bathe only once a week. The desired time ranged from 5:00 A.M. to bedtime. Preferences for tub bath or shower were divided about equally. Giving patients a choice about personal hygiene seems to be one way to minimize the loss of identity and control associated with hospitalization. Although offering patients this choice may raise staffing problems, the overall time for bathing is not increased by changing the hour.

The physiologic and psychologic significance of food for the ill person is undisputed. Yet the best food does not nourish the patient who fails to eat because he dislikes it or because he cannot chew it. Information about food likes and dislikes, and about conditions which affect his eating makes it possible to foster good nutrition and patient satisfaction. Two questions were particularly illuminating. One asked whether the patient considered himself underweight, overweight, or about right. The fact that nurse perceptions of a patient's weight and his perceptions of his weight do not always agree cannot be discounted if she must help in weight control.

Inquiring what foods were eaten primarily revealed some glaring deficiencies. For example, a 19-year-old girl with chronic ulcerative colitis "mostly ate macaroni, french fries, dill pickles, and vanilla ice cream." The patient's knowledge of his hospital diet, his past experiences with a special diet, along with what he expects when he goes home, all provide clues to his teaching needs.

Inquiry into elimination habits showed that what patients considered normal and the means used to facilitate bowel evacuation were highly individual. One patient dosed herself with "salts" at bedtime if she did not have two bowel movements each day. The influence of habit on elimination was demonstrated by the maternity patient who regularly had a cigarette and Coke immediately after breakfast. This practice could be followed in the hospital only if the nurse knew of it and took deliberate steps to enable the patient to do so. A 68-year-old woman, confined to bed with a fractured hip, reported that she normally had one bowel movement a week and only with the help of an enema. Because the nurse knew the effects of prolonged inactivity and knew the patient's elimination pattern soon after admission, she could institute measures to prevent a fecal impaction. Interviews documented widespread use of laxatives—a fact with clear teaching implications.

Questions pertaining to sexuality explored the effects of illness on the sexual role, as well as specific sexual functioning. While some patients did not choose to discuss this subject, others welcomed the opportunity to express concern about their inability to lead normal sex lives.

Some patients answered the nurse's questions pertaining to allergy by giving a history of allergy although they had not mentioned this to the physician. In response to the last, open-ended question, most patients did not wish to tell the nurse anything more. However, a few gave further information. One man wanted the nurse to know he "got mean" when he had pain, "cussed and everything," but that he really did not mean what he said. It appeared important to him for the nurse to understand his behavior.

CONCLUSIONS

Our testing indicates that the nursing history form is not only valuable for identifying individual patient needs, but for establishing early nurse-patient rapport. In general, patients responded cooperatively to the interview and many of them voiced appreciation for the nurse's interest in them as persons. During follow-up visits, patients consistently picked up the discussion of their concerns where the previous conversation had ended. One patient with diarrhea for which no organic cause could be found spoke freely about recent crises in her life but denied vehemently that these could be related to her symptoms. On each successive visit she immediately began to talk about what had happened to her. After several visits with the nurse, she concluded there probably was a relationship between her recent experiences and symptoms, and added, "I've gone through enough in the past few months to give anyone diarrhea." Thus it appears that the nursing

history interview, besides yielding vital information, also broadens the nurse's therapeutic effectiveness.

Must one use a nursing history form to identify needs? Obviously, no, but the form facilitates gathering data early in hospitalization. Only 30 minutes spent with the patient soon after admission yields quantities of information valuable throughout his stay. One nurse commented, after taking her first history, that she probably would have obtained almost all the information had she cared for the patient for several days. Since the length of the interview may raise a question about using this form in busy patient services, it is worth noting that while interview time can be measured readily, it is much harder to measure the time spent resolving problems which could have been prevented had information been available earlier. Priority use of the nurse's time is something that must be faced realistically. The nurse's comments about obtaining information in 30 minutes by interview which ordinarily would have taken several days of caring for the patient underscores the time value of a systematic approach to the nursing history.

So far, we have used the nursing history form only to collect data about individual nursing needs. However, the form lends itself equally well to collecting epidemiologic data relevant to the needs of a patient population. Nurses are frequently astute in their observations about individual patients, but the development of a nursing science has been impeded by the lack of data about groups of patients and their statistical analysis for characteristics common to a patient population. Plans are under way to use the nursing history form to collect epidemiologic data which will contribute to nursing knowledge.

UNIVERSITY OF KENTUCKY
COLLEGE OF NURSING

Nursing History

Date _____   Medical Diagnosis: _____
Name _____   _____
Hospital Number _____   _____
Address (city or county) _____   _____
Age _____ Sex: M _____ F _____   Information obtained from Patient: _____
Occupation _____   Other: _____
Religion _____   Relationship: _____
Race/National Origin _____   History needs to be rechecked at later date
_____

I. Patient Perceptions and Expectations Related to Illness/Hospitalization

1. Why did you come to the hospital? (or go to the doctor?) _____
_____

2. What do you think caused you to get sick? _____
_____

3. Has being sick made any difference in your usual way of life? If so, how? _____
_____

4. What do you expect is going to happen to you in the hospital? _____
_____

5. What is it like for you being in the hospital? _____
_____

6. How long do you expect to be in the hospital? _____
7. With whom do you live? _____
8. Who is the most important person(s) to you? _____
9. What effect has your coming to the hospital had on your family? (or closest person?)
_____

10. Are any of your family (or close persons) able to visit you in the hospital? _____
_____

11. What do you enjoy doing for recreation? (to pass the time) _____
_____

12. How do you expect to get along after you leave the hospital? _____
_____

II. Specific Basic Needs

1. Comfort, Rest, Sleep
   a. Pain/Discomfort
      1) Have you had any pain or discomfort since admission?   Yes _____
                                                                      No _____

(Nursing History Form continues)

If yes, describe _____

_____

2) Did you have any pain or discomfort before coming to the hospital?   Yes _____
   No _____

   If yes, describe _____

   _____

   How long? _____
   What did you do to relieve the pain/discomfort? _____
   Was the pain/discomfort relieved by treatment?   Completely _____
   Partially _____
   Not at all _____

3) If you have pain/discomfort while in the hospital what would you like the nurse to do
   to relieve it? _____

   _____

b. Rest/Sleep
   1) Are you having any trouble getting enough rest or sleep since you came to the
      hospital?   Yes _____
      No _____

      If yes, describe _____

      _____

   2) Do you usually have trouble going to sleep?   Yes _____
      No _____

      Do you usually have trouble staying asleep?   Yes _____
      No _____

      If yes, describe _____

      _____

      What have you done in the past to help you get enough rest or sleep? _____

      _____

      Was it effective?   Always _____
      Usually _____
      Sometimes _____
      Never _____

   3) What would you like the nurse to do to help you get the rest and sleep you need while
      in the hospital? _____

      _____

c. Personal Hygiene
   1) Do you need help with your bath while in the hospital?   Yes _____
      No _____

      If yes, describe _____

      _____

   2) Do you need help with brushing your teeth?   Yes _____
      No _____

      If yes, describe _____

      _____

(<u>Nursing History Form continues</u>)

3) Is your skin usually

Dry _____
Oily _____
Normal _____

4) What, if anything, do you use on your skin?

Face _____
Body _____

5) How often do you prefer to bathe?

Morning _____
Afternoon _____
Evening _____
No preference _____

6) Do you prefer a

Tub bath _____
Shower _____

This question is not pertinent _____

2. Safety
   a. Locomotion
      1) Do you have any difficulty walking about?

Yes _____
No _____

If yes, describe _____

_____

2) Did you have difficulty in walking before you came to the hospital?   Yes _____
No _____

If yes, describe _____

_____

How did you manage? _____

_____

3) Has anyone said anything to you about staying in bed (or getting out of bed) since you came to the hospital?

Yes _____
No _____

If yes, what? _____

_____

What do you think about staying in bed? (or getting out of bed?) _____

_____

4) Do you expect to have any difficulty getting about after you leave the hospital?

Yes _____
No _____
Don't know _____

If yes, how do you expect to manage? _____

_____

   b. Vision
      1) Do you have any difficulty in seeing?

Yes _____
No _____

If yes, describe _____

_____

2) Do you wear glasses?

Yes _____
No _____

(Nursing History Form continues)

3) If #1 is yes, in what way does your limited sight handicap you? _____

_____

How do you manage? _____

_____

c. Hearing
1) Do you have any difficulty in hearing?   Yes _____

                                                                       No _____

If yes, describe _____

_____

2) If yes, do you wear a hearing aid?   Yes _____

                                                                       No _____

3) If #1 is yes, in what way does your limited hearing handicap you? _____

_____

How do you manage? _____

_____

3. Fluids
1) Has the amount of fluid you usually drink been changed since you got sick?

                                                              Increased _____

                                                              Decreased _____

                                                             Unchanged _____

2) What fluids do you like to drink?
Water _____   Coffee _____

Milk _____   Tea _____

Fruit juice _____   Soft drinks _____

_____   _____

3) What fluids do you dislike? _____

4. Nutrition
a. Teeth/Mouth
1) What is the condition of your teeth?   Good _____

                                                                Cavities _____

                                                                  Other _____

2) Do you wear dentures?   Upper _____

                                                                  Lower _____

                                                                 Partial _____

3) Is eating limited by the condition of your teeth?   Yes _____

                                                                       No _____

If yes, describe _____

_____

4) Do you have any soreness in your mouth?   Yes _____

                                                                       No _____

If yes, does it interfere with your eating?   Yes _____

                                                                       No _____

(Nursing History Form continues)

b. Do you consider yourself to be   Overweight _____   How much _____
                                            Underweight _____   How much _____
                                            About right _____

c. Appetite/Food Preference
    1) Has being sick made any difference in your eating?   Yes _____
                                                                  No _____

        If yes, describe _____

                                                                 _____

    2) What foods do you eat mostly? _____

                                                                  _____

    3) Are there any foods you do not eat?   Yes _____
                                                        No _____

        If yes, which food do you not eat and why? _____
                                                                   _____

d. Diet
    1) Are you on a special diet?   Yes _____
                                           No _____

        If yes, what kind _____

    2) Were you ever on a special diet before you came to the hospital?   Yes _____
                                                                  No _____

        If yes, what kind _____
        Did you have any problems with your diet?   Yes _____
                                                         No _____

        If yes, describe _____

                                                                  _____

    3) Have you had any problems with your food since you came to the hospital?
                                                                              Yes _____
                                                                              No _____

        If yes, describe _____

                                                                  _____

        If yes, what do you think would correct the problem? _____

                                                                  _____

    4) Do you expect to be discharged on a special diet?   Yes _____
                                                                  No _____
                                                          Don't know _____

        If yes, how do you expect to manage? _____

                                                                  _____

5. Elimination
   a. Bowels
       1) Has being sick changed the way your bowels function in any way?   Yes _____
                                                                                   No _____

           If yes, describe _____

                                                                     _____

(Nursing History Form continues)

2) Do you usually have

Constipation _____
Diarrhea _____
Neither _____

3) How often do you usually have a bowel movement? _____

4) What time of day do you normally have a bowel movement? _____

5) Do you take a laxative Regularly _____   or an enema? Regularly _____
Frequently _____   Frequently _____
Occasionally _____   Occasionally _____
Never _____   Never _____

If yes, what kind? _____
_____

6) Do you do anything else to help you have a bowel movement?

Yes _____
No _____

If yes, describe _____
_____

7) Do you expect to have any problem with your bowels after you leave the hospital?

Yes _____
No _____

If yes, how do you expect to manage? _____
_____

b. Bladder
1) Have you had any difficulty in passing your urine (water) since you came to the hospital?

Yes _____
No _____

If yes, describe _____
_____

2) Did you have any difficulty with your urine before you came to the hospital?

Yes _____
No _____
Don't remember _____

If yes, describe _____
_____

How did you manage? _____
_____

3) If #1 is yes, what do you think would help you pass your urine (water) while in the hospital? _____
_____

4) Do you expect to have a problem with your urine after you leave the hospital?

Yes _____
No _____

If yes, how do you expect to manage? _____
_____

(Nursing History Form continues)

6. Oxygen
    1) Has being sick caused any change in your breathing?   Yes _____
                                                                     No _____

       If yes, describe _____
       _____

    2) Did you have any difficulty with your breathing before you came to the hospital?
                                                                     Yes _____
                                                                     No _____

       If yes, describe _____
       _____

       If yes, how did you manage? _____
       _____

    3) If #1 is yes, what do you think would make it easier for you to breathe while you are at
       the hospital? _____
       _____

    4) Do you expect to have any difficulty with your breathing after you leave the hospital?
                                                                     Yes _____
                                                                     No _____
                                                                     Don't know _____

       If yes, how do you expect to manage? _____

7. Sexuality (Ask according to marital status and appropriateness to the patient.)
    1) (If Married) Has being sick made any difference in your being a
           husband _____   wife _____   Yes _____
           father _____   mother _____   No _____
       If yes, describe _____
       _____

       (If single and appropriate) Has being sick made any difference in your relationship
       with other people, particularly the opposite sex?   Yes _____
                                                                     No _____
       If yes, describe _____
       _____

    2) (If appropriate) Has being sick caused any change in your sexual functioning (sex life)?
                                                                     Yes _____
                                                                     No _____
       If yes, describe _____
       _____

    3) Do you expect your sexual functioning (sex life) to be changed in any way after you
       leave the hospital?   Yes _____
                                                                     No _____
                                                                     Don't know _____

       If yes, describe _____
       _____

(Nursing History Form continues)

4) Do you expect your ability to function as a husband, wife, father, mother, or in a social relationship to be changed in any way after you leave the hospital?

Yes _____

No _____

Don't know _____

If yes, describe _____

_____

III. Other

1. Do you have any known allergies?

Yes _____

No _____

If yes, what kind? _____

_____

How have you managed? _____

To what extent does the allergy handicap you? _____

_____

2. How far did you go in school? _____

Can you read and write? (Ask only if indicated)

Yes _____

No _____

3. Is there anything else you wish to tell me that would help us with your nursing care?

_____

_____

_____

IV. Nurse's Impressions and Suggestions

1. In your judgment which word(s) best describe this patient?

Alert _____	Homesick _____
Angry _____	Hyperactive _____
Answers questions readily _____	Hypoactive _____
Answers questions reluctantly ____	Lethargic _____
Anxious _____	Nonquestioning _____
Confident _____	Nontalkative _____
Confused _____	Passive _____
Cooperative _____	Questioning _____
Critical _____	Quick to comprehend _____
Demanding _____	Secure _____
Depressed _____	Seeks support _____
Disoriented _____	Slow to comprehend _____
Distrustful _____	Talkative _____
Embarrassed _____	Trustful _____
Euphoric _____	Unable to comprehend _____
Fearful _____	Withdrawn _____

(<u>Nursing History Form continues</u>)

2. Summary of findings that are significant for nursing care. _____
_____
_____
_____
_____

Chapter 2

Observation and Listening

This chapter, with its discussion of observation and listening, begins to build the foundation of skills needed to carry out the nursing process. Observation and listening are key skills that are used by the nurse in every facet of work. Because they appear to be such simple skills, however, they are sometimes quickly discounted. Yet, these two skills are vital in providing health care—particularly in providing individualized, humanistic health care.

Observation and listening can be thought of as lifeline skills, for it is through their use that the caregiver can determine a client's physiologic and emotional status, as well as changes in a client's status. Both formal and informal observation and listening are a continual part of the nursing process and have ever-changing results. These skills are essential in all phases of the nursing process but are particularly valuable in assessment and evaluation.

Observation involves constant, alert interest and attention paid to all the various systems and to the changes in those systems. Listening involves more than hearing; it includes the ability to be attuned to people and to the environment and to the meanings of things that are unspoken, as well as those that are spoken. Both observation and listening are skills that can be very difficult at times.

A conceptual framework for understanding these skills involves a study of perception and empathy. Following the discussion of these concepts, the chapter delineates the physical and emotional factors in nursing care that mandate use of these skills. Feedback as a means of validating observation and listening concludes Chapter 2.

CONCEPTUAL FRAMEWORK

The framework for understanding observation and listening skills predominantly includes concepts of perception and empathy. These are important facets of a caregiver's humanistic skills.

Perception

Perception is that organizing process by which one comes to know objects in their appropriate identity (Garrett, 1955). It means recognizing something, having insight into it, understanding it, and being able to interpret and explain it. An object, place, person, or event is recognized and perceived by the use of receptors (receivers): exteroceptors, interoceptors, and proprioceptors. Langley, Cheraskin, and Sleeper (1974) defined *exteroceptors* as those sensitive to stimuli outside the body and *interoceptors* as those sensitive to stimuli inside the body. Those receptors focusing on movements of the body are called *proprioceptors*. Marriner (1983, p. 179) defined perception as "a conscious awareness of the environment".

In order to perceive, one must always observe first, but the time interval between observing and perceiving seldom is noticed (Smeltzer, 1962). One pays attention in three ways—voluntarily, involuntarily, and habitually (Smeltzer, 1962)—with perceptions being the interpretations given to sensory experience within oneself. Since physical organisms are

capable of receiving a broad range of sensory experiences, it follows that people are capable of developing a broad range of perceptions. Perception is, therefore, a dynamic and learned process (Hilgard, Atkinson, & Atkinson, 1979). It involves comprehending a present situation in the light of past experience, always within the unique world of the observer.

One's awareness of self and the world around depends on sense organs and the stimuli that excite them. The sense organs are commonly referred to as eyes, ears, nose, mouth, and skin (seeing, hearing, smelling, tasting, and touching), with Kelley (1947) designating vision as the most important. Using all of one's sense organs, one constructs and reconstructs the world in accordance with how one perceives and knows it.

Perception, however, is selective, and since one selects what one perceives, the perceptual field of each individual is unique. Sense organs are constantly bombarded with stimuli, some of which are perceived and others of which are blocked. Much of what is allowed to enter depends upon *mental set*—that is, on what one is geared to perceive. Jarvis and Gibson (1965, p. 36) stated that "reception of stimuli in consciousness can be cut out." A sudden stimulus, however, might make one attend to it involuntarily. This is termed "attention getting factors in the stimulus" (Garrett, 1955, p. 157). Mental sets and, therefore, perception are influenced by past experience. Thus, interest and training can lead one individual to perceive certain aspects and details of a stimulus that escape others (Hilgard, Atkinson, & Atkinson, 1979). Jarvis and Gibson (1965) further explained this point by saying that the way one sees is learned. Finally, Frieze and Bar-Tal (1979), applying attribution theory, explained that people first form an idea about something or somebody and then collect data to support that idea. Sociologic factors, therefore, play a primary role in one's perceptual field.

Factors Governing Perception. Research has suggested that there are many external factors governing what one attends to and, hence, what is perceived (Senger, 1974). For example, intensity and size affect what is perceived (Matheson, 1975); if two stimuli are competing for attention, the most intense or largest will be the first one noticed. Also, change causes one to shift attention (Smeltzer, 1962), and repetition of a certain stimulus can increase sensitivity or alertness to the stimulus (Matheson, 1975). Human beings, for example, are quite sensitive to objects that move in their field of vision (Smeltzer, 1962), with anything unusual or novel catching one's attention. It has been noted, too, that perception can be determined by direct or subtle suggestions as well as by curiosity. One also views objects as members of a common group when they are similar but not identical; *Gestalt* psychologists term this phenomenon *similarity* (Matheson, 1975).

Another factor governing what is perceived is *closure*; closure is the tendency to fill in gaps of stimulation so that the whole is perceived, rather than parts (Matheson, 1975).

Individual needs and values also strongly influence what is perceived. Since needs and values (motivation) affect perceptual intake, Maslow's (1970) hierarchy of needs can be applied in understanding perception. For example, if one is hungry (physical need), the sights, sounds, and smells of food become priority items to the exclusion of other items.

Perceptual organization also encompasses the *Gestalt* concept of the *figure-ground* relationship. When a simple, definite object is placed on a background, it is immediately perceived as a figure, even though it may not be recognized or identified (Matheson, 1975). Another example is that letters on a textbook page are perceived as black letters on a white background. It is not common to think of a black background with white letters.

Shape, size, and color are *perceptual constancies* (Jarvis & Gibson, 1965). This is a phenomenon in which objects are perceived as they really are, rather than according to the stimulation received from them. In *shape constancy*, there is a strong tendency for the perceived shape of

familiar objects to remain the same, irrespective of the position or condition in which the shapes are viewed. Furthermore, if cues of depth perception are operative, an image will look smaller in a positive relationship to its distance; this is termed *size constancy*. Finally, color is usually constant regardless of any abnormal condition present in the object (Matheson, 1975).

Visual cues are usually threefold: *Monocular* cues are depth cues when one eye is looking, and *binocular* cues depend on two eyes. Kinesthetic impulses from eye muscles signaling the brain regarding their position and tension form the third visual cue, commonly referred to as *accommodation* (Matheson, 1975).

Tools of Perception.   Words, signs, symbols, and functions of objects are called *tools of perception* (Smeltzer, 1962). A considerable part of life's learning time is devoted to the names of objects, and signs and symbols are used to shorten the stimulus presentation for perceptual processes. Moreover, the functions and uses of objects usually make up the largest area of perceptual tools. Thus, giving attention to something is most often followed by interpretation of what it is for, what it will do, and how it works (Smeltzer, 1962).

Anomalies of Perception.   Illusions, hallucinations, and delusions are seen as anomalies (deviations) of perception. An *illusion* is a common misinterpretation of a stimulus. Sensory experiences without relevant or adequate sensory impulses are called *hallucinations*. *Delusions* are false opinions or beliefs that cannot be shaken by reason (Matheson, 1975). Hallucinations and delusions are often evident in psychotic behaviors.

Extrasensory Perception.   Extrasensory perception (ESP) is a rapidly growing science that involves one's ability to obtain information about an object or person when sensory input (as far as we know) is nonexistent. It may involve intuition, precognition, clairvoyance, and/or telepathy. With expanding affirmative documentation of a reality-base (Ostrander & Schroeder, 1971; Rao, 1966), this area of perception must be noted and considered.

Theoretic Model of Perception.   Three decades ago, Ittelson and Cantril (1954) developed a theoretic model for perception composed of three major features. It is useful for actualizing the concept of perception.

The first feature of the perception model is the concept of *transactions*. According to Ittelson and Cantril, "the facts of perception always present themselves through concrete individuals dealing with concrete situations. They can be studied only in terms of the 'transactions' in which observed" (Ittelson & Cantril, 1954, p. 2). It is impossible to isolate and study a perception without seriously distorting its meaning. Since no perception stands alone, it follows that it must be studied in terms of the situation in which the phenomenon takes place; perceptions are context bound. This requires application of a systems approach as well as a sociologic perspective for studying perceptions. The term *transaction* indicates that all parts of a situation have an active role in affecting perception, and perception owes its existence to this active participation; neither the parts of a situation nor perception exists separately.

The second feature of the theoretic model is the *personal behavior* center. Each person gives and takes personal experiences in a given situation, with each party engrossed in a situation reflective of his own personal experience (Ittelson & Cantril, 1954). Thus, two people in different professions may have varied perceptions and experiences relative to a given object or phenomenon, while two people in the same profession may have common experiences and perceptions. This point is the basis for all social activity. Nevertheless, each person's perceptions are still unique to the individual observer.

The last feature of the model is *externalization*. This is the actual means by which a person puts together a transaction (Ittelson & Cantril, 1954). The experience of perception is exter-

nally oriented; that is, the things heard, tasted, seen, and touched are experiences outside the self. Yet, they possess the characteristics that one individually creates in light of past experience and one's personal world of objects and events.

Application in Nursing.   Why is it important in nursing to understand the theories of perception? It is known that one's perceptions are comprised, formed, and realized individually and that they are based on thoughts, feelings, philosophies, values, desires, behaviors, and experiences (see PELLEM Pentagram, Chapter 17). If one desires to observe and listen for client information to plan individualized nursing care, how can one get past one's own selective perceptions in order to have truly a clean slate and pick up what is important in the client's world? The absolute answer to this question is that it is an impossible event, for one cannot disengage self from self for the sake of others. The nurse must move from a deterministic model to a probabilistic model and pose the questions: How can one move closer to another's world? How can one gain greater insight into another perceptual field while realizing the self exists? These questions can be answered, and they involve three components: (1) awareness of one's own perceptual motivations facilitated by the consciousness-raising activities of the PELLEM Pentagram,* (2) having empathy, and (3) establishing reliability for perceptions by checking them with others to note similarities and differences (feedback).

Empathy

The concept of empathy (discussed more fully in Chapter 15 and in the selected readings in that chapter) is generally viewed as an ability to place oneself mentally and emotionally in the world of the person with whom one is inter-

---

*Chapter 17 provides a discussion of this model.

acting (Rogers, 1961). More recently, based on research findings, the definition of empathy has been expanded: empathy is perceiving the feelings in a client's world and responding to the client in a way that acknowledges the perceived feelings; the client must then perceive that the helper has understood (La Monica, 1979a, 1979b, 1981; La Monica & Karshmer, 1978). However, it is necessary to free one's mind of self to accomplish this task. Logical reasoning dictates the impossibility of freeing oneself from anything unless one is aware of what one is to be freed from (on other words, "I cannot put away what I do not know I have!"). This point emphasizes the need for self-awareness. It also frees one to perceive another, and this is best done when the perceiver takes all information known about another and constructs a fantasy. The guiding questions asked of self are: Given the points known and what has been said, how would I feel in this situation? What would I feel if I were in the other's shoes? What would I want, need, and think? What would be helpful to me? This process involves understanding and interpreting self-perceptions with emphasis on another's world. It also involves using self purposefully and with awareness, rather than attempting to repress or blot out one's own perceptual system with the delusion that one can disengage self from the other person. Involved is an owning or meeting of oneself as a means to understand others. If one knows self, there is greater probability that one can move closer to knowing and understanding another since the art of exploring the self is similar to the art of exploring another's individuality and perceptual field. Conversely, when one is unable to look at oneself for whatever reason, how could one ever truly perceive an array of aspects in another without being oppressed in selected areas? Masserik and Wechsler (1959) termed the process *interpersonal perception* (subtitled *empathy revisited*); it is the process of understanding people.

Now that we have examined the conceptual framework involving perception and empathy, we can look at observation and listening as skills necessary in nursing.

OBSERVATION AND LISTENING IN ACTION

Perhaps the most succinct and articulate definitions of the observation and listening skills are by Webster. He viewed observation as the act of perceiving, noticing, and watching attentively. Listening he described as attending closely, with the sense organ being the ear—that is, making a conscious effort to hear. Looking at the organs of perception, the following becomes evident in terms of these skills: observing involves the senses of sight, touch, and smell; listening involves the sense of hearing.

The act of talking becomes important when providing feedback on or seeking clarification or affirmation of what has been observed and heard. Logic tells one, therefore, that observation and listening come first, talking second—unless, of course, one wishes to be observed and heard first, which would imply that one's own agenda is of primary importance and the client's of only secondary importance. However, when seeking to discover priorities in the client's world in order to uncover areas needing assistance, a helping nurse must place the client's agenda—what the client needs to have taken care of—in the foreground. In later stages of the nursing process, and in line with the model presented in Chapter 9 for implementing nursing care, the agenda of the nurse may be foremost at times, but certainly not always. Of course, the nurse often initiates the observation and listening process by talking and asking leading questions to elicit information that requires further observation and needs to be heard. It is important to remember, however, that professional expertise is only a guide to giving care; it should not be an end in itself. An individual client's agenda is paramount. Davis (1981) provided 10 guides for effective listening.

TEN GUIDES FOR EFFECTIVE LISTENING

1. *Stop talking!*
   You cannot listen if you are talking.
   Polonius (Hamlet): "Give every man thine ear, but few thy voice."

2. *Put the talker at ease.*
   Help the person feel free to talk.
   This is often called a permissive environment.

3. *Show the talker that you want to listen.*
   Look and act interested. Do not read your mail while someone talks.
   Listen to understand, rather than to oppose.

4. *Remove distractions.*
   Don't doodle, tap, or shuffle papers.
   Will it be quieter if you shut the door?

5. *Empathize with the talker.*
   Try to help yourself see the other person's point of view.

6. *Be patient.*
   Allow plenty of time. Do not interrupt the talker.
   Don't start for the door or walk away.

7. *Hold your temper.*
   An angry person takes the wrong meaning from words.

8. *Go easy on argument and criticism.*
   This puts people on the defensive, and they may "clam up" or become angry.
   Do not argue: Even if you win, you lose.

9. *Ask questions.*
   This encourages the talker and shows that you are listening.
   It helps to develop points further.

SOURCE: *Human Behavior at Work: Organizational Behavior,* 6th Ed., by K. Davis. Copyright © 1981, 1977, 1972, 1967, 1962, 1957, p. 413. Reprinted by permission.

10. *Stop talking!*
    This is first and last, because all other guides depend on it.
    You cannot do an effective listening job while you are talking.

- Nature gave people two ears but only one tongue, which is a gentle hint that they should listen more than they talk.
- Listening requires two ears, one for meaning and one for feeling.
- Decision makers who do not listen have less information for making sound decisions.

Categorically speaking, there can be two basic kinds of data regarding a client that must be observed: physical aspects and emotional aspects.

Physical Aspects

The area of physical aspects refers primarily to the physiologic signs and symptoms that a professional nurse should be alert for and accurately report so as to facilitate understanding with other health personnel. The list of signs and symptoms provided in Table 2-1 is not meant to be exhaustive but, rather, provides a framework. Physical-assessment skills are necessary in many of the areas.

Emotional Aspects

The nurse is constantly listening for and observing emotional aspects of the client. These are the individual's feelings. Perception of these feelings is closely entwined with the verbal and nonverbal communications of the client, an area covered in the next chapter. For our purposes here, it is necessary only to look broadly at the perception of feelings. Gazda, Asbury, Balzer, Childers, and Walters (1977) have divided feelings into two dimensions: surface and underlying. Surface feelings are those that are explicitly expressed by the client; they are obvious by the words or way a person says something.

Table **2-1**   Physical Symptoms to Be Observed
and Terms to Use in Reporting Them*

	Observation	Term to Use
Abdomen	1. Hard, boardlike	1. Hard, rigid
	2. Soft, flabby	2. Relaxed, flaccid, soft
	3. Appears swollen, rounded	3. Protuberant
	4. Hurts when touched	4. Sensitive to touch
	5. Filled with gas	5. Distended, tympanites
	6. Note area of abdomen observed	
Areas		1. Epigastric
		2. Right lumbar
		3. Umbilical
		4. Left lumbar
		5. Right iliac
		6. Hypogastric
		7. Left ilias
Belch	Belching	Eructation
Bleeding	1. Spurting of blood	1. In spurts
	2. Very little	2. Oozing
	3. Nosebleed	3. Epistaxis
	4. Blood in vomitus	4. Hematemesis
	5. Blood in urine	5. Hematuria
	6. Spitting of blood	6. Hemoptysis
	7. When bleeding is stopped	7. Hemorrhage controlled
	8. Color	8. Bright red, dark red, frothy
Breathing	1. Breathing	1. Respiration
	2. Act of inhaling	2. Inspiration
	3. Act of exhaling	3. Expiration
	4. Difficult breathing	4. Dyspnea
	5. Short periods when breathing has ceased	5. Apnea
	6. Inability to breathe lying down	6. Orthopnea
	7. Normal breathing	7. Eupnea
	8. Rapid breathing	8. Hyperpnea
	9. Increasing dyspnea with periods of apnea	9. Cheyne-Stokes respiration
	10. Snorting breathing	10. Stertorous breathing
	11. Large volume of air inspired or expired	11. Deep breathing
	12. Small volume of air inspired or expired	12. Shallow breathing
	13. Abnormal variation in rhythm	13. Irregular respiration

Table **2–1**   (continued)

	Observation	Term to Use
Chill	1. Blanket applied to help warm the patient 2. Type as to severity 3. Duration	1. External heat applied 2. Severe, moderate, slight 3. Lasting number of minutes
Coma	1. Partly in coma 2. Deep in coma	1. Partially comatose 2. Profound coma
Convulsion	1. Continuous shaking 2. Shaking with intervals of rest 3. Begin without warning	1. Duration and description 2. Duration and description 3. Sudden onset
Cough	1. Coughs at all times 2. Coughing over a long period of time 3. Coughs up material 4. Short, hard cough	1. Continuous cough 2. Persistent cough 3. Productive cough, describe 4. Hacking cough
Defecation	1. Bowel movement material 2. Bowel movement (act of) 3. Excessive defecation 4. Gray colored stool 5. Dark brown liquid 6. Formed, yet soft stool 7. Formed, yet hardened stool 8. Infrequent bowel movements 9. Black stool	1. Feces, stool 2. Defecation 3. Diarrhea, describe 4. Clay colored liquid stool 5. Highly colored liquid stool 6. Soft formed stool 7. Hard formed stool 8. Constipation 9. Black, tarry stool
Dizziness	Dizziness	Vertigo
Drainage	1. Watery, from nose 2. Containing pus 3. Bloody 4. Consists of feces 5. Of serous fluid 6. Containing mucus and pus 7. Tough, sticky 8. From vagina (after delivery)	1. Coryza 2. Purulent 3. Sanguineous 4. Fecal 5. Serous 6. Mucopurulent 7. Tenacious 8. Lochia
Dressings	1. A second dressing added to the first 2. Dressing removed, another applied 3. Drain tubes cut off 4. Drain taken out	1. Dressing reinforced 2. Redressed 3. Drain tubes shortened (number of inches) 4. Drain removed
Emesis	1. Produced by effort of patient 2. Ejected to a few feet distant 3. If blood is only noticeable	1. Induced 2. Projectile 3. Blood tinged

Table **2-1**   (continued)

	Observation	Term to Use
	4. Material vomited	4. Vomitus, emesis
	5. Contents	5. Describe color, odor, appearance, consistency
Eyes	1. Sharpness of vision	1. Visual acuity
	2. Yellow in color	2. Jaundiced
	3. Puffy	3. Edematous
	4. Motionless	4. Staring
	5. Sensitive to light	5. Photophobia
	6. Double vision	6. Diplopia
	7. Squinting	7. Strabismus
	8. Abnormal protrusion of eyeball	8. Exophthalmus
	9. Inflammation of conjunctiva	9. Conjunctivitis
Faint	Fainting	Syncope
Fever	1. Without fever	1. Afebrile
	2. Temperature above normal	2. Pyrexia
	3. Temperature greatly above normal	3. Hyperpyrexia
	4. Temperature suddenly returns to normal	4. Crisis
	5. Temperature gradually returns to normal	5. Lysis
Gas	1. Gas in the digestive tract	1. Flatus
	2. Having gas in the digestive tract	2. Flatulence
	3. Swelling of abdomen	3. Distention
Hallucination	1. Of hearing	1. Auditory hallucination
	2. Of sight	2. Visual hallucination
	3. Of smell	3. Olfactory hallucination
	4. Of taste	4. Gustatory hallucination
Head	1. Forehead	1. Frontal region
	2. Region over temple	2. Temporal region
	3. Back of head	3. Occipital region
	4. Base of skull	4. Basilar region
Joints	1. Bending	1. Flexion
	2. To straighten	2. Extension
	3. Turn inward	3. Inversion
	4. Turn outward	4. Eversion
	5. Revolve around	5. Rotation
	6. Move away from median line	6. Abduction
	7. Move toward median line	7. Adduction
Lice	1. Head, body, pubic	1. Pediculi
	2. Condition of lousiness	2. Pediculosis

Table **2–1**   (continued)

	Observation	Term to Use
Nourishment	1. Very small amount of water	1. Sips water
	2. Small pieces of ice	2. Chipped ice
	3. Drink of water	3. Water (number of ccs)
	4. Given through tube into stomach	4. Lavage
	5. Given by enema	5. Nutritive enema, fluid and amount
Odor	1. Not unpleasant	1. Aromatic
	2. Like fruit	2. Fruity
	3. Very unpleasant	3. Offensive
	4. Belonging to a particular drug, and so forth	4. Characteristic
	5. Like feces	5. Fecal
Pain	1. Great pain	1. Severe
	2. Little	2. Slight
	3. Spasmodic; period of great pain followed by period of little or no pain	3. Paroxysmal
	4. Spreads to distant areas	4. Radiating
	5. Started all at once	5. Sudden onset
	6. Hurts worse when moving	6. Increased by movement
Paralysis	1. Of the muscles of the face	1. Facial
	2. Of the legs	2. Paraplegia
	3. Of one side of the body	3. Hemiplegia
	4. Of a single limb	4. Monoplegia
	5. Both arms and legs	5. Quadriplegia
Perspiration	1. Large amount	1. Profuse diaphoresis
	2. Small amount	2. Scanty
Pulse	1. Number of beats per minute	1. Rate
	2. Rhythm	2. Regular or irregular
	3. Beats missed at intervals	3. Intermittent
	4. Over 100 beats per minute	4. Rapid
	5. Very rapid, beats indistinct	5. Running
	6. Slow in rate	6. Slow
	7. Scarcely perceptible	7. Thready
	8. Small, rapid and tense	8. Wiry
Skin	1. Normal	1. Healthy
	2. Pink, hot	2. Flushed
	3. Blue in color	3. Cyanotic
	4. Very white	4. Extreme pallor

Table **2-1**   (continued)

Observation		Term to Use
	5. Shines	5. Glossy
	6. Raw surface	6. Excoriation
	7. Yellow in color	7. Jaundiced
	8. Torn	8. Lacerated
	9. Containing colored areas	9. Pigmented
	10. Wet	10. Moist
	11. Scraped	11. Abraded
	12. Black and blue mark	12. Ecchymosis
	13. Cold, clammy	13. Cold, clammy
Unconsciousness	1. Complete unconsciousness	1. In comatose condition
	2. Partial unconsciousness	2. In stuporous condition
	3. Pretended unconsciousness	3. Feigned unconsciousness
Urination	1. To urinate	1. Void, urinate
	2. No control over urination	2. Involuntary, incontinent
	3. Burning when voiding	3. Burning sensation on urination
	4. Large amount of urine voided	4. Polyuria
	5. Total suppression of urine	5. Anuria
	6. Frequent voiding at night	6. Nocturia
	7. Painful urination	7. Dysuria
	8. Pus in urine	8. Pyuria
	9. Blood in urine	9. Hematuria
	10. Hemoglobin in urine	10. Hemoglobinuria
	11. Glucose in urine	11. Glucosuria
	12. Albumin in urine	12. Albuminuria
	13. Acetone in urine	13. Acetonuria
	14. Bile in urine	14. Choluria
	15. Scantiness of urine	15. Oliguria
	16. Sugar in urine	16. Glycosuria
Weight	1. Overweight	1. Obese
	2. Thin, underweight	2. Emaciated
Wounds	1. Deep	1. Deep
	2. Slight, surface only	2. Superficial
	3. Not infected	3. Clean
	4. Discharging pus	4. Suppurating
	5. Infected	5. Infected
	6. Torn	6. Lacerated

*SOURCE: These descriptions were derived from materials compiled by an anonymous source.

Example:	(Pale, listless client to nurse, in weak voice) "I am not feeling like my usual self—my energy seems gone."
Feelings expressed:	weak, listless, lacking in energy, sick, unhappy, down

Gazda et al. (1977) further described underlying feelings as a content interpretation of what a client says; these feelings may not have been overtly verbalized, but a nurse can read between the lines and also consider the feelings in relation to previously observed data.

Example:	(Same situation as before, plus the following information) The nurse knows the client is one day post-operative of abdominal surgery.
Underlying feelings:	washed-out, sicker than she thought she'd feel, wondering whether these feelings are normal

It is important to note that verbal ability and appropriate use of the language can facilitate accuracy in responding to surface and underlying feelings. Therefore, included in the suggested-reading portion of Chapter 3 is an article by Moorhead (1972) containing a list of words used to describe feelings. Gazda et al. (1977) also contains an appendix of affective adjectives. Referring to these sources may be helpful.

Feedback

It follows that after one perceives the physical and emotional dimensions of the client, it is necessary to establish the validity of these because one's perceptual field is guided by the self. Clients must sense that the helper or nurse has been empathic—that is, has accurately perceived their feelings. This process involves feedback to the client and to colleagues.

Knowledge and experience enable the nurse to rest with more security on perceptions of physical signs and symptoms than on perceptions of emotional ones. If unsure of these physical signs, however, it becomes the nurse's responsibility to check findings with one who is more experienced. This process usually involves asking for an opinion or consultation. It parallels what physicians do when they request expert consultation. When two people agree, the perception is more reliable; conversely, if disagreement occurs, clarification and discussion become necessary.

This same process is carried into the client's emotional domain, but here consultation with the client is necessary. Orlando (1961, p. 1) described the task of the nurse as distinguishing "between the understanding of general principles and the meanings which she must discover in the immediate nursing situation in order to help the patient." In order to accomplish this, the nurse must understand the meanings in the client's world and then exercise his or her professional functions with relation to the client's needs. In essence, this involves perceiving the client's feelings and validating these perceptions with the client.

Validation requires stating what was heard from the client, reflectively and in one's own natural words. It means building a response to the client which conveys that one heard the expressed feelings and understood the underlying feelings, all of which personifies empathy. Cash, Scherba, and Mills (1975) proposed five steps meant to assist the helper in the aforementioned process of building empathic responses:

1. Identify the mood.
2. Specify the feelings—surface and underlying.
3. Decide the intensity level of the feelings—high, low, moderate.
4. Select words that are analogous with the expressed feelings.
5. Verbalize a sentence incorporating perception of items 1–4.

Gazda et al. (1977) further pointed out guidelines for building responses:

1. Verbal and nonverbal behavior should be the focus of the helper.

2. The helper should formulate responses of empathy in a language and manner that is most easily understood by the helpee.

3. The tone of the helper's response should be analogous to that of the helpee.

4. The helper should actively use empathy in responding to the helpee.

5. The helper should concentrate on what the helpee is expressing and also be aware of what is not being expressed.

6. The helper must accurately interpret responses to the helpee and use them as a guide in developing future responses.

Using the same example previously explicated, a natural response that incorporates these guidelines would be:

Example: (Same situation as before, evoking natural response of the nurse) "You sound as if you are feeling extremely weak and exhausted, possibly even wondering if you will ever feel like yourself again."

In this example, the nurse has communicated that what the client expressed was heard and that what the client did not express also was understood. In addition, the nurse is communicating interest in and concern for the client and has granted the client permission to express personal feelings. This latter factor alone is paramount in building a trusting nurse/client relationship. It opens the door for further client-centered communication.

Validation of perceptions by the client is possible because the client has an avenue through which to respond, knowing that the nurse cares and will listen. Because the nurse does not ask questions at this time (nurse's agenda), the client has freedom to respond with her own agenda, and the nurse can then obtain client-centered data. Closure of the interaction is predominantly guided by the client.

SUMMARY

The skills of observation and listening were presented using a conceptual framework involving perception and empathy. Physical and emotional dimensions were discussed, and the use of feedback was presented as a method for validating perceptions.

REFERENCES

Cash, R., Scherba, D., & Mills, S. (1975). *Human resources development: A competency based training program* (Trainer's manual). Long Beach, CA: Author.

Davis, K. (1981). *Human behavior at work: Organizational behavior* (6th ed.). New York: McGraw-Hill.

Frieze, I., & Bar-Tal, D. (1979). Attribution theory: Past and present. In I. Frieze, D. Bar-Tal, & J. Carroll (Eds.), *New approaches to social problems.* San Francisco: Jossey-Bass.

Garrett, H. (1955). *General psychology.* New York: American Book Company.

Gazda, G., Asbury, F., Balzer, F., Childers, W., & Walters, R. (1977). *Human relations development: A manual for educators* (2nd ed.). Boston: Allyn and Bacon.

Hilgard, E., Atkinson, R., & Atkinson, R. (1979). *Introduction to psychology* (7th ed.). New York: Harcourt Brace Jovanovich.

Ittelson, W., & Cantril, H. (1954). *Perception: A transactional approach.* Garden City, NY: Doubleday.

Jarvis, J., & Gibson, J. (1965). *Psychology for nurses.* Oxford, England: Blackwell Scientific Publications.

Kelley, E. (1947). *Education of what is real.* New York: Harper and Brothers.

La Monica, E. (1979a). Empathy in nursing practice. *Issues in Mental Health Nursing, 2,* 1–13.

La Monica, E. (1979b). The nurse and the aging client: Positive attitude formation. *Nurse Educator, 4*, 23–26.

La Monica, E. (1981). Construct validity of an empathy instrument. *Research in Nursing and Health, 4*, 389–400.

La Monica, E., & Karshmer, J. (1978). Empathy: Educating nurses in professional practice. *Journal of Nursing Education, 17*, 3–11.

Langley, L., Cheraskin, E., & Sleeper, R. (1974). *Dynamic anatomy and physiology* (4th ed.). New York: McGraw-Hill.

Marriner, A. (1983). *The nursing process: A scientific approach to nursing care* (3rd ed.). St. Louis: Mosby.

Maslow, A. (1970). *Motivation and personality* (2nd ed.). New York: Harper and Row.

Masserik, F., & Wechsler, I. (1959). Interpersonal perception. *California Management Review, 1*, 36–46.

Matheson, D. (1975). *Introductory psychology: The modern view*. Hinsdale, IL: Dryden Press.

Moorhead, T., Jr. (1972). *Communication for educational problem-solving*. Melbourne, FL: Human Dynamics.

Orlando, I. (1961). *The dynamic nurse-patient relationship*. New York: Putnam's.

Ostrander, S., & Schroeder, L. (1971). *Psychic discoveries behind the Iron Curtain*. New York: Bantam.

Rao, K. (1966). *Experimental parapsychology*. Springfield, IL: Charles C. Thomas.

Rogers, C. (1961). *On becoming a person*. Boston: Houghton-Mifflin.

Senger, J. (1974). Seeing eye to eye: Practical problems of perception. *Personnel Journal, 53*, 744–751.

Smeltzer, C. (1962). *Psychology for student nurses*. New York: Macmillan.

Chapter 3

Communication

Communication is of paramount importance in nursing, pervading every phase of the nursing process. Essentially, everything one does involves communication—with clients, with colleagues, and with oneself—and spoken and unspoken messages are the guides for accomplishment of each and every intent.

Chapter 3 closely follows the material presented in the previous chapter on observation and listening. The specific focus of this chapter, however, is the nurse's communications. The overall purpose of this chapter is to present a broad perspective on the communications concept, thereby providing a basis and rationale for an individual practitioner to develop a personal philosophy and conceptual framework for communication that can be heightened further through experience.

This chapter responds basically to the following questions:

1. What is communication?

2. Is there a theoretic model for communication?

3. What are the purposes of communication in nursing?

4. How does the nurse communicate?

5. What does a nurse communicate?

WHAT IS COMMUNICATION?

In one sense, communication is everything, for no human being exists in an autonomous vacuum, going through life in an impermeable cell and reaching only to self to fulfill needs. Even though one would suspect from Slater's (1976) exposition of American culture, for example, that one positive goal of life is to be independent of others, this outcome is never purely achieved and is considered an aberration; humans are social beings. Groups have developed spoken languages by which to reach out to closely related others, and body language is often considered to be universally understood.

Shannon and Weaver (1949) provided an early definition of communication when they said that it encompasses all that occurs between two or more minds. They included written and spoken language, art, music, theater, and *all* of human behavior. It can be concisely stated that behavior is communication and that all communication produces behavior. Gibran (1951) included in his discussion of talking a message that identified verbal speaking as a way of also communicating with self. Johnson (1981) defined communication as a means for one person to relay a message to another with the goal of receiving a response. Although the others add to our view of the complexity of communication, it is this latter definition that leads to formation of a theoretic model of communication.

THE THEORETIC MODEL

Theorists have developed an almost universally accepted model for communication processes. Berlo (1960) and Miller (1966) made major contributions to Hein's (1980) presentation of the model in nursing. Hein described six elements (Johnson, 1981, closely paralleled these steps in his portrayal of the model):

1. the reason for communicating, or referent

2. the sender, or source-encoder

3. a message that involves content

4. method(s) of communicating, or channel(s): verbal and/or nonverbal

5. the receiver, or decoder

6. feedback

Figure 3–1 portrays the model.

It is easy to see from the rather simplistic example in the figure that the model is dynamic; senders become receivers, and vice versa, until the communication ceases. Even though patterns of communication are rarely as simple as denoted, the example is meant to illustrate the model. All communications can then be studied within this framework.

The feedback process is the same validational procedure described in Chapter 2. Berlo (1960) emphasized the point that what and how one communicates relate to the attitudes, knowledge, and sociocultural system of the individual. Therefore, what is received relates to the same. Effective communication necessitates discovering a relatively positive wavelength between sender and receiver; the goal is congruence between the message intended and that received.

PURPOSES OF COMMUNICATION IN NURSING

The purpose for communicating with clients and colleagues specifically relates to one's definition of nursing and the reasons for care. As has been elucidated in earlier portions of this book, nursing involves facilitating clients' movement toward fulfillment of their health potential; when nurses intervene in this movement, it is toward this same goal. Specific assistance or interventions are required of the nurse to restore the client to health and, in doing so, erase nursing diagnoses. It becomes necessary, therefore, to narrow communication in nursing practice and to speak of "therapeutic

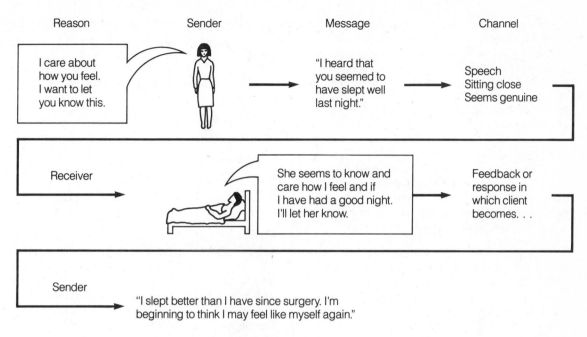

Figure 3–1

Theoretic Model of Communication

communication," a phrase mentioned by Goldin and Russell (1969) and Hein (1980), "effective communication" (Johnson, 1981), or "purposeful, effective communication in response to the client" (this author). Communications with colleagues or health personnel should be directed toward the same purpose, with the client being the major concern.

Johnson, Dumas, and Johnson (1967) and Peplau (1960) suggested that skillful nurse/client interactions are the essence of care. If one were to operate under the basic assumption (and this author does!) that all nurses—as well as all other health professionals—care about their clients, then it becomes necessary to explain why there is a growing body of literature pointing to consumers' perceived inhumane treatment by health care professionals. Nevertheless, it would be folly not to operate with the positive assumption. After all, if nurses do not care, what is there to prove? What is there to

strive for and why bother? It becomes a death wish. You see, if the author believes nurses do not care, the author, being a nurse, is most specifically pointing at self. Responsibility for the profession rests within the individual first! Moving from this slight digression, the explanation for the consumers' perceived qualities of non-caring, inhumaneness, abruptness, or whatever must rest within the effective/ineffective communication process, for *communication is behavior*, and behavior is all that anyone can perceive. Furthermore, communication is defined only as what is perceived by others. If there is a discrepancy between one's attitudes of caring and one's perceived behaviors of caring, the fault must lie in communication. Conversely, and positively speaking, if a nurse's attitudes are consonant with caring—that is, desiring to help another grow and actualize self (Mayeroff, 1971)—and the client so perceives this, it can be only a result of purposeful and effective communications. Thus, the need for effective communication becomes explicit: it is our only means for fulfilling our responsibilities, relating to either physical or emotional dimensions of care and guided by the desire to facilitate a positive experience for all members of the interaction. This relates to achievement of the client's physical goals as well as the emotional ones.

Ponthieu (1977) stated characteristics of an authentic communicator. Even though Ponthieu's perspective is from a manager's viewpoint, his thoughts nevertheless are deemed pertinent to discuss within a nursing framework. According to Ponthieu,

1. *Communication should not be determined by a role.* This requires that the nurse be genuine, rather than wear the mask of the "professional." It means meeting people on an adult-to-adult level (Berne, 1978), according to a transactional analysis model. Questions of hierarchy have no place in the communication process.

2. *The communicator must be aware of and in touch with his or her own attitudes (feelings, beliefs, and values).* Dissonance between a sender's attitudes and behaviors can be and usually is perceived by the receiver. If one's goal is to communicate clearly, it follows that one must be clear on what one wishes to communicate. Therefore, factual content and emotional overtones of the communication should correspond—words and music should go together.

3. *The communicator must be self-confident and accepting.* Remembering that the nurse is a unique person first, it is vital to recognize that the nurse's feelings *are* valid; this facilitates self-acceptance. Since the nurse further desires to enable a client to accept self, given different stages of health and illness, the best way may be as a role model. This involves recognition of both one's strengths and one's weaknesses.

Hewitt (1981) delineated specific purposes for which communication processes are used. However, the following purposes are rarely, if ever, used in isolation of one another.

1. To learn or to teach something
2. To influence someone's behavior
3. To express feelings
4. To explain one's own behavior or to clarify another's behavior
5. To relate to others
6. To untangle a problem
7. To accomplish a goal
8. To reduce tension or to resolve conflict
9. To stimulate interest in self or in others

METHODS OF COMMUNICATION

There are two types of communication: verbal and nonverbal. Within each category, the communication may be either one-way or two-way. Figure 3–2 illustrates these points.

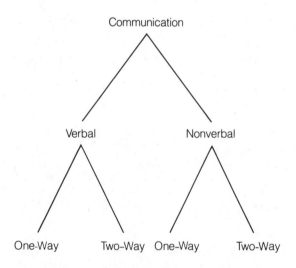

Figure 3–2

Types of Communication (SOURCE: *Nursing Leadership and Management: An Experiential Approach,* by E.L. La Monica. Copyright © 1983 by Wadsworth, Inc. Reprinted by permission of the publisher, Wadsworth Health Sciences Division, Monterey, California.)

Verbal communication generally includes all that is spoken and written. Verbal interactions between nurse and client, between nurse and nurse, between nurse and other health professionals, and so forth, form the basis for this primary area. Secondary sources of verbal communication include messages sent by one person to another and may be directed toward a specific person or toward parts of the health-care system. These secondary sources include the nurse's notes, discharge summaries, memoranda from all sources, and similar items.

Nonverbal communication involves all that is implied by body language, which is also behavior. Included are gestures, eye contact, facial expressions, posture, and space variations between the interactors. These communications generally amplify or detract from verbal statements but can stand alone in communicating meanings of silence. Very often, dissonance between attitudes and verbal behaviors are perceived through nonverbal messages. Table 3–1 portrays various nonverbal attending skills and ineffective and effective uses of each (Walters, 1983).

Two-way communication involves feedback; one-way does not. Johnson (1981) continued this definition by saying that one-way communication is when the sender is unable to discover how the receiver is perceiving or decoding the message. Two-way communication is when the sender receives feedback or validation. Obviously, both types of communication are used in health care, as in the following:

1. Sender gives message and does not provide avenue or time for feedback (one-way).
Example: Physician writes stat order and leaves.

2. Sender gives message and provides avenue for feedback, but receiver does not comply with request, at least verbally (one-way).
Example: Nurse: "You look like you're hungry."
   Client: Silence

3. Sender gives written message and waits for or requests a reaction (two-way).
Example: Head nurse sends a written memorandum requesting reactions to the introduction of staff-development programs on the unit and to the content of these programs. Space is provided on the memorandum to respond.

4. Sender gives verbal message and waits for response; receiver replies to message (two-way).
Example: Nurse: "Your record states that this is your third admission to this unit."
   Client: "Yes. I was admitted two years ago with the same problem. I didn't know that was important right now."
Nurse picks up on client's implied message and goes on with conversation.

The literature is replete with broad and specific discussions of methods used during communication processes. For this reason, our discussion here has not been lengthy. Building from the information presented, however, it becomes important to look at *what* a nurse communicates.

WHAT A NURSE COMMUNICATES

In addition to the content involved in nurse/client and nurse/nurse interactions, there is a pattern of communication which is unique to the helper and which should be reflective of counseling. Using this technique, interactions are based on a personal philosophy and a conceptual framework. It should be noted that purposeful, effective communication is a nursing goal with and for the client. Counseling is an interchange of opinions, feelings, and the like with the planned purpose and design of assisting or facilitating others to help themselves. In clinical nursing practice, communication often is counseling.

Whether a nurse's communication involves the practice of one theory or of several theories of counseling, the counseling should indeed be based on an application of theory. The individuality of the helper remains, however, regardless of what theory is used (Arbuckle, 1974).

Table **3-1**   Attending Skills*

Ineffective Use	Nonverbal Modes of Communication	Effective Use
Doing any of these things will probably close off or slow down the conversation.		These behaviors encourage talk because they show acceptance and respect for the other person.
Distant; very close	Space	Approximate arm's length
Spread among activities	Attention	Give fully to talker
Away	Movement	Toward
Slouching; rigid; seated leaning away	Posture	Relaxed but attentive; seated leaning slightly toward
Absent; defiant; jittery	Eye contact	Regular
You continue with what you are doing before responding; in a hurry	Time	Respond at first opportunity; share time with them
Used to keep distance between the persons	Feet and legs (in sitting)	Unobtrusive
Used as a barrier	Furniture	Used to draw persons together
Sloppy; garish; provocative	Dress; grooming	Tasteful
Does not match feelings; scowl; blank look	Facial expression	Matches your own or other's feelings; smile
Compete for attention with your words	Gestures	Highlight your words; unobtrusive; smooth
Obvious; distracting	Mannerisms	None, or unobtrusive
Very loud or very soft	Voice: volume	Clearly audible
Impatient or staccato; slow or hesitant	Voice: rate	Average, or a bit slower
Apathetic; sleepy; jumpy; pushy	Energy level	Alert; stays alert throughout a long conversation

*SOURCE: "The Amity Book: Exercises in Friendship and Helping Skills," by R. Walters. In G. Gazda, F. Asbury, F. Balzer, W. Childers, and R. Walters (Eds.), *Human Relations Development: A Manual for Educators,* 3rd Ed. Boston: Allyn and Bacon, 1983. Reprinted by permission of the author.

There are a number of counseling theories that pattern the process of communication for a helper. The theory of Carl Rogers (1961, 1965), later researched and documented as effective by Carkhuff (1969), will be discussed presently, and the reader is referred to a broader presentation of this client-centered approach in Chapter 15. The steps of the counseling process are the foci at this point.

Carkhuff (1969) delineated eight core conditions, previously explicated by Rogers (1961, 1965), that the helper must facilitate in the communication process. They involve two phases: understanding and action.

UNDERSTANDING PHASE

1. Empathy—getting inside another's skin and understanding the world as the other perceives it to be[1]

2. Respect—believing in another; respecting the other's world and rights, as well as the validity of the other's unique feelings

3. Warmth—caring; being concerned and loving

4. Concreteness—being specific, succinct, and clear

5. Genuineness—being a real human being; being honest and true

6. Self-disclosure—being able to communicate one's own humanness; sharing feelings

ACTION PHASE

7. Confrontation—pointing out conflicts, discrepancies, or problems; saying constructively what one observes

8. Immediacy—focusing on the here-and-now; looking at what seems to be happening between the helper and the helpee

Both Rogers (1961, 1965) and Carkhuff (1969) pointed out the need for both of these phases to occur within a relationship. If one

---

[1]Descriptions are adapted from the work of Gazda, Asbury, Balzer, Childers, and Walters (1977).

goes to a helper because one is unable to meet the problems faced and one requires intervention, the helper becomes an expert—one who possesses the knowledge and experience needed to assist. The understanding phase is meant to build a relationship between nurse and client; the action phase is the content phase, possibly requiring changes in the client's habits, routines, and behavior patterns. Thus, the understanding phase precedes the action phase, with empathy being the key ingredient (Carkhuff, 1969).

The following example is intended to clarify this process: Suppose you are a client, meeting a nurse for the first time in a clinic. You enter wearing green pants and an orange shirt. The first statement from the nurse is: "Green and orange do not match. You would look much better if you wore complementary colors!"

What would your reaction be? One of my feelings would be: "Who are you to tell me what to wear?" You see, the nurse doesn't know why you wore what you did. It may be that those were your best clothes or even your only ones. Who knows except you? The tendency at this point is for the client to block the nurse's statement and have a negative reaction to the nurse.

Now, further suppose that you had been going to this nurse for six months; you trust her and know she is interested in all that is best for you; she cares about you. If she made the same statement as before, would you be likely to listen? Would you think she was trying to help? If your green pants were treasured by you, would you be likely to tell her?

In this situation, the trusting, cared for, understood person will have a greater probability of listening and maybe changing, if the change is appropriate or needed in the client's world.

Carrying this example into practice, nursing involves facilitating change within the client, teaching, and dealing with lifestyles and attitudes. (Remember that *change* is synonymous with *learning*.) It follows, therefore, that an understanding relationship must be developed prior to taking any action. Time in a relationship is a significant variable because one must meet the demands and priorities reflected in the nursing diagnoses (discussed in Chapter 6). The understanding phase can be compressed into a five-minute, meaningful interaction or lengthened over years; it corresponds to needs and to the time available to meet them. In each phase, however, perceptions should be validated, and messages should require feedback. This is all a part of communication.

SUMMARY

This chapter focused on communication, moving from a broad perspective to one that is pertinent in nursing practice. Communication was illustrated with a theoretic model. Purposes and methods for communicating in nursing were discussed. Nonverbal and verbal patterns were presented, and one-way/two-way processes exemplified. The chapter concluded with what a nurse communicates; this was built on the counseling theory of client-centered and humanistic helping relationships.

REFERENCES

Arbuckle, D. (1974). The practice of the theories of counseling. *Counseling Education and Supervision, 13,* 214–222.

Berlo, D. (1960). *The process of communication.* New York: Holt, Rinehart and Winston.

Berne, E. (1978). *Games people play.* New York: Ballantine.

Carkhuff, R. (1969). *Helping and human relations: A primer for lay and professional helpers* (Vols. 1 and 2). New York: Holt, Rinehart and Winston.

Gazda, G., Asbury, F., Balzer, F., Childers, W., & Walters, R. (1977). *Human relations development: A manual for educators* (2nd ed.). Boston: Allyn and Bacon.

Gazda, G., Asbury, F., Balzer, F., Childers, W., & Walters, R. (1983). *Human relations development: A manual for educators* (3rd ed.). Boston: Allyn and Bacon.

Gibran, K. (1951). *The prophet.* New York: Knopf.

Goldin, D., & Russell, B. (1969). Therapeutic communication. *American Journal of Nursing, 69,* 1928–1930.

Hein, E. (1980). *Communication in nursing practice* (2nd ed.). Boston: Little, Brown.

Hewitt, F. (1981). Introduction to communication. *Nursing Times, 77,* center pages.

Johnson, D. (1981). *Reaching out: Interpersonal effectiveness and self-actualization* (2nd ed.). Englewood Cliffs, NJ: Prentice-Hall.

Johnson, J., Dumas, R., & Johnson, B. (1967). Interpersonal relations: The essence of nursing care. *Nursing Forum, 6,* 324–334.

La Monica, E. (1983). *Nursing leadership and management: An experiential approach.* Monterey, CA: Wadsworth.

Mayeroff, M. (1971). *On caring.* New York: Harper and Row.

Miller, G. (1966). *Speech communication: A behavioral approach.* Indianapolis: Bobb-Merrill.

Moorhead, T., Jr. (1972). *Communication for educational problem-solving.* Melbourne, FL: Human Dynamics.

Peplau, H. (1960). Talking with patients. *American Journal of Nursing, 60,* 964–966.

Ponthieu, J. (1977). Open communication: The key to self-actualization and success. *Health Services Manager, 10,* 8–9.

Rogers, C. (1961). *On becoming a person.* Boston: Houghton-Mifflin.

Rogers, C. (1965). *Client-centered therapy.* Boston: Houghton-Mifflin.

Shannon, C., & Weaver, W. (1949). *The mathematical theory of communication.* Urbana: University of Illinois Press.

Slater, P. (1976). *The pursuit of loneliness.* Boston: Beacon Press.

Walters, R. (1983). *The amity book: Exercises in friendship and helping skills.* In G. Gazda, F.

Asbury, F. Balzer, W. Childers, & R. Walters (Eds.), *Human relations development: A manual for educators* (3rd ed.). Boston: Allyn and Bacon.

SELECTED READING

The suggested reading for this chapter is by Moorhead (1972). This article provides a rich discussion of the communication process. Although Moorhead specifically discusses communication in education, his remarks apply equally well to communication in nursing. Examples are given for listening, validating perceptions, and giving information (describing behavior and feelings to others). The author also includes a word list that is helpful in building responses that can accurately reflect the feelings of others.

Communication for Educational Problem-Solving

Ted B. Moorhead, Jr.

Communication is from the Latin *communis*, common. When we communicate we are trying to get something in common between us. You may know a fact which I do not know. In some way you make that fact known to me; then you and I both know that fact: We have it in common.

So, through communication processes we share facts, ideas, attitudes, opinions, and feelings. Thus we learn from each other and come to understand one another, if communication is effective. If it is ineffective, learning is blocked and misunderstandings occur.

We tend to assume we communicate well. If we are misunderstood, it's because someone else is stupid. We also tend to assume we receive and understand the communication of others well. If we don't understand someone, it's because he can't talk straight.

Actually, communication is a very complicated process. There are many points in this process at which breakdowns can occur, even between highly intelligent persons. Also, few of us have opportunity to develop and check out our communication skills in a structured program. The purpose of these sessions is to give you such an opportunity.

Let's look at communication between two persons:

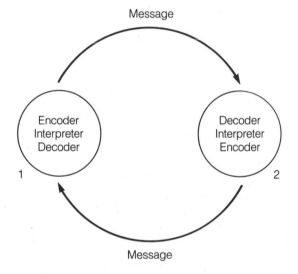

Suppose person 1 initiates communication. He must decide what it is he wants to communicate, how to do it, and how it is likely to be received by person 2. Let's say person 1 communicates a message with words (including vocal inflections, tones, and volume), facial expressions, hand gestures, and body position. Person 2 must receive all this data, decode the symbols, interpret what the total message means, decide on a response, encode that response, and send the message.

This is actually a simplified diagram. It does not take into account the interplay of the emotional and rational processes within an individual which influence his communication. But it should be clear that the communication process we often take for granted is indeed intricate. And it requires maintenance if it is to be kept intact.

Communication can break down at any point in the process. Person 1 may not understand himself well, or what he wants to communicate, or what kind of response he is trying to get from person number 2. In this case, he stands a strong chance of putting his foot in his mouth.

Then there is the problem of semantics. A word may mean one thing to person 1 but something entirely different to person 2. So the decoder doesn't match the encoder.

And any of the other communication symbols can be misinterpreted. Some people "sound" angry all the time. Others "sound" happy all the time. Until you get to know them and can pick up other clues, it is difficult to understand their feelings.

When a message is sent and another sent back, the return process is called *feedback*. By paying close attention to our feedback, we can learn a lot about how our messages are being received and interpreted. And we can make adjustments and develop our communication skills.

COMMUNICATION FOR SOLVING PROBLEMS

All of life can be viewed as a series of problems to be solved. The word "problem" is used here not in a negative sense of situations to be avoided, but in a positive sense as the very process of life. My basic problems are how to get the food, air, water, and affection I need to survive. As an infant, I communicated these needs by crying, squirming, and cuddling. My mother and other meaningful persons helped me solve these problems by responding to my communication. Sometimes they became confused as to what my problem was and how they could help, because my communication was not clear. We have a better chance of solving problems when communication is clear.

Educational processes are also a series of problems to be solved. A person needs to learn to perceive himself, others, and life situations accurately. He needs to learn behavior which will enable him to function responsibly and productively in meeting his own needs and as a member of society.

Communication is the key to solving these and other problems. And by communication I mean action as well as words, for we communicate by what we do and by what we say.

Through communication *helping relationships* are built. These are relationships in which each helps the other to solve problems of mutual concern. This is an ideal teacher–pupil relationship. A pupil has a problem: He needs to improve his reading skill. The problem is of concern to the teacher: He has responsibility for helping pupils improve reading skill, feels for the pupil in his need, and wants to help. So the teacher does what he can do to help the pupil solve the problem.

In a helping relationship, each person must help the other. The problem may be identified as primarily belonging to the pupil. And the teacher may see the pupil as the one receiving help, and himself giving. But unless the teacher also receives help from the pupil, he cannot give help to the pupil. The pupil must help the teacher understand what the problem is. The teacher needs to receive information from the pupil, without which the teacher will be unable to give help. Also the pupil must help the teacher by cooperating with whatever strategy is developed to solve the problem.

So two-way communication is essential to the educational problem-solving process. And the more effective this communication is in bringing about sharing of information relevant to a problem, the better the chance of solution.

Let's say a child is behaving disruptively. This is a problem for the child (hindering his learning and socialization), for the teacher (hindering his efforts to maintain a climate for learning), and the class (hindering their learning and socialization). In order to help solve the problem, the teacher must understand the nature of the problem. Is the child bored, confused, restless, frustrated, hostile, desiring attention, or what? He must decode and interpret the message sent by the child in his behavior and respond helpfully. That response must be a message which is clear enough to be decoded and interpreted accurately by the child.

So in the educational problem-solving process, clarity and accuracy of two-way communication is important.

Also vital is an openness of communication lines between persons so that the necessary information can be exchanged. If the child feels constrained in communicating with a teacher, through fear of rejection or punishment, the teacher is not likely to get much needed information from the child.

Let's say Johnny is struggling with reading. Teacher says, "Johnny, I see you are having a hard time in reading. What's the problem?" Johnny says, "I don't know. I just don't like to read." This is a crucial point at which a helping relationship can either grow or be squelched. The teacher can react defensively: "Well, you'd better learn to like to read because there's plenty of it all the way through school." Interpreted by Johnny, this means his feelings don't matter; school must be accepted as hateful work because that's the way it is. And he is not likely again to give his teacher such information about how he feels. But on the other hand, the teacher can respond openly: "I'm sorry you aren't enjoying reading. I'd like to help. Tell me more about how you feel when you read." This opens the way for a further exchange of information and a possible revelation of the root of the problem.

There are certain communication skills which can facilitate a maximum exchange of information needed to solve problems. These skills are not common. The lack of their use hinders classroom communication and problem solving. But these skills can be learned and used by teachers, pupils, and administrators. The result is a cultural change away from destructive game-playing and toward the problem-solving communication of helping relationships.

SKILLS IN RECEIVING INFORMATION

Reflective Listening

Listening is a vital skill for building helping relationships between persons. Perhaps the most vital.

Reflective listening is a method for clarifying what one hears. It can facilitate effective communication and can help ensure accuracy of understanding.

Also, this can be supportive and affirmative to the person who is talking. It says you care enough about him to listen to what he says and to make sure you understand. It communicates acceptance of him as a person, whether or not you agree with what he says.

Furthermore, this style of listening opens the way for maximum reception of needed information. The person sending information tests, consciously or unconsciously, to see how he is being heard. He sends a message. If the response indicates misinterpretation by the receiver, he may try again or give up. If the receiver indicates indifference to the message, the communication line is damaged. If the receiver gives back defensiveness, communication is blocked. But if the receiver is interested and open, giving out data indicating he is hearing and understanding or wants to understand, the sender is reinforced in giving more data.

Look at an example: Mary, who is making poor grades, has her head on the desk while teacher is giving an assignment.

> Teacher: "Mary, will you look up please. You are missing an important assignment."
> Mary: "Aw, I'm tired of this class."
> Teacher: "Your problem, Mary, is you're lazy. Now sit up and listen."

What did Mary communicate? She could have meant she was tired at this moment in time. Past data (grades) would indicate the problem is more chronic. But does she see the subject matter as irrelevant, herself incompetent, the teacher incompetent, or what? The teacher will not learn for sure what the problem is—he has already assumed it is Mary's laziness. By pinning this label on her, he confirms his negative perception of her, which may be also a confirmation of her own low self-esteem. This transaction is not likely to be helpful. If I see myself as lazy and no-good and you tell me I am lazy and no-good, I am likely to act out our mutual perception in an interpersonal relationship.

Now look at another way the transaction could have occurred:

Mary: "Aw, I'm tired of this class."

Teacher: "Do you mean you're not interested in what we are doing?

Mary: "Yeah, I don't see any sense in all this work we're doing. It doesn't mean anything to me."

Teacher: "You mean you don't see any way that what we're studying applies to your life right now?"

Mary: "Yeah, that's it."

Teacher: "Perhaps some others have this same problem. I'd like to know how some of the rest of you feel about this."

This opens the way for others as well as Mary to give the teacher information vitally needed to solve problems. One result could be modification of curriculum or teaching methods to make the learning process more relevant. Another result could be the disclosure of reasons why the present material is relevant— reasons which would have special appeal to Mary, coming from her peers. Or additional discussion could reveal hidden problems, such as interpersonal conflicts, which were behind Mary's disinterest.

At any rate, Mary has been heard rather than cut off. This in itself affirms her and supports her self-esteem. Being heard may in itself motivate her to do better work. It gives her a feeling of being a more valuable person, one whose opinions are worth listening to. And it gives her a perception of the teacher as a person who cares enough to listen.

Some teachers say they do not have time for this kind of discussion or individual attention in a classroom. This reflects the condition of getting so locked into content that the process of instruction cannot be dealt with. When process is ignored, content will inevitably get bogged down. The task as well as interpersonal relationship will suffer. It would pay in the long run to take the time necessary to do "processing," as in the above example between the teacher and Mary.

Also remember that when you are engaged in a meaningful exchange with one person others are also learning. Others, as well as Mary, were learning something about the relevance of the curriculum. They were learning about the teacher as a helping person, and about themselves as being able to communicate with this adult. Most of all, they were learning they could participate in making decisions and solving problems. They could share in educational responsibilities, rather than having these all handled exclusively by the teacher. Thus, they could begin to see themselves as responsible persons, and behave accordingly.

The key to true "reflective listening" is empathy. Put yourself mentally and emotionally into the place of the person to whom you are listening. Think with him and feel with him until you understand what he is thinking and feeling.

Another important element is suspension of evaluation or judgment of what is being said until understanding has occurred. Carl Rogers said, ". . . the major barrier to mutual interpersonal communication is our very natural tendency to judge, to evaluate, to approve or disapprove, the statement of the other person, or the other group."* Our listening pattern is typically to judge first and clarify understanding second, if at all. This pattern must be reversed in order to practice "reflective listening" and to facilitate understanding.

Note that there is a difference between

---

*Carl R. Rogers, *On Becoming a Person* (Boston: Houghton Mifflin), p. 330.

understanding and agreement. I may listen to your opinion and check my interpretation of what you are saying until I fully understand, yet still disagree with you. Agreement is much more likely when this quality of communication is taking place. But understanding is the essential goal. Two persons may have a mutual helping relationship and yet disagree in many areas. But they cannot have such a relationship without understanding each other.

There are several techniques which may be employed in "reflective listening."

One way to make sure you received a message clearly is to repeat it word for word: "I do not like what is happening."—"I heard you say 'I do not like what is happening'." The sender has a chance to confirm or correct what you heard. And he knows you are listening. But he does not know how you are *interpreting* his message. You have verified the words you have heard, but not your understanding of the words.

Another response could be, "What do you mean by that?" This puts the entire burden of clarification on the sender, and may draw a defensive reaction. It implies that you have no idea of what he is trying to communicate and that he is failing completely to get through to you. A better response, if indeed you have no comprehension of what is being said, is to admit you are having a problem understanding and ask the person to repeat the message. If the communication is vague, ask for an example.

An excellent technique for "reflective listening" is to *paraphrase* what you think the person means. Reflect back your interpretation of his message, putting what he said in your words: "I do not like what is happening."—"Do you mean you are uncomfortable with what we are doing?" This gives the sender an opportunity to hear how you interpret what he says and to decide whether or not you understand. Also, this opens the way for him to confirm or correct and increase your understanding of his message by further communication.

"Do you mean . . . ?" is a good preface to paraphrase. Others are, "Are you saying . . . ?", "Let me check my understanding . . .", "You

mean . . . ?", "This means . . . ?", and "In other words . . . ?"

A paraphrase may be quite direct, with only a key word or two changed: "I am happy we solved that problem."—"You mean you are happy we worked that out?" This is a safe reflection and can frequently open the way for further communication. It is not likely to get a "no" response. However, it does not give back much data on the depth of your understanding. So the direct paraphrase is useful, but limited.

An amplified paraphrase contains more interpretation of the message: "I am happy we solved that problem."—"Do you mean you are relieved and glad that a difficult problem is solved?" Such an amplification could be based on data in addition to the words spoken. The listener may be aware of background information which gives clues to meaning. Non-verbal and verbal signals provide data on the intensity of feelings, which can be reflected in the paraphrase. Facial expressions, gestures, body positions give impressions. And tone, volume, and velocity of voice are all a part of the message. The amplified paraphrase gives back much data on your understanding. It is more difficult to do, and more frequently subject to challenge since it is more subjective.

A reverse paraphrase can help clarify understanding: "I am happy we solved that problem." —"Do you mean that problem was bothering you quite a bit?" Here both sender and receiver can take a look at a communication from another perspective: A positive statement can be restated negatively, or a negative statement can be restated positively. Either way could be helpful: "If only we could work together, things would go better."—"Do you mean there are ways we are not working together which are preventing things from going better?" "Things are going terribly."—"Do you mean you would like for things to go better?"

An "alternatives" paraphrase can help differentiate between two or more possible meanings: "I don't like this course."—"Do you mean you are dissatisfied with the content or the method of preparation?"

The type of paraphrase to use can usually be played by ear so long as the listener is effectively practicing empathy and suspending evaluation.

Obviously, one need not paraphrase every incoming message. This method is especially helpful in these conditions:

1. When there is a possibility of misunderstanding, and to understand is important.

2. When the other person may be helped by the assurance he is understood (by feeling accepted as a person and cared for).

3. When an incoming message carries heavy emotional weight (such as in a conflict).

"Reflective listening" has benefits beyond simple verification and clarification of communication. It can help remove blocks to understanding in heavy emotional situations. Frequently, in conflict persons become so intent on defending a position that neither one is actually hearing the other. Paraphrasing requires listening to each other and breaks through such blocks. Thus, it is an important skill in conflict resolution.

Also, it can help a person understand himself. As he hears his communication reflected back as interpreted by another, he clarifies his own understanding of what he means. Often one will find his feelings about a matter moderating as another listens receptively. He hears irrational elements in his message as it is reflected back. If the receiver is not defensive, the sender's need to be defensive is minimized. Faulty opinions are more likely to be changed under these conditions.

And, most helpfully, "reflective listening" to a person can facilitate his self-acceptance and self-esteem. When someone listens, understands, and accepts his feelings, a person can better accept himself. When someone values him as a person enough to listen and understand his communication, a person can better see himself as having worth. Such self-acceptance and self-esteem are basic essentials to growth and actualization of one's potential as a person.

Carl Rogers describes the "helping relationship" which can occur when communication skills such as "reflective listening" are used effectively. He says the following:

> I am by no means always able to achieve this kind of relationship with another, and sometimes, even when I feel I have achieved it in myself, he may be too frightened to perceive what is being offered to him. But I would say that when I hold in myself the kind of attitudes I have described, and when the other person can to some degree experience these attitudes, then I believe that change and constructive personal development will *invariably* occur—and I include the word "invariably" only after long and careful consideration.*

Perception Check

A "perception check" is another way to verify information received. This is a question by which you check your perception of the feelings of another person. It is useful when a person is sending verbal and/or non-verbal signals about his feelings which are not completely clear or direct. Also, the "perception check" can help a person become conscious of feelings which he is communicating but which are beneath his level of awareness.

Let's say Johnny is scratching his head, frowning, and not writing when the class is supposed to be working on a written assignment. Teacher, picking up these non-verbal signals, says, "Johnny, are you having difficulty with the assignment?" (perception check). This tells Johnny you are aware of his having a problem, but that you aren't making assumptions about the nature of the problem without checking with him. It opens the way for Johnny to help teacher understand the nature of his problem so as to be helpful to him.

---

*Ibid., p. 35.

Mary says, "This is a stupid course." She is not talking about her feelings. She is giving an evaluation of the course. But feelings are evident in her voice and body expressions. Teacher picks this up, and says, "Mary, are you feeling angry about having to do this work?" (perception check).

> Mary: "Yes, I think it's stupid and I don't like it."
> Teacher: "You mean you don't understand the purpose of what we are doing and get tired of doing it?" (reflective listening)
> Mary: "Yes."
> Teacher: "I'm sorry you're having problems with it. I want to help you. Can we work on it?" (description of feelings and offer to help solve problem)

Helping relationships are built as persons communicate on a "feeling" as well as intellectual level. Teacher could have had an intellectual debate with Mary on the merits of the course and accomplished nothing. By being aware of and checking out what Mary was feeling, accepting her feelings, and going on to share her own feelings and an offer to help, teacher practiced effective problem-solving communication.

In making a "perception check," it may be more helpful to actually check your perception with a question rather than assume your perception is accurate and make a statement about it.

You see someone getting red-faced and talking loudly. NOT—"You are getting angry. What's wrong with you?" BUT—"*Are* you getting angry with me?"

It is helpful in making a "perception check" to pinpoint the object of feelings, like "Are you getting angry *with me?*" The person could be angry with someone else or about something apart from you. Clarification could result from such a check.

After making a "perception check," communicate acceptance rather than judgment toward the feelings. NOT—"Are you getting

angry with me?" "Yes." "Well, that's too bad. You better cool off." BUT—"Are you getting angry with me?" "Yes." "I see. Can we work on the problem? What's bothering you?"

A pupil needs to learn to be aware of, accept, own, and describe his feelings. He needs to learn that feelings are internal to himself, not out in the external environment where he may tend to project them. The fact is not that the course is stupid. That is an opinion. But the fact is Mary is feeling disturbed in the course. Mary needs to learn to differentiate between an opinion she has of the course and her disturbed feelings, which are a more vital component of the problem. Teacher's perception check can help her learn this differentiation and how to accept and cope with negative feelings—an important element of emotional development.

So far, checking perception of negative feelings has been discussed. Also valuable is the "perception check" of positive feelings. Johnny, who has been struggling in language arts, comes up to teacher with face aglow and says, "I got a B on my test!" NOT—"I know, I graded it." BUT—"Say, you're happy about that, aren't you?"

The "perception check," as well as verifying perceptions of others' feelings, says you care and are aware of how they feel—that you feel with them in their pain and joy. With this, you come through a real person and a sincere helper. You can give the kind of emotional support and aid to effective development needed by many children.

SKILLS IN GIVING INFORMATION

So far we have focused on listening and checking perceptions. Now we look at the sending side of the communication cycle.

How can you be sure the messages you send are clear and accurate? How can you assure a congruent signal, readily understood, rather than mixed messages, which can be confusing? How can you differentiate between facts and opinions, and communicate objective observations rather than inferences, when this is important? How can you cope with and communicate your own emotional feelings, both positive and negative, to pupils?

These are vitally needed kinds of communication to be exchanged in the helping relationship of a classroom. But unusual communication skills are required for such transactions. Skills of giving information so as to maximize the reception and effectiveness of such information can be developed.

Describing Behavior

In order to have satisfactory relationships, people must consider how their behavior affects other people. If someone is doing something that damages the relationship between you and him, he must know what that action is if he is to consider changing it. On the other hand, if someone's behavior is enhancing the relationship, it is more likely to continue if identified and affirmed.

But many people do not describe behavior clearly enough for others to know what they mean. Instead of describing behavior, often inferences are made about feelings, motivations, and attitudes. Also, a lot of value judgments are passed off instead of behavior descriptions.

Example   Behavior description, combined with description of feelings and establishment of authority: "Johnny, you threw a paper wad. I am angry because this disrupted the class. You must not do such a thing again."

Value judgment and inference: "Johnny, you are a bad boy. You are trying to show off for the whole class."

The skill of behavior description depends on accurate, objective observation. It requires being able to distinguish between an objective observation of fact (what you actually saw and heard) and inferences you may have drawn from the observation. People often become so accustomed to making inferences they are unaware of the actual behavior from which the inference was drawn.

Example   "Hey, why are you so gloomy?" "What makes you think I'm gloomy?" "I don't know, you just seemed gloomy." "No, I'm just tired."

Also, an objective behavior description is nonevaluative. It does not imply that what happened was good or bad, right or wrong.

Examples
Behavior descriptions

"Mary, you interrupted Joan while she was talking."

"Larry, you did not complete your assignment."

Evaluative or inferential statements

"Mary is rude."
"Mary wasn't interested in what Joan was saying."

"Larry, you work too slowly."
"Larry, you are playing when you should be working."

Now let's see what difference the use of this skill can make in communication.

Suppose you see me do something and you say to me, "You are acting bad. Stop it." I may not know specifically what the behavior is that you are talking about. Furthermore, I may not agree with the opinion that what I was doing was bad. I may stop it so as not to incur your wrath, but there has been minimal learning and our relationship may have been damaged, and has not been helped by this transaction. There is no basis for increased understanding.

But suppose you tell me, "You are talking when I am talking. Stop it." I know exactly what I am doing that drew your reaction. There is no question of whether it was good or bad. It obviously affected you adversely and you wanted it stopped. If I care about you as a person, I am responsive to this kind of communication. At any rate, you have given me clearer data on my behavior, which gives me a better chance to learn and change my behavior.

So, in order to develop skill in describing behavior you must sharpen your observation of what actually occurs and carefully distinguish this from inferences and value judgments. As you practice this you may discover how much your own feelings affect the way you react to others. You may discover persons who have no observable behavior patterns which should affect you. But, for some reason you do not like them. This could indicate that you are stereotyping people and projecting your own feelings and motives onto them.

Description of behavior can be helpful in educational problem-solving, particularly when combined with other communication skills.

> Teacher: "Johnny, you have not turned in your work for three successive days." (description of behavior, rather than an inference, such as, "You are getting quite lazy about your work.") "I am wondering if you are having a problem."
>
> Johnny: "I don't understand this work you have assigned us."
>
> Teacher: "Do you mean you don't know how to do the work?" (reflective feedback)
>
> Johnny: "Yes."
>
> Teacher: "Would you like to work with someone who is getting it?"
>
> Johnny: "OK."
>
> Teacher: "If you continue to have problems or if something like this happens again, please let me know. I want to help. And I like for you to keep up in your work. OK?" (suggestion of alternate behavior, description of own feelings, clarification of expectations and check for commitment)

Skill in behavior descriptions can help solve problems in these ways:

1. It can give persons more specific data on behavior which affects you and increase the possibility of change.

2. It can prevent your drawing hasty and unfounded inferences about people's behavior.

3. It can prevent your projecting your feelings and value judgments on the behavior of others.

4. Particularly when combined with a description of your feelings it constitutes an effective message with high learning potential for the receiver. He is getting clear feedback on his behavior and the way it is affecting you.

5. Particularly when combined with a description of alternate behavior and request for commitment to try alternate behavior, it helps pupils to learn more responsible and productive behavior.

6. It helps pupils differentiate between behaviors and self-worth: it is not that one is a bad person, but that he is behaving in a way which is not helping himself or others.

7. Description and affirmation of productive behavior reinforce this behavior and make recurrence more likely. Example: "Johnny, you participated in our class discussion for the first time today. I am pleased to hear you speak up and appreciate what you said."

Describing Your Feelings

A feeling is an inner signal of a need, or the satisfaction of a need. If I feel hungry, this tells me I need something to eat. When I feel full, this tells me I have eaten enough.

A strong case can be made for the theory that anything one does is in response to a personal need. So even action to help others arises from an inner need to help others.

If this is true, our feelings are very important factors in our behavior. Feelings signal us that we have needs and motivate us to take action to meet these needs. Other feelings indicate to us we have been successful in meeting these needs.

This is not to say that our behavior cannot be modified by thinking. A child may feel hungry and want to eat a cookie. But if mother has said no, the action prompted by the feeling can be restrained by thought and will. Of course, in this case other feelings come into the picture: fear of what will happen if mother is disobeyed, and some frustration and anger perhaps.

Training and conditioning help us to control feelings which could be destructive if unleashed in our complex society. But this also can cause us to lose touch with our basic feelings. We then tend to respond automatically, like trained animals, rather than as thinking, feeling persons.

Also, feelings which are suppressed rather than communicated in some way tend to have an effect anyway. These feelings may affect a person physically with psychosomatic illness. And feelings may be expressed deviously. Person 1 says something and person 2 feels hurt by it. Person 2 does nothing at the time to communicate his feelings of hurt. But later when person 1 offers a suggestion in a meeting, person 2 blocks it and starts an argument. Or feelings may be misdirected. You may feel angry because the children have misbehaved in class, but express this feeling toward your spouse or children at home.

So feelings do affect us and the ways in which we relate to others. It is important to be able to communicate feelings clearly and appropriately. This is difficult to do. Often people tend to blame others, rationalize their actions, deny feelings, project their feelings to others, and do everything but clearly communicate what they are feeling. This leads to confusion and unresolved conflict between persons.

Feelings are communicated in many different ways: actions, words, tone of voice, bodily changes, and facial expressions. Sometimes these messages are difficult to decode. And even if you think you got the message, there is still a question about whether the sender knows what he is communicating, how the feeling is likely to affect his behavior, and how you are likely to respond.

One way to communicate more clearly is to *describe what you are feeling*. We usually try to convey our thoughts accurately. But description of feeling is frequently neglected. Often we talk about "feeling" something when what we really mean is that we "think" something. I may say, "I feel this lesson is too long." What I really mean is, "I feel bored. I think this lesson is too long."

In order to describe your feelings, you must be able to recognize what you are feeling. This in itself is difficult. Your actions may be affected by feelings of which you are unaware. One way to get in touch with your feelings is to notice what is happening to you physiologically and interpret this in terms of feelings.

Here are some ways that feelings can be described to someone else:

1. Identify the feeling with words. "I feel annoyed." "I feel happy." At the end of this section is a sample list of words which may be used to describe feelings.

2. Use figures of speech. "I feel full of sunshine." "I feel as though a storm were raging inside me."

3. Tell what kind of action the feeling urges you to do. "I feel like walking out of the room." "I feel like staying here all day."

4. Tell what is happening to you physiologically. "My heart is pounding." "My palms are moist."

It is both possible and healthy to be able to identify and describe your feelings objectively. To do this you must be able to "own" your feelings. That is, you accept your feelings as being a part of you, rather than blaming yourself or someone else. NOT—"You make me angry." BUT—"When you did this, I became angry." The first statement imputes blame to someone for making you angry. The second statement associates the feeling of anger with the action of another person, but does not necessarily blame the action of another person. It is an objective statement of fact: "You did that; I became angry." This leaves an opening to explore factors in both of us which may have caused the reaction, without imputing blame to anyone. To "own" your feelings means also that you accept it as OK to have and admit having any feeling. Otherwise, much denying of feeling is done. This serves only to submerge feelings, making their effects more devious and difficult to cope with.

The purpose in describing your feelings is to start a dialogue which can improve understanding. Unless you make your feelings known,

WORDS TO DESCRIBE FEELINGS

Positive		Negative	
happy	intelligent	hurt	dominated
pleased	clever	angry	manipulated
joyful	attractive	afraid	used
exuberant	beautiful	scared	controlled
exhilarated	well	insecure	shut-out
refreshed	bright	irritated	shut-in
stimulated	confident	annoyed	incompetent
invigorated	assured	put down	unworthy
enthused	certain	aggravated	confused
relaxed	cleansed	frustrated	mixed-up
affectionate	triumphant	disgusted	dull
loved	free	discouraged	bored
cared for	liberated	inadequate	uneasy
loving	comfortable	depressed	uncomfortable
secure	at ease	hopeless	lonely
safe	calm	hostile	rejected
accepted	rested	violent	sad
included	soothed	furious	grieved
united	relieved	hate	embarrassed
trusted	healed	guilty	ugly
trusting	open	hostile	misunderstood
appreciated	honest	jealous	foolish
respected	real	defensive	stupid
self-esteem	alert	defeated	bad
self-reliant	aware	excluded	lost
worthy	interested	powerless	undecided
reinforced	excited	sick	unsure
satisfied	exciting	impotent	tired
successful	potent	helpless	rushed
fulfilled	virile	weak	up tight
understood	pleasant	crushed	strung out
competent	self-controlled	exasperated	tense
together	whole	hysterical	hungry
strong	rewarded	uncontrolled	thirsty
rational	important	exhausted	dirty

another person cannot accurately consider them in his relationship to you. And unless you know what another person is feeling, you cannot accurately consider his feelings in your relationship to him.

Suppose you are having negative feelings toward someone. These are signals that the relationship between the two of you is not satisfactory. What will you do about these signals and the relationship? You may ignore the signals or deny them, but they are still there. Or you may assume that the other person is at fault and begin pinning blame on him. Or you may assume that you are at fault and begin kicking yourself for having such feelings.

Instead, by describing your feelings objectively you can avoid casting blame in either direction. His feedback to you may show you that your feelings resulted from a misinterpretation of him. In this case, your feelings would probably change because of new understanding. Also, your feedback to him may help him to see that his behavior is bringing responses from you of which he was not aware. He may recognize a behavior pattern which should be changed.

But description of feelings should not be used to coerce someone into changing to accommodate your feelings. It is a statement of fact, without judgments, about what you are feeling.

It is the kind of information that must be communicated if two people are to understand each other and build a relationship.

The clearest communication occurs when the message is conveyed *congruently* (with all elements of communication in agreement). If I say I am angry, but am smiling, you have a difficult message to decode. You are getting a mixed signal. But if I say I am happy and am smiling, have a pleasant and enthusiastic voice, and perhaps some body and hand movement, you are getting multiple signals, all conveying the same message. This is easily understood and more believable. When I am angry, I need to communicate this with words, tone and volume of voice, and body expressions which make the message clear to the receiver.

A teacher's describing his own feelings in key situations can help in several ways to solve problems.

1. It identifies teacher as a real human being who has and is willing to admit having feelings. This tends to break through the stereotype "teacher" role and facilitates person-to-person classroom relationships.

2. It establishes a classroom norm in favor of accepting, rather than denying, feelings and in favor of describing feelings, rather than acting out feelings in disruptive behavior.

Examples of describing feelings

"I feel embarrassed"
"I feel pleased"
"I feel annoyed"

"I feel angry"
"I'm feeling shut out"
"I'm worried about this"
"I feel hurt"

"I enjoy her sense of humor"
"I respect her ability"
"I like her"

"I am getting bored"
"I feel angry with myself"
"I am angry with you"

**Examples of expressing feelings
without describing them**

Blushing and saying nothing
Blushing and smiling
Blushing and frowning

Arguing, talking loudly
Becoming silent in a group
Blaming, arguing, and frowning
Making cutting remarks

"She's funny"
"She's an able person"
"She's a wonderful person"

"You are talking too much"
"I always goof up"
"You are acting foolishly"

It is acceptable to say, "I am angry with you," but not to hit.

3. It establishes a classroom norm in favor of owning, rather than projecting, feelings. It is acceptable to say, "I am angry with you," but not to call someone a liar.

4. It gives pupils information on how their behavior adversely affects teacher. This breaks up the game of "let's drive teacher crazy" by exposing the game and insisting on an authentic rather than manipulative game-playing relationship. Example: "I am angry right now. Several of you are talking in the back of the room while I am giving instructions. If you need to speak, raise your hand. If not, be quiet while I am speaking."

5. It gives pupils information on how their behavior positively affects teacher. This reinforces problem-solving behavior as teacher expresses positive feelings about such behavior. Example: "I am so pleased with the work you have just done. It's a pleasure for me to try to help you learn when you respond like that."

6. Such a "feeling" statement can be more effective than an "evaluative" statement, either positive or negative. "I feel very annoyed when several of you are talking at the same time." NOT—"This is a thoughtless class. You constantly interrupt each other." "I feel pleased at the report you made." NOT—"You are a good student."

Of course, most pupils may appreciate a positive evaluation like, "You are a good student." But some will not find this believable because of low self-esteem. A "feeling" affirmation is more credible than the evaluation, especially if expressed with genuine feeling, a smile, and a pat on the shoulder.

THE PROBLEM SOLVING PROCESS

The communication skills which have been discussed can facilitate the process of solving problems.

Several steps in this process can be identified:

1. Statement of the problem.

2. Gathering data bearing on the problem.

3. Clarification of the problem.

4. Consideration of alternative solutions.

5. Commitment to try one or more alternatives.

6. Evaluation of attempted solutions.

7. Implementation of continued action.

The following example illustrates how the communication skills are used in the problem-solving process.

Mr. Tate teaches low-phase high school students. His course is Comparative Political Systems. He has had severe discipline problems and low achievement in past classes. This semester, after learning some new communication skills, he decides to try to apply them in classroom meetings as well as in person-to-person transactions.

Desks are arranged in a tight circle as class begins.

Mr. Tate: "I am concerned about what we are going to accomplish here this semester and how we will get along." (description of feelings, statement of the problem) "I want to know how you feel about being in this class and what you hope to get out of it." (request for data bearing on the problem)

Long silence. Further encouragement from teacher to speak up.

Mike: "I don't expect nothin' from this class except maybe a passing grade. It's a drag I've heard from other kids. But we're required to take it."

Mr. Tate: "You mean you don't expect to learn anything worthwhile in here, but you want to make a passing grade because it's required?" (reflective listening feedback)

Mike: "Right. It's just something you have to put up with."

Joan: "I think there are helpful things in this course. I would like to learn more about politics and why different nations do the things they do."

Betty: "Yes. It's important to understand how governments work. That's the only way to change things."

Ben: "Baloney! You can't change anything. And all you'll get in here is a lot of propaganda."

Mr. Tate: "Ben, you think I'm here to give you propaganda?" (reflective listening)

Ben: "Yes. This course is just supposed to brainwash us to fit the system."

Jerry: "I don't agree with that. We can disagree with what's taught if we want to."

Ben: "Not if you want to make a grade."

Mr. Tate: "Let me check my understanding so far. Some of you are saying you see no value in the course, others that you do see value in learning what's going on in different governmental systems, and some are concerned about being given propaganda and forced to accept it. Right?" (summary of reflective listening, clarification of problem, and question for verification)

Some heads nod approval.

Mr. Tate: "OK, I want to deal with those concerns. I will try to help you learn about different political systems presently operating. There is factual information I will expect you to know, such as the way the government of the Soviet Union is organized. As to opinions of the way a system works, we will freely explore various opinions and the reasons for these opinions. You are welcome to your opinion. You will not be penalized for having opinions different from mine, so long as you know the facts." (consideration of alternative solutions)

Mike: "But if our opinions are different don't expect a good grade on a test."

Mr. Tate: "Mike, are you feeling doubtful about what I am saying?" (perception check, opening way to verify feelings expressed indirectly)

Mike: "Yeah, I doubt that I can make as good a grade by disagreeing with you as I can by agreeing."

Mr. Tate: "OK. If at any time anyone thinks he is being graded down for an opinion different from mine, I want to know about it. I am willing to consider such a case with the whole class and to get help from the class in making an adjustment." (consideration of alternative solution)

At this point several persons begin speaking to each other while one person speaks out more loudly than they and to the teacher.

Mr. Tate: "Hold it! Several of you are talking and I am getting annoyed. I cannot hear more than one of you at a time. I want to hear what you have to say, so please speak one at a time." (description of behavior, description of feelings, description of alternative behavior)

Mr. Tate: "All right, now I want someone to repeat back to me what I have said about this course and let me know how you feel about it."

Jerry: "You have said we will study various governments. You expect us to know some facts about them. And we can have our own opinions, which we will not be graded down on."

Mr. Tate: "Right. Now, how do you feel about that?" (checking for commitment to solution)

Mike: "That sounds OK to me, if it really happens."

Mr. Tate: "You are still somewhat doubtful?" (perception check)

Mike: "Yeah, but I'm willing to go along."

Mr. Tate: "How about the rest of you?"

Most heads nod in approval. (commitment to solution)

Mr. Tate: (Smiles and leans back more relaxed) "I'm feeling better already about working with you this semester. I really appreciate this discussion, and I hope we can be happy together." (description of feelings) "We will have discussions like this frequently to evaluate our progress and make adjustments." (provision for evaluation and further implementation)

Mr. Tate used reflective listening to demonstrate an openness which encouraged pupils to give him information. They soon sensed they would not get a defensive or punishing reaction to what they said. This maximized their input of data. Also, this technique enabled him to verify and clarify data received. And it enabled pupils to hear his interpretation of what they were saying and clarify and perhaps modify their own thinking! He set a norm for open, nonjudgmental listening which should greatly help the classroom climate. The listening model is a good one for pupils to emulate, and they should pick it up as the class progresses.

He checked his perception of feelings of others, thus verifying his perceptions and helping pupils to become aware of feelings they were expressing. This also communicated his willingness to accept feelings, even when hostile. And this helped him to come through as a sensitive, perceptive person. Such a person tends to receive respect because he gives respect to others.

He described his own feelings, both positive and negative, appropriately and congruently. This gave pupils data on how their behavior affected him, for better or worse. It helped establish person-to-person caring relationships, and helped eliminate possible manipulative game-playing in which feelings are hidden or projected through blaming tactics.

He described behavior and set limits on behavior which adversely affected the class task. He described alternate behavior and got commitment to try it. He demonstrated effective use of communication skills in a problem-solving process. The problem was identified. Data was gathered. The problem was clarified. Solutions were considered. Commitment was made to alternatives. And provision was made for evaluation and on-going action.

Chapter 4

Interviewing

While useful in other phases of the nursing process, the interview is the primary procedure used in assessment and specifically in data collection. It is especially important in the gathering of information from the primary source—the client—but is also appropriate with secondary sources such as the family, social workers, friends, and others. The gathering of data related to the nursing history also is done by means of an interview. Interviewing is a skill built on other skills, so some skills discussed in previous (and subsequent) chapters are important in carrying out an interview: observation, listening, and communication are particularly essential.

WHAT IS AN INTERVIEW?

Bermosk (1966) denoted the interview as a special time when the nurse focuses particular attention on the client and/or the client's system with the purpose of understanding the client's world of experience, feelings, beliefs, attitudes, and behavior. Hein (1980) simply stated that interviewing is a human interaction during which information is requested and/or shared.

The eventual purpose of this process, according to Keltner (1970), is determined by the people involved in the interview process. Bermosk and Mordan (1973) noted the interpersonal nature of the interview but also identified it as a developmental procedure. Their rationale for this description was based on their belief that the interview involves sequenced, directed, and progressive changes in all participants of the interview process, especially the nurse and the client.

In many areas of the literature, the interview is recognized as a strategy. Kahn and Cannell (1964) conceived the interview as purposeful conversation; Schatzman and Strauss (1973) agreed with this description even though their perspectives were as field researchers in the areas of sociology and anthropology.

PURPOSES FOR AN INTERVIEW

Perhaps the primary purpose for an interview that relates to our definition of nursing has been explicated by Hein (1980): In nursing practice, verbal communication is used to interrelate with a client with the intent of facilitating restoration of the client's fullest health potential. It is, therefore, a strategy for data collection to help the nurse discern the client's world, recognize areas requiring nursing assistance, and plan individualized care that is aimed toward alleviating nursing diagnoses. Marriner (1983) termed the interview as goal-directed communication.

It is evident that the interview must be specific to the client by dealing with the client's system and world. Categories of information that may be obtained during the interview process have been delineated by Hein (1980). These areas follow those of the PELLEM Pentagram (Chapter 17):

1. description of the happening

2. perceptions of client regarding the event

3. behaviors

4. attitudes and beliefs

5. feelings

6. values

Questions and statements by the nurse or interviewer should have the purpose of generating information on the categorical guidelines above. They should describe and elaborate, clarify, validate, substantiate, interpret, and compare. In a sense, the interviewer's comments should be levers by which the interviewee can find further self-expression.

CONDITIONS AND PRINCIPLES OF INTERVIEWING

Kahn and Cannell (1964) viewed the interview as a lengthy conversation in which there are three conditions for success: accessibility, cognition, and motivation. The first requires that the information received by the interviewer be in a conscious, clear, and relevant form. It must relate to the purposes of the interview for each unique client. Cognition requires that the person interviewed understand his role, and the reasons for data collection. Finally, motivation, or willingness to interact, is the major requirement for a successful interview.

Since client motivation has been observed as a paramount and necessary condition, much research by social scientists has been devoted to the area. In one example, Kahn and Cannell (1964) postulated both instrumental and intrinsic factors in their motivational framework (Figure 4–1).

It is easy to observe that the interview can and should be regarded as a complex social phenomenon. *Instrumental factors* of motivation focus heavily on the interviewee's belief that the results of the interview will have some positive effect on what happens to him. The second type of motivation factors, *intrinsic* (Kahn & Cannell, 1964), reflect the qualities of the interviewer. Receptiveness, warmth, understanding, and interest are all important. It is also pertinent to note that Carl Rogers's (1961)

Respondent Attributes   Interviewer Attributes

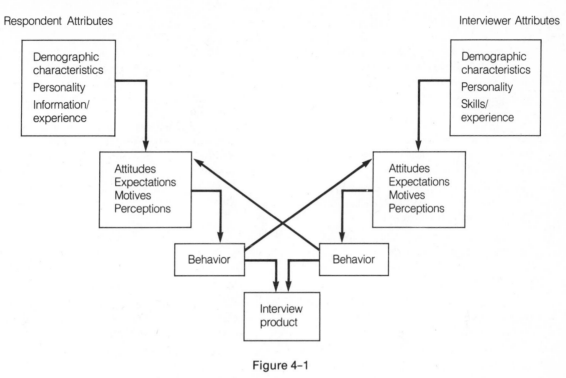

Figure 4-1

Motivational Model of the Interview as a Social Process

(SOURCE: *The Dynamics of Interviewing,* by R. Kahn and C. Cannell.
Copyright © 1964 by John Wiley & Sons, Inc. Reprinted by permission.)

ingredients of a meaningful counseling relationship, which were discussed in Chapter 3,
were noted by Kahn and Cannell (1964) as
equally valid for a productive interview. This
confirms the importance of effective communication skills in all of a nurse's interactions.

Certain principles for an effective interview
must be integrated into the technique. Hein
(1980, p. 26) explicated the following essentials:

1. An interview is effective to the degree that
   the nurse creates an atmosphere that encourages and supports the patient's freedom of expression.

2. An interview is effective to the degree that
   the nurse clearly establishes and understands the nursing goals in the interview.

3. An interview is effective to the degree that
   the nurse can relate to the patient without
   using value judgments.

4. An interview is effective to the degree that
   the nurse examines, encourages, and clarifies mutual thoughts and feelings that may
   affect nursing care.

5. An interview is effective to the degree that
   the nurse consistently evaluates patient
   needs, nursing goals, and the behavioral
   responses of the patient to his nursing care.

6. An interview is effective to the degree that
   the nurse is able to evaluate her communication behavior objectively in relation to the
   patient's needs and behavioral responses to
   the care he receives and the nursing goals.

7. An interview is effective to the degree that the nurse employs and encourages the use of feedback with patients in conveying, implementing, and evaluating nursing goals.[1]

In addition, Bermosk (1966, p. 207–210) stated other requisites:

8. The climate the nurse creates within the patient-nurse interaction influences the substance of the interview.

9. Professional attitudes of warmth, acceptance, objectivity, and compassion are essential for effective interviewing.

10. The identification and clarification of conflicting thoughts and feelings of the patient and of the nurse lead toward a harmony of goals in the interview.[2]

The social process involved in the interview can again be noticed by studying the principles; the interpersonal facet involves the nurse interviewer, the client, and the interaction of both.

DESIGNS AND CONTINGENCIES OF THE INTERVIEW

The interview can be structured or nonstructured. *Structure* implies that specific questions related to topic areas are posed by the interviewer; the nursing-history guide in Chapter 1 is an example of a structured interview since the same questions would be asked of all clients. *Nonstructure* relates to the fact that the interviewer's wording of questions is not specified prior to the interview. Questions flow spontaneously from the interview context, so different clients could be asked different questions.

The purposes of the interview, however, are a constant in both.

Formal and *informal* are words used to further classify interviewing. Formality broadly represents the fact that time, place, and content are arranged prior to the interaction. It generally involves a longer period for interviewing than does the informal interview. Informal interviewing can be anything from a lengthy, unplanned talk to a five-minute, spontaneous interaction in which data are collected.

Schatzman and Strauss (1973) stated various contingencies that shape the interview's form and content:

1. Expected duration: How long is it expected to last? Will it be interrupted? Can it be extended or shortened as guided by the interaction?

2. Single interview versus a series: Is this the only one? Is there a series? Where in the series does this one fall?

3. Setting: Is this a public or private place? What does the environment feel like? Is this feeling conducive to the interview's purpose? Is a specific conversational style more appropriate than others in this setting?

4. Identities: Is the interviewer an outsider or insider to the client's system? Can the interviewer and interviewee be seen as part of the same group?

5. Style of the respondent

In addition to these, this author includes the following:

6. Style of the interviewer

7. Harmony between respondent's style and that of the nurse

It is important to note that a nonstructured interview, be it formal or informal, usually requires greater experience on the part of the interviewer. Nursing students usually begin learning how to interview using a specified

---

[1]From *Communication in Nursing Practice*, by E. Hein. Copyright © 1980 by Little, Brown and Co., Inc. Reprinted with permission.

[2]Reprinted with permission from *Nursing Clinics of North America*, 1966, Vol. 1, No. 2. Refer to the selected reading at the end of this chapter.

procedure with explicit questions. This tends to diminish interviewer anxiety. Clients, however, may feel overcome with questions, especially in a short, intense interview. Carnevali (1983)[3] offered alternative forms of interviewer behavior that can elicit information from the client without questioning. These nonstructured techniques may be integrated into a structured format, but only if it is comfortable for the interviewer to do so.

> *Reflection:* A technique that became so overused that it was caricatured. It is a response in which one picks up a central or terminal word or phrase and repeats it in a rather tentative tone of voice. The client says, "I've been having so much trouble sleeping at night." And the interviewer continues, "trouble sleeping . . . ." It shows that the interviewer has tuned in to the message and is interested in hearing more. (p. 130)

> *Clarification:* Restating the client's ideas in different words to allow him to hear your version and validate, modify, or expand on the ideas. The client says, "I just don't know how I can manage to rest in the afternoon." The interviewer may say, "You have too many things to do to be able to lie down for an hour after lunch . . . ." Again, the tone of voice is tentative rather than declarative. (p. 130)

> *Giving an Opinion:* At times offering an opinion yields data. A lady who was inquiring about a low calorie diet in the course of discussing her nutrition patterns said she drank orange juice for vitamin C. The nurse gave the opinion that tomato juice would yield vitamin C with a lower number of calories. To

which the lady responded, "But I'm on a low salt diet and tomato juice has salt in it." A whole new line of data opened up. (p. 130)

> *Sharing of Yourself:* While this technique carries some risk of personal exposure for the interviewer, it can be very useful where the client is uncomfortable or the area under discussion is sensitive. Comments such as, "Being treated that way would make me angry," or "I'd be uncomfortable with such a situation," or "I didn't find it easy to . . . ." (p. 130)

> *Describing What You See:* Putting into words your impressions permits the client to validate or modify your observations. "It seems to me you hear better on your left side." "You're rubbing your breastbone again; the pain must be returning." "It appears to me from what you've said that you're a pretty independent person who would rather not ask for things." "That joint feels stiffer than the other one." (pp. 130–131)

> *Requesting Information:* Someone once said that a question is only a disguised demand for information. A logical variation, then, would be to request information. This technique is useful in starting an interview or in shifting from one area to another. "I'd be interested in knowing about . . . ." "It would help in planning for your care if you would tell me about . . . ." "Please tell me how . . . ." "I'd like to know more about . . . ." (p. 131)

> *Rewarding Responses:* Any interviewer response that shows approval will tend to encourage continuation of the behavior—for instance, such remarks as "That's interesting," "good," "uhm," and "I see." Nonverbal behavior such

---

[3]From *Nursing Care Planning: Diagnosis and Management*, 3rd Ed., by D. Carnevali. Copyright © 1983 by J. B. Lippincott. Reprinted by permission.

as nodding, leaning forward, and looking interested also indicate that one is listening. (p. 131)

Silence: It has been said that human beings want closure. For this reason, perhaps, people often feel impelled to fill silences with words. In an assessment interview, pauses can encourage a respondent to continue to share information unless he is quite withdrawn, or has become aware of the technique and is playing competitive games with you. (p. 131)

Unfinished Sentences: The human need for closure can be used to draw the client out in another way. The nurse responds to his initial statement with an unfinished sentence and allows him to fill in the missing information. This technique takes practice, but here is an example. The client says, "I've been working the evening shift for years. I get home around midnight and unwind with the paper and a bite to eat, so I get to bed about 1 or 1:30 in the morning." The nurse then responds, "Well in the morning then you . . ." again trailing off on the last word. (p. 131)

SUMMARY

It becomes clear that interviewing is a complex social process involving the principal interactors, purposes guided by principles of interviewing, and many extraneous variables that also must be considered.

REFERENCES

Bermosk, L. (1966). Interviewing: A key to therapeutic communication in nursing practice. *Nursing Clinics of North America, 1,* 205–214.

Bermosk, L., & Mordan, M. (1973). *Interviewing in nursing.* New York: Macmillan.

Carnevali, D. (1983). *Nursing care planning: Diagnosis and management* (3rd ed.). Philadelphia: Lippincott.

Hein, E. (1980). *Communication in nursing practice* (2nd ed.). Boston: Little, Brown.

Kahn, R., & Cannell, C. (1964). *The dynamics of interviewing.* New York: Wiley.

Keltner, J. (1970). *Interpersonal speech-communication: Elements and structures.* Belmont, CA: Wadsworth.

Marriner, A. (1983). *The nursing process: A scientific approach to nursing care* (3rd ed.). St. Louis: Mosby.

Rogers, C. (1961). *On becoming a person.* Boston: Houghton-Mifflin.

Schatzman, L., & Strauss, A. (1973). *Field research: Strategies for a natural society.* Englewood Cliffs, NJ: Prentice-Hall.

SELECTED READING

Bermosk's classic article is included here for further study of the interviewing process. She sees interviewing as a key in therapeutic communication and comprehensively discusses five principles for interviewing in nursing practice.

Interviewing: A Key to Therapeutic Communication in Nursing Practice

Loretta Sue Bermosk, B.S., M. Litt.

Interviewing in nursing is a specific kind of communication which is in operation when the professional person (the nurse) focuses her attention on the patient (client, subject, group, family) and attends to the business of helping this person to better understand what is happening or what has happened to him at a particular moment in a particular situation. She encourages him to describe his actions and to express his thoughts and feelings so as to identify needs and to establish goals which will help him to regain, maintain, or improve his health status. With the acceptance of the interpersonal relationship as the context within which the actions of nursing are performed, and wherein the nurse functions as a counselor, teacher, technician, and socializing agent, it seems imperative that patient-centered, purposeful, and goal-directed communication be initiated and maintained by the nurse.

Principles of interviewing and supervised practice in applying these principles are currently seen as essential content in undergraduate and graduate nursing curricula. The specific content which provides the knowledge necessary for the implementation of the interviewing process has been derived from the theories and concepts of social psychology, personality, growth and development, normal and abnormal behavior, humanities, linguistics, and psychiatry. The supervised practice within

the performance of nursing care in a variety of situations, with the intent of making the conversational aspect of the nurse-patient interaction purposeful and meaningful, allows nurse and supervisor and/or student and teacher to scrutinize both verbal and nonverbal responses and evaluate their effect on the patient. From this learning experience, the nurse is enabled to develop a nursing approach to each patient which incorporates an organization of verbal and nonverbal actions directed toward promoting a relationship with the patient in which the messages exchanged are patient-centered, clear, mutually understood, and goal-directed.

As she experiences working with patients who present deep-seated difficulties or are faced with overwhelming problems in adjusting to life or death situations, the nurse grows in her understanding and ability to recognize patient needs, and develops increased skill in selecting those verbal and nonverbal responses that will be most helpful to the patient. Thus, she reaches a point in her administration of nursing care when the *communication* between professional person and patient is of a therapeutic nature and truly comprehensive in intent.

In this paper, the five principles of interviewing described by Bermosk and Mordan are presented as knowledge that becomes a key to open the door and bring the nurse to the threshold where she can communicate therapeutically as a psychiatric nurse practitioner. These principles guide the nurse's actions in relation to (1) the climate for the interview, (2)

Reprinted with permission from *Nursing Clinics of North America*, 1966, Vol. 1, No. 2, pp. 205–214.

the nurse's attitudes and role, (3) and (4) the content of the interview, and (5) evaluation of the interview and the nurse-interviewer.

Although the psychiatric nurse has been chosen as the exemplar here, for the reason that the interview is a vital tool in her particular metier, the principles and examples cited can all be applied to the broad field of general nursing care. In all verbal interchange with patients, nurses can find application of one or more of these principles.

PRINCIPLES OF INTERVIEWING IN NURSING

1. *The climate the nurse creates within the patient-nurse interaction influences the substance of the interview.*

Climate is composed of those immediate conditions, circumstances, and influences which surround and affect people interacting with each other. The physical, emotional, external, and internal factors are seen as dynamic forces which cause the climate within which the interview is conducted to change in relation to the specific areas or subjects being explored. The physical setting, the day's experiences, interactions with other patients and staff, and physical and emotional status affect the thoughts and feelings of patient and nurse. The expectations the patient has for himself and for the nurse, and the expectations the nurse has for herself and for the patient, are an influence on climate.

A graduate student, working with a woman patient who had many neurotic and psychophysiological complaints, expressed dissatisfaction, boredom, and loss of interest in this patient, because "nothing's happening. The patient says that everything's going great since she has this new boy friend. Neither her kids nor boss bother her anymore."

Instr.: You're bored with what she tells you?
G.S.: I think I should be spending my time with a patient who really needs me.

Instr.: You're saying this woman doesn't need your help.
G.S.: Not as much as some others.
Instr.: What would you like her to talk about in your sessions?
G.S.: Well, it would be nice if she thought she was getting some help from the clinic.
Instr.: From you?
G.S.: Well, yes. I have been seeing her for some time. I do want to help her, and I think I have, but she attributes any change in her mood to her boy friend.
Instr.: And now you find yourself losing interest in her because she isn't meeting your expectations of her.
G.S.: Seems that way. I'm not meeting my own expectations either with this lady —she jumps from one topic to another so quickly that I am unable to keep her focused on any subject long enough to identify what the problem really is. She makes me feel inadequate.

In exploring the situation, we find that the nurse's feeling of inadequacy in relation to her interviewing skills (not meeting expectations of self) was emphasized when she thought that the patient was saying that she (the patient) was being helped more by the boy friend than by the nurse (patient not meeting nurse's expectation that patient would recognize that nurse was helping her). This heightened feeling of inadequacy influenced the climate of the interview so much that the nurse was consciously aware of being bored, disinterested, and dissatisfied with the patient's responses. The patient may have kept the substance of the interview centered on her boy friend who wasn't bored, disinterested, and dissatisfied with her responses as a defense against the nonverbal communication of the nurse. Discovering the impact of her feelings of inadequacy on the climate of the interview and on the developing relationship between patient and nurse, the nurse can put more of her energies into developing her interviewing skills. Meanwhile, she goes into her next interview with her patient with a greater awareness, a little more objectivity, and a strenghtened intention to focus on the patient.

How does the nurse create and maintain a climate which reflects her intention of helping the patient so that he will come to believe that she wants to help him, and will trust her and talk about those actions, thoughts, and feelings that concern him?

Knowledge of the concept of climate within the interview will increase the nurse's awareness of and sensitivity to those factors in the immediate surroundings that may enhance or interfere with the interaction between patient and nurse. Her intention must be sincere or the patient will sense the masquerade and avoid her.

In her initial contact, whether the patient is interested or not, actively verbal or passively nonverbal, the nurse approaches the patient in a relaxed, unhurried manner, introduces herself so that he knows who she is (name, discipline, and echelon)—so he can fit her into some frame of reference; tells him what she will be doing that concerns him (talking with him, going to activities, etc.); and arranges with him for a time to meet that will be mutually agreeable (hour, day, length of each conference, extent of total period of nursing therapy—if feasible at this time). She screens the bed unit, or seeks an alcove, a room, or an out of doors area for the conference where privacy, confidentiality, and relative freedom from noise and interruptions are possible. She provides comfortable chairs that can be arranged in such a way as to facilitate ease of listening and responding. She attends to both the verbal and nonverbal expressions of the patient, encourages him to tell her about his experiences and concerns, and helps the patient organize the telling by asking the who, where, what, and when of each incident. Thus, she demonstrates her interest and intent and the patient experiences an interaction wherein he is the center of attention and his concerns are listened to and responded to in an attempt to understand their import and meaning.

2. *Professional attitudes of warmth, acceptance, objectivity, and compassion are essential for effective interviewing.*

The development of these professional attitudes is dependent upon how well the nurse is able to work through her personal attitudes arising from her life experiences and sociocultural milieu. Identification of these attitudes and recognition of the strength of their influence on her behavior is an on-going process, and, when started early in the nursing curriculum through analysis of nurse-patient interactions in a variety of clinical settings, allows the nurse to experience her reactions to both subject matter and patient behavior. Comprehensive discussions of such subjects as pain, fear, sexual identification, masturbation, promiscuity, infidelity, birth control, abortion, unwed mothers, birth anomalies, race, religion, suicide, dying, and death, all of which relate to the nature of man and his adaptations to living and dying, are essential to achieving some degree of objectivity in relating to all patients. Identification and working with such personal feelings as shock, helplessness, inadequacy, heterosexual and homosexual attractions, anxiety, rejection, or dependency also become part of the learning experience. If the nurse is to communicate therapeutically with the psychiatric patient, she must be clear in her understanding of the dynamics of behavior so as to help the patient whose intrapsychic and social communications are distorted and impaired to arrive at some organization and clarity of ideas. Conscious awareness of her personal attitudes and how they have developed prepares her to respond to the patient's attitudes in terms of helping him to understand how his attitudes developed and how they influence his behavior.

How does the nurse demonstrate the professional attitudes of warmth, acceptance, objectivity, and compassion?

The nurse demonstrates *warmth* when she is kind, gentle, and thoughtful. She shows respect for the patient as a person by addressing him by name, and by remembering his personal preferences, idiosyncracies, and problems.

She demonstrates the attitude of *acceptance* when she views the patient's behavior as purposeful, meaningful, and a method arrived at for handling a stressful situation. She attempts to learn to identify the need being expressed, and to take appropriate action. Behavior that is helpful and behavior that is harmful to the patient or to others is recognized in terms of the needs being expressed, and the nurse intervenes either to facilitate or to inhibit the action. If the patient says he is going to kill himself, she accepts this statement as an expression of a need, but in light of her responsibility to help the patient through this stress period, she institutes precautions to protect the patient from this action against himself.

Complete *objectivity* is an impossibility, but the nurse works at being relatively objective—relatively free from bias and prejudice—when she bases her assumptions on the collected data gathered in the reality of the situation—that which is seen and heard—and attempts to validate her conclusions with the patient and with other professionals in the situation.

The nurse demonstrates *compassion* when she has reached the point where she is truly working with the patient within the sphere of his feelings and needs. She has learned to tolerate and harbor the impact of the emotion expressed by her patient with sufficient absorption that she can accept its meaning and enter into a feeling of fellowship with him. This implies that she has arrived at a point where she herself is comfortable with the feeling being expressed, and can move forward into translating the attitude of compassion into nursing action.

3. *Defined needs and goals (for the patient and for the nurse) determine the purpose of the interview.*

There is a time sequence involved in developing the ability to define needs and goals. Theory related to growth and development and the dynamics of human behavior orients the nurse to the existence of needs and to the physical, psychic, and social forces that generate these needs. Through the supervised practice of interacting with patients of all ages with varying degrees of illness, and the careful analysis of process recordings describing the words and actions of patient and nurse within these interactions, the nurse learns to recognize the overt and covert ways in which she and the patient express their needs. At the same time, she learns to recognize elements within each situation that threaten the security of patient and nurse, and works toward diminishing or removing the threatening element. She also experiences the sequence of phases found in the nurse-patient interaction—orientation, identification, exploitation, and resolution—and learns that her role in each phase will change as the patient becomes clear in his thinking and gains sufficient strength from the relationship to progress on his own.

4. *The identification and clarification of conflicting thoughts and feelings of the patient and of the nurse lead toward a harmony of goals in the interview.*

The patient will become clear in his thinking only as the nurse is able to become organized and clear in her thinking and can give direction to the communication that she shares with the patient. In her role of therapeutic agent, the nurse identifies the area in which the patient's conflict lies—in his thought processes, or at a deeper emotional level. She helps the patient describe events that happened to him and works toward a logical and sequential description of time, place, people, and event, so that the chaos of thoughts causing the patient's confusion has a time sequence, a beginning and an end, a cause and an effect, and can be looked at by patient and nurse as an experience that has meaning to the patient. She helps the patient to separate "this is what I was doing" from "this is what I was thinking" and from "this is what I was feeling," so that he can gain some perspective and objectivity in looking at his behavior during the particular event. He learns to distinguish between action, thought, and feeling along with discovering their relationship to each other. The conflict itself becomes less threatening as patient and nurse discuss it objectively. The conflict is visualized by both patient and nurse and the way is clear for setting up a goal to deal with this conflict which is mutually understood and accepted by each.

The actions of the interview that help the nurse to define needs, to identify and clarify thoughts and feelings, and to arrive at a harmony of goals with the patient are observation, listening, verbal and nonverbal responses, interpretation of data, and recording of data.

Observation   Observation that is planned, specific, and oriented in time, place, people, and events and associated with a particular patient behavior provides data about the patient which help the nurse learn the patient's reaction to stress, and to make assumptions about the degree of anxiety experienced by the patient and his methods of handling it. As the nurse learns the patient's habitual behavior patterns, she assesses the degree of organization and/or disorganization, his awareness or unawareness of others around him, his appearance, dress, stature, and walk, and carefully notes when a change appears and looks further to note what in the situation may account for the change. She also notes her own behavior and assesses its influence on the patient.

Listening   Listening accompanies observation, and adds words and greater meaning to the observed actions. It adds another dimension in learning about the patient—the pitch, tone, harshness or softness of his voice, his vocabulary and choice of words, his hesitancy or intensity in speaking. The nurse listens to the patient's words and attempts to identify those themes that are stressed and those that are vaguely hinted at; those that indicate healthy aspects of the patient's personality, and those that indicate the areas where he experiences the most conflict and disturbance.

Nonverbal responses   Nonverbal responses include all the methods by which one communicates other than by the spoken word, e.g., gestures, body movements, sweaty palms, limp handshake, pushing away from a person or moving closer, physical appearance, and choice of make-up and clothing. Silence may be an indication of many emotions or complete apathy, the exact meaning of which must be explored with the patient.

Verbal responses   Verbal responses include questions, statements, and those words that indicate that one is listening, such as "yes," "go on," "uh huh." Questions and statements that contain a single idea will elicit the clearest responses. The "what," "where," and "who" open-ended questions related to a specific topic introduced by the patient aid in helping the patient get the specific event organized so that he and the nurse are able to explore it together. Learning to focus on an event so as to see the relationship to the patient's thoughts and feelings becomes the intent and purpose of the nurse for communicating with the patient. She helps the patient look more closely at his strengths in particular situations and, in looking at his failures, provides him with information to consider in handling the situation differently the next time. For the most part, she encourages the patient to organize his thoughts, reconstruct situations, take a look at what really did happen and what the patient thought happened.

In working with psychiatric patients, the nurse learns to become aggressive in intervening in the stream of words issuing from the patient in an effort to break into the stereotyped thinking, the rigid, the biased, the prejudiced, the judgmental, the self-effacing, and to introduce new ideas to increase or decrease the amount of reflected light on the subject, to separate the real from the fantasy, to clear up the dark areas—the unknown, the frightening, the prohibited, the unexplored—to help the patient obtain a different, new, or altered perspective of himself and the "others" in his world.

Interpretation of data   Interpretation of data within the interview is an on-going intellectual function of the nurse. She listens and observes and from her knowledge of behavior relates principles and facts to her collected data. She interprets the meaning of the patient's behavior to herself and makes certain assumptions about his needs. She then can do one of three things: she can respond to the data and test her assumption, she can ignore the data and change the subject, or she can physically retreat from the situation. Her decision directs her action. Whatever her action, her recognition of the selected action and its influence on the nurse-patient relationship will dictate her next approach.

In learning to interpret behavior and to respond appropriately (constructively), the nurse learns to test her assumptions and the validity of her interpretations. She may err. Her intention of helping the patient is not lost; this gets communicated nonverbally. Aware of her error, she reviews and evaluates the process of thinking that led to the incorrect assumption. This too is learning. To err is human, and for the nurse to discuss her error with the patient sometimes paves the way for the patient to talk freely with her about his inadequacies and/or failures. In the role of professional practitioner, the nurse assumes the responsibility for the results of her nursing actions whether she attempts to meet the patient's needs or to ignore them.

Recording of data   Recording of data follows two patterns, each with a specific purpose: (1) the recording of raw data—the content of the interview—so as to study the behavior of patient and nurse, to obtain a record of patient progress and learning, and to assess the skill of the nurse as an interviewer and psychiatric nurse practitioner; and (2) the recording of certain aspects of her interaction with the patient for other team members through written nurses' notes and verbal conferences to contribute toward continuity of patient care.

In recording the actual interview, nurses are becoming adept in using a notebook and pencil and/or a tape recorder. The most accurate reproduction of verbal content will be gained by using the recorder. However, the nurse also needs to note and remember the nonverbal

responses. With the notebook and pencil, the nurse develops a code for herself so she can keep pace with the patient and herself, as well as noting silent periods and other nonverbal responses. Recording the action of the interview after one leaves the patient allows memory loss and distortion to enter the record, and if this method is used, the recording should be done as soon after the event as possible.

One great advantage of recording by tape or writing during the interaction is the opportunity to review content with the patient. The nurse may play back certain sections of the tape to help the patient hear the anger in his voice when talking about a particular person or situation, or hear the words he used in describing a person or place. With the notebook, she can refer accurately to some of the patient's statements in an attempt to help him clarify meaning or sequence of time and events.

5. *Continuous and terminal evaluations of the interview are made in terms of behavior changes in the patient and in the nurse related to the defined needs and goals.*

In the activity of the interview, in concentrating upon the patient's behavior, each observation and response of the patient is attended to by the nurse. She is continuously trying to ascertain whether or not the words used are conveying the meaning each intends, to search for meaning in each exchange, to assess the level of anxiety, to keep the focus on a particular subject matter until it is explored and understood, and to make associations between events the patient chooses to introduce. She is continuously in the process of evaluating, making a quick judgment, and then selecting her own response to the patient based on this judgment. Sometimes her responses bring her and the patient closer to their goal and sometimes they do not. Often, she may be able to reword, rephrase, or retract her response on the spot if she is immediately aware of the situation. Other times, it is only in retrospect as she reviews her recording of an interchange that she becomes aware that she and the patient were miles apart. Then she attempts to reconstruct the sequence of exchanges within the interaction to pinpoint the ideas, feelings, or behavior which interfered or interrupted the patient and the nurse in working toward their defined goal. She reviews data from other interactions with this patient to support or negate her assumptions about patterns of behavior which indicate her own difficulties in handling certain behavior or situations. She confers with her professional colleagues both to gain other points of view and to be as objective as possible in reading her data. She peruses the literature to add to her knowledge of behavior and psychiatric nursing.

Learning to communicate with the psychiatric patient in a therapeutic manner evolves from the application of interviewing principles and psychiatric nursing principles practiced within the context of the nurse-patient relationship. When the principles of interviewing and guided experiences are introduced early in the nurse's education, and she is both encouraged and expected to expand her interviewing knowledge and to develop her interviewing skills in each clinical situation as she progresses from relatively simple to more complex health problems, she possesses a key to open the door to therapeutic communication in her nursing practice.

REFERENCES

1. Bermosk, Loretta Sue, and Mordan, Mary Jane. *Interviewing in nursing.* New York: Macmillan, 1964.

2. Peplau, Hildegarde. *Basic principles of patient counseling.* 2nd ed. Philadelphia: Smith, Kline & French Laboratories, 1964.

3. Reusch, Jurgen. *Therapeutic communication.* New York: Norton, 1961.

4. Spiegel, Rose. Specific problems of communication in psychiatric conditions. In Arieti, S., Ed.: *American handbook of psychiatry.* New York: Basic Books, 1959, Chap. 46.

Humanistic Exercises

Exercise 1

Nursing-History Interview Format

Purposes
1. To develop a personal nursing-history interview format based on one's individual philosophy of practice.
2. To experience using the format with peers.

Facility
A large room where participants can form dyads and interview one another.

Materials
Paper and other writing materials.

Time Required
One hour.

Group Size
Unlimited dyads.

Design
1. As a homework assignment, have participants read Part I and other nursing-history articles and written materials.
2. With the information gleaned from the above, request that each student bring to class a nursing-history interview format that is based on individual beliefs concerning this area. Interview techniques to be used should be explained and should reflect the individual's experience and needs concerning this skill.
3. Request members to form into dyads and use their nursing-history formats on each other. The student being interviewed should then provide feedback on the process, if requested by the interviewer.
4. Personal reactions of the interviewer and interviewee may be shared.
5. Nursing-history interview formats can now be reevaluated and changed by the interviewer, based on the results of this experience.
6. Reform into a total group and discuss the experience.

Variations
This exercise can be done completely as a homework assignment. Further, learners may use their formats in the clinical laboratory or with their clients.

Exercise 2
Observation

Purposes	1. To sharpen observational skills.
	2. To increase perception of nonverbal behavior.
Facility	A classroom large enough to accommodate participants.
Materials	None.
Time Required	Twenty minutes.
Group Size	Unlimited pairs.
Design*	1. Members should form pairs.

Design*

1. Members should form pairs.
2. Pairs should sit facing one another for two minutes, each person observing everything about his/her partner. If necessary, it can be suggested that certain items be noted, such as posture, eye contact, placement of hands and feet, facial expressions, dress, jewelry, and so forth.
3. Then members of each pair should turn back-to-back with the agreed-upon partner changing five things about herself or himself.
4. When changes have been accomplished, members should once again face each other. The observing partner attempts to verbalize the noticed changes.
5. Roles are reversed.
6. Discuss the experience.

Variations

The exercise can be lengthened by using the same pairs and requesting members to change five more things about themselves. This occasionally poses a problem, and people often do not know what to change further. During discussion, ask participants whether they thought of asking for help from another close member of a pair who was also searching for changes. If they did, how did they feel about needing help on a seemingly simple task? If they did not request assistance, why not?

---

*The idea for this exercise came from Kenneth Blanchard, School of Education, University of Massachusetts, 1973.

Exercise 3

Observation of Body Talk

Purposes

1. To increase awareness of how different emotions can be expressed nonverbally.
2. To interpret perceptions of nonverbally expressed emotions.
3. To validate perception of nonverbally expressed emotions.

Facility

Large enough room to accommodate participants sitting around tables or on the floor in a circle.

Materials

Small pieces of paper. Two hats or baskets.

Time Required

Thirty minutes or more, depending on group size.

Group Size

12 to 15 is ideal; two or more groups may be formed if group is large.

Design

1. In a large group, ask participants to verbalize emotions/feelings. Write one each on a slip of paper; fold the papers and place them in a hat.
2. Repeat step 1, except this time ask that participants verbalize parts of the body that can be used to express emotions/feelings. Place these slips of paper in a second hat.
3. A person from the group should then distribute the slips of paper or have participants pick a slip of paper from each hat.
4. Request each participant who has picked an emotion and body part to role-play the emotion nonverbally, primarily using the designated body part.
5. Group participants should then try to guess what feeling is being expressed.
6. Discussion follows.
7. Role-players should place papers back in each respective hat and steps #3 through #6 should be repeated. This should be done until all members have a chance to role-play.

Variations

If two or more groups of twelve are possible, equalize the number of emotions and body parts for both groups, and time how long it takes for groups to carry out the task. Then have groups work against one another; all role-plays should result in the group accurately diagnosing the emotion and body part used in expression. Only then may they proceed to the next role-play. The group finishing first has the sharpest observational skills of those present.

Exercise 4
Perception

Purposes	1. To increase awareness of the variety of perceptions that can be elicited from a given situation.
	2. To raise self-awareness regarding individual perceptual fields.
Facility	Room to accommodate class size in groups of six.
Materials	Worksheet A: Scenarios Paper and pencils.
Time Required	One hour.
Group Size	Unlimited groups of six.
Design	1. Have participants individually read Scenario 1 and write down their perceptions and reactions concerning what happened, their feelings in the situation, and what conclusions they reach.
	2. Ask that participants share these notations with their small group.
	3. Observe and discuss perceptual differences, possible reasons for such, and rationale for conclusions. Dichotomous differences between members should be studied more fully.
	4. Repeat the design with Scenario 2.
Variations	Participants can develop their own scenarios based on actual or hypothetical experience. They can then share them with their small group and follow the design for as many scenarios as time permits.

Exercise 4

Scenarios

Worksheet **A**

Scenario 1: It is 11:15 A.M. Ms. Blue, a supervisor, is making rounds on a surgical unit. She observes a patient with traction of the right leg, a basin of water on the bedside table, a stripped bed, a gown placed over the patient's chest, and the patient, Ms. Green, reading a book. As the supervisor enters the room, the patient explains that the student nurse assigned to assist her with a bath had struck his head against the crossbar of the traction frame at 10:30 A.M. and that the nursing instructor had taken him to the emergency room. On the way to the nurse's station, the supervisor notices several nursing personnel, including the head nurse, drinking coffee in the utility room. As she begins calling the Nursing School office to report that a nursing student and instructor had left a patient unattended, the head nurse comes in to tell her about the accident.

Scenario 2:* The setting is a general hospital unit in an urban city. Three people are involved: Ms. King, the new head nurse of the medical unit; Ms. James, the director of Nursing Services; and Ms. Carmichael, the day supervisor of the building. Ms. King gives the patients' nursing care file a last-minute check to be sure all patients' activities, treatments, medications, and so forth are taken care of or are in process. Then she checks the patients, going from room to room. "It's going pretty well," she thinks. She is particularly satisfied with the way Ms. Garcia is responding to the care plan now. She has spent a great deal of time working with Ms. Garcia. "Certainly," Ms. King thinks, "Ms. James can find nothing wrong here; the patients are all receiving excellent care." Ms. King has heard a lot about these "spontaneous rounds" by Ms. James. Shortly thereafter, Ms. James and Ms. Carmichael arrive on the unit by the backstairs, so it is some time before Ms. King even knows they are there.

During the "rounds" with Ms. James and Ms. Carmichael, Ms. King makes several attempts to comment on certain patients and their progress. Ms. James ignores the attempts and starts to jot down notes on her clip board. Ms. James and Ms. Carmichael maintain a general conversation about the unit while they finish the rounds. No attempt is made to draw Ms. King into the conversation. After rounds are completed on the unit, Ms. King asks whether there is any additional information they need. Ms. James says, "No. However, there are a few small items I would like to call to your attention, Ms. King. The shelves in the medicine cupboard are rather dusty, and the utility room is very cluttered. Will you please see that these things are taken care of?" With that, Ms. James and Ms. Carmichael leave the unit.

On the way to the next unit Ms. James remarks to Ms. Carmichael, "On the whole, I think Ms. King is doing a good job with her unit. She should make a fine head nurse."

---

*This scenario was received by this author at the College of Nursing, University of Florida, 1966. Author unknown.

Exercise 5

Communication in Counseling

Purposes	1. To focus on the verbal and nonverbal cues that may be emitted in a counseling situation.
	2. To validate messages received with messages sent.
	3. To become aware of the intent of one's own communications as perceived by others.
Facility	Large enough room to accommodate participants seated around tables or in a circle on the floor.
Materials	None.
Time Required	One hour or more, depending on group size and number of volunteers.
Group Size	Unlimited groups of 12.
Design	1. Paired volunteers should be given a couple of minutes to develop a hypothetical counseling situation. They should decide which of them is to be the counselor and which is to be the counselee. (A hypothetical counseling situation is a made-up story in which the counselee is seeking help/advice from the counselor. These should not be personal.)
	2. The pair should then role-play the counseling situation, with instruction being given to the counselor that he or she should decide whether to be effective or ineffective in the role. Only the counselor should be aware of what is decided.
	3. Following the role-play, players and the group members should receive feedback on their reactions and perceptions of what was nonverbally and verbally communicated. Players should reveal their intent after group members give feedback.
	4. Discuss the experience.
Variations	1. The instructor can prepare the scenes to be role-played prior to class. Situations from Carkhuff's Index of Communication, *Helping and Human Relations,* Vol. 1, 1969, pp. 95–99, may be used.
	2. Learners may be given a homework assignment to prepare a scene prior to the class in which the exercise will take place.

Exercise 6

Communication—Process Recordings

Purposes
1. To raise self-awareness on communicative interactions with peers and clients.
2. To validate perceptions with peers and instructors.
3. To validate one's effective use of communication skills with peers and instructors.

Facility
Access to interactions with clients and peers in any setting.

Materials
Worksheet A: Process Recording Sheets. Pen or pencil.

Time Required
Variable.

Group Size
Dyads composed of instructor and learner or two peers.

Design
1. Using the Process Recording Sheet (Worksheet A), have participants engage in an interaction with a chosen and agreeable peer. Notes can be taken either during the talk or immediately following it.
2. Process recordings can then be discussed with another peer or a teacher. Rationale for perceptions, the thoughts and feelings of the student during the interaction, and communication skills all should be in focus. Alternatives in communicating may be suggested by both parties.
3. Repeat design using clients.

Variations
This exercise can be done only with clients. The nursing-history interview also can be done and studied using this format.

Exercise 6   Worksheet **A**

Process Recording Sheet

What the client/peer communicates (verbal and nonverbal)	What the nurse communicates (verbal and nonverbal)	Perceptions of or about client/peer	Thoughts and/or feelings about these perceptions

Part II

Analyzing: Identifying Needs

Beryl Skog, R.N., M.A., C.C.R.N., was the clinical
consultant for the case analysis used in this book. She is
the Assistant Director of Nursing for Critical Care at St.
Vincent's Hospital and Medical Center of New York.

Chapter 5

Data Processing

The guiding goal in nursing care is to give holistic care that encourages the client to meet maximum health potential (Bower, 1982). As was discussed in Chapter 1, when a client needs assistance, the nurse's responsibility is to provide help while maintaining the individuality of the client and the client's system. To accomplish this, the nurse collects data with the intent of discovering what is necessary in order for the nursing-care consumer to fulfill and further individual potential. Simply, the nurse is a helper.

Data processing is the step following data collection in the nursing process, and it is a tool used to assist decision making by both nurse and client. Data processing is an important part of the analyzing phase and is necessary to integrate scientifically knowledge about clients and their systems with the responsibilities and knowledge of professional nursing, as well as nursing personnel. Data processing is the act of interpreting collected data; it is the procedure of analyzing and examining information in relation to other information in the client's system. The purpose of data processing is to ensure that nursing care responds to the individual needs and wants of the client. This concept of data processing is similar to discussions by Bower (1982), Gordon (1982), Simms and Lindberg (1978), Sundeen, Stuart, Rankin, and Cohen (1981), and Watson (1979), among others.

Similar to data collection, data processing is a continuously occurring event. Each piece of information that an individual receives or even blocks from consciousness becomes a part of past learning, experiences, values, beliefs, and goals. Because research suggests that behavior results from attitudes, motives, and goals, for the nurse to become more aware of the reasons for client behavior and the client's condition and for the nurse to integrate the different perceptions of others concerning the client, data processing is an important tool. In addition, it is a valuable aid in communicating requirements of client care to other members of the health team. It also organizes data for suitable storage and retrieval (Simms & Lindberg, 1978). Let us look again at the equation presented in Chapter 1.

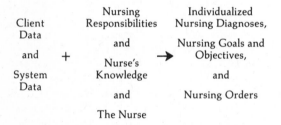

The first segment of the equation involves the collection of client and system data. The second segment of the equation involves data processing. The elements of this segment—nursing responsibilities, the nurse's knowledge, and the nurse—act upon the collected information, interpreting it and translating it into a useful care plan comprised of individualized nursing diagnoses and nursing orders. Again, data collection is a tool of the assessment phase of the nursing process, and data processing is the first aspect of analyzing. It should be noted that many authors—for example, Marriner (1983)—included data processing and establishing nursing diagnoses as parts of assessment. However, the National Council of State Boards of Nursing (1982) included "Analyzing" as a distinct step of

the nursing process, and this book is based on the Council's delineation and descriptions of the nursing process. A discussion of data processing follows.

AREAS OF NURSING RESPONSIBILITY

According to theories of professionalism (see Chapter 15), there are three essential components of the nursing profession: areas of responsibility, autonomy, and authority. The first component, areas of responsibility, makes up the basis of nursing actions and is important in processing information. Many of these responsibilities have been assigned to nurses ever since Florence Nightingale (1860/1969) established the framework of nursing practice in 1859. The following areas of responsibility, many of which were first written about by Nightingale and later discussed by Henderson (1966), are considered in data processing because they reflect nursing goals to be included in the total care plan. The areas of responsibility are as follows:

1. comfort
2. nutrition
3. exercise
4. personal hygiene
5. sleep, rest patterns
6. diversional activities
7. socializing and privacy
8. elimination
9. safety
10. environmental considerations
11. teaching
12. spiritual comfort and/or assistance
13. prevention of complications
14. assurance of physiologic status—health maintenance and promotion
15. emotional support, counseling

The areas of responsibility are usually presented as part of a beginning-level nursing course. Subsequent courses and experiences of the practitioner amplify the understanding of these responsibilities, and different client-care situations supply the nurse with more information about these responsibilities. Thus, the nurse grows in the understanding of responsibilities through experience. This learning process is similar to Hall's (1964) model of nursing practice, which portrayed nursing functions as moving from simple to complex. Growth through experience requires that the funnel of knowledge always expand, even though the basic concepts are grounded in nursing practice. A nursing theory that frames practice can further amplify and describe areas of nursing responsibility.

THE NURSE'S KNOWLEDGE AND THE NURSE

To process data while considering the areas of nursing responsibility, a solid body of knowledge is required, so knowing the theory framing each responsibility is important. For example, in dealing with the area of nutrition, it is necessary to study the physiology of the gastrointestinal (GI) system; physiologic responses of the GI tract to stress; normal diets; diets that are specific for certain physiologic or psychologic alterations; and the psychomotor skills and social aspects of feeding. In addition, the area of nutrition is related closely to elimination since overlap exists in many areas. Thus, it is important to develop knowledge not only of specific areas of concern but also of the areas of overlap to assist in processing and planning care.

Nursing knowledge and the individual nurse are, of course, closely interrelated. Nursing knowledge revolves around the areas of responsibility and combines with the values, beliefs, and experiences of the individual nurse to produce nursing diagnoses and orders. Lewis (1968) stressed that nursing care should be designed to provide interventions that meet the clients' needs in an individual manner. According to Sundeen et al. (1981), the nurse is a member of a client-oriented profession; the nurse seeks to identify the unexpressed and expressed needs of the client, find meaning in the client's coping responses, and maximize the client's strengths.

Data processing provides the bridge between (1) the nurse's knowledge and experience concerning what the client needs, including the medical diagnosis and orders, and (2) the needs as expressed by the client. The manner in which the client is most apt to receive care depends on the individual nurse. In data processing, the nurse asks, "What is it necessary for me to know about the client and the client's system so that I can make nursing diagnoses relative to my areas of responsibility?" The nurse's response to this question reflects the nurse's body of knowledge and experience, the nurse's perception of responsibilities, and the nurse's reaction to the client.

A CASE STUDY

The following case study is presented to facilitate learning how to process collected data. This case study also will be used to follow the other steps of the nursing process in Chapters 6, 7, 9, and 11 in order to illustrate the process in action. Refer to Box 5-1.

Box 5-1

Mr. Munson, the client, is a married, 52-year-old, white male who entered the hospital through the emergency room on June 30. Diagnosis: possible myocardial infarction. The professional nurse's first contact with him took place the morning following admission in the coronary-care unit on July 1. On July 7 he was transferred to an intermediate-care unit and then to an ambulatory-care unit on July 15. On July 23 he was discharged to return home.*

---

*The case material used in this section was modified from that presented by Eugene Kresco, University of Massachusetts, 1975.

Data collection started with the nurse's first contact and continued throughout admission. Primary nursing care was the organizational model used in the facility. The nurse taking care of Mr. Munson was a baccalaureate nursing student who wished to become a coronary-care specialist. The first step in the nursing process was to explore the purpose of nursing care; see Box 5–2.

Box 5–2

Although it was not definite that Mr. Munson had a myocardial infarction, he nevertheless seemed susceptible, based on presenting symptoms. Data were collected and analyzed to discover facts about him and his habits and to decipher bits of information that might lead to the clarification of behaviors associated with the disease process. At the same time, strict monitoring of the client was indicated to prevent further heart damage or progression of symptoms.

It should become obvious that if nursing care were concerned just with physiologic factors and prevention of complications, expansive data collection and processing would not be necessary. These factors, however, are only one segment of comprehensive nursing care. Furthermore, physiologic nursing care generally is standardized. It would be difficult to individualize the technic of taking an electrocardiogram (ECG) or of monitoring the electrical impulse of the heart in a coronary-care unit; however, it is possible and desirable to individualize how the client is prepared for the procedure.

In processing data, remember that predominant elements of a system change. Figure 5–1 shows the foci of Mr. Munson's system in the coronary-care unit. These change in response to his recovery and movement to different environments. Progressive examples are shown in Figures 5–2 and 5–3. It should be remembered, however, that the figures are only examples

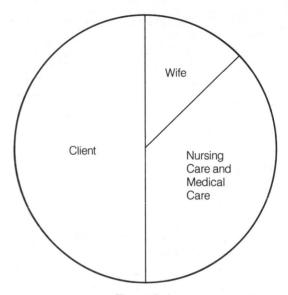

Figure 5–1

Foci of a Client's System While in a Coronary-Care Unit

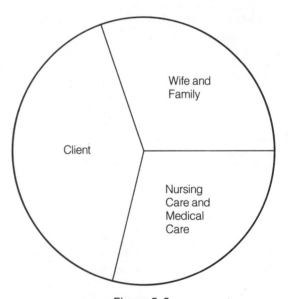

Figure 5–2

Foci of a Client's System While in an Intermediate-Care Setting

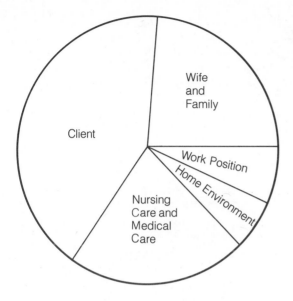

Figure 5-3

Foci of a Client's System While
in an Ambulatory-Care Setting

that are used to portray the concept of change through levels of care. The pies can be sliced differently in response to the needs of individual clients.

It should be pointed out that the quantity of medical care decreases as physical illness abates. Nursing care also can decrease as the client's home environmental factors come into play and the client requires less professional help. During the ambulatory phase, the client's work position and responsibilities also must be considered. Just as the system changes, so does the purpose. This point is cogently expressed by Hornstein, a social psychologist, who says:

> Purposive behavior varies with circumstance; it is not a consistent, robot-like reaction that is unmindful of changing conditions. Warnings are purposive if they are made *only* when another animal is endangered and they stop when the other is safe. In short,

the act's beginning and end must be determined by the other's condition of distress. (1976, p. 72)

A METHOD OF DATA PROCESSING

Once data are collected, one must write or list the information in any usable framework for oneself and others who may need access to it. One method is to divide the data into five categories: physiologic factors, psychologic factors, sociologic factors, the medical regimen, and laboratory reports. Referring back to the case presented (Boxes 5–1 and 5–2), the following data will be used to clarify the technique of data processing (see Box 5–3). Data processing will be done on those data collected during the beginning of the client's hospitalization.

Box 5-3

DATA BASE

Physiologic Data

1. Male, 52 years old

2. Admitted with chest pain; nonrecurrent

3. Admitted through emergency room

4. Low, substernal pain without radiation on admission

5. Pain was described as "dull" with "a feeling of fullness"

6. History of intermittent dyspnea with stress

7. No respiratory distress noted

8. Normal color; circulation appears normal

9. Warm, dry skin

10. Denies nausea or dizziness

11. Controlled, mild diabetes for five years

12. Takes Dymelor at home, 500 mg QD

Box 5–3 (continued)

13. History of smoking 2 to 3 packs of cigarettes a day for 23 years

14. Quit smoking three months prior to admission

15. States he follows a haphazard diet at home

16. Seems muscular and robust, but states he tires easily

17. Height: 6'0"; weight: 200 lbs

18. Underwent a cholecystectomy 12 years prior to admission

19. Oldest brother has diabetes

20. States his appetite is usually good, even with the diabetic diet

21. Prefers to eat 9–2–7; hospital serves 8–12–5

Psychologic Data

22. He is on the cardiac monitor

23. CCU standing order places all patients on "danger list"

24. Vital signs are all within normal limits; no PVCs

25. Desires definite diagnosis; MI currently not confirmed

26. Wife appears to be extremely concerned, nervous, and protective

27. Left school after completing eighth grade because of father's death

28. At 15 years of age, sought employment in order to support family

29. Has worked full time since he was 15

30. Father died suddenly; cause is unknown to client

31. Mother died at a young age, following what the client calls a "thyroid problem"

32. Appears anxious concerning hospitalization

33. Sleeps well at home on one pillow with the exception of the last month

Box 5–3 (continued)

prior to hospitalization, when he noted mild chest pain during the night and occasionally used two pillows

34. Verbalizes his desire to be at home with his family; they are separated only rarely

35. Seems to be outgoing, pleasant; has a good sense of humor

36. Seems to be sensitive to the feelings of others, especially his family

37. Appears to be extremely independent and questioning

38. Maintains neat appearance

39. Demonstrates good hygiene; insists on caring for self

40. Questions why he is in the coronary unit

41. Seems to have limited understanding about diabetes, or possibly does not want to be concerned with it since he states he has no problems

42. Dislikes the food served and the times it is served; occasionally refuses to eat

43. Does not seem to like being in a private room; wanders out to visit other patients often; occasionally sits at nurse's station

44. States that he dislikes being inactive

Sociologic Data

45. One previous hospitalization for gall bladder surgery

46. Unaware of purpose of coronary-care unit or why he is in it

47. Married for 30 years; wife works as dietary aid in hospital

48. Three children: two sons and one daughter

49. Elder son and daughter are married; one son in college

Box 5-3 (continued)

50. Avid sportsman: likes sailing, water skiing, scuba diving, and tennis

51. Captain of bowling league, which meets twice a week

52. Plays golf frequently

53. Takes flying lessons; expects to be licensed in about one year

54. Is a karate instructor; holds a black belt

55. Drinks alcohol rarely and only socially

56. Works as a foreman at Smith & Wesson in quality control

57. Believes that his job is secure

58. Visiting hours are restricted to ten minutes every hour

Medical Regimen

59. Defibrillate for ventricular fibrillation, PRN

60. Lidocaine 50 mg IV, for PVCs greater than 6/min or coupling

61. Atropine 0.5 mg IV for sinus bradycardia below 40/min or less than 60/min associated with B/P less than 80 systolic

62. O^2 PRN (via nasal cannula) at 4 liters/min

63. Record intake and output; OOB with commode privileges

64. Vital signs as per CCU routine

65. On 2000 calorie diabetic diet: 3 eggs per week; no added salt; no coffee, tea, soda; may have decaffeinated coffee

66. MS 2 mg IV for chest pain

67. Peripheral IV, keep vein open, D_5W Lidocaine 2 Gm 500 D_5W at 2 mg/min × 24 hours then DC

68. Colace 100 mg QD

69. Urine for clinitest and acetone-AC and HS

Box 5-3 (continued)

70. Dalmane 30 mg PO QHS PRN

71. Valium 5 mg PO QID

72. S/A urine coverage (with regular insulin-U-100)

    4+ = 10 units
    3+ = 5 units
    2+ or 1+ = no insulin

73. Daily FBS and 3 pm blood sugar

74. ECGs QD

75. Cardiac enzymes Q8h × 3 then QD until normal

76. Electrolyte Profile QD

77. Baseline CBC and clotting studies

Laboratory Reports

78. Negative chest x-ray

79. CBC: within normal limits

80. Electrolytes: within normal limits

81. Admission urine analysis: 4+ sugar and small amount of acetone

82. FBS 286 on 7/1

83. Cholesterol 270 on 7/1

84. Cardiac enzymes on 7/1: within normal limits

85. FBS 220 on 7/2

86. Cardiac enzymes on 7/2: within normal limits

87. Blood sugar and cholesterol levels are elevated

88. ECG changes consistent with subendocardial ischemia; 6/30

89. ECG: comparison shows continued STT wave changes in inferolateral leads consistent with ischemia; 7/1

90. ECG: shows continued STT wave changes over the inferolateral leads consistent with subendocardial ischemia; 7/2

One method of integrating these client data with the areas of nursing responsibility is to number each datum and then look at each nursing responsibility in terms of the applicable data (see Table 5-1). Place the number associated with each piece of pertinent datum alongside each area and then summarize these data. In this way, data are categorized and organized for easy reference, and areas of overlap can be seen. You may locate possible problem areas by referring to the number of a potentially troublesome bit of information and by determining under which area(s) of responsibility this number occurs.

This process can be equated with a computer system. The input is client/system data, the program and memory bank correspond to areas of nursing responsibility, and the output involves the integration of data and responsibility, yielding conclusions or nursing diagnoses.

With the results of data processing, the nurse has a profile of the individual client broken down according to the areas of nursing responsibility, thus facilitating the development of nursing diagnoses and subsequent orders that are based on the uniqueness of the client. Chapter 6 will use these data in the next step of the nursing process. It should be noted, however, that experience in using the presented data-processing technique will enable one to use the format with greater ease. It may become unnecessary, for example, to write out this process in the lengthy detail described. In initial steps of learning, however, the author believes that detail while learning the process is necessary so that subsequent shortcuts can provide the same comprehensive, individualized care.

Table **5-1**   Data Processing in the Case Study

Areas of Nursing Responsibility	Applicable Data	Data Summary
Comfort	2, 4, 5, 6, 7, 16, 21, 22, 32, 33, 37, 44	Admitted with low, substernal, nonrecurrent chest pain; pain described as "dull" with "a feeling of fullness"; history of intermittent dyspnea when stressed; no respiratory distress evident; muscular, robust, but tires easily; eats at 9-2-7—hospital serves at 8-12-5; on cardiac monitor; appears anxious concerning hospitalization; sleeps well at home with one pillow but last month noted mild chest pain during night and occasionally used two pillows; seems independent and questioning; dislikes inactivity
Nutrition	11, 12, 15, 17, 18, 20, 21, 32, 41, 42, 55, 63, 65, 68, 69, 72, 73, 81, 82, 83, 87	Controlled, mild diabetes for five years; takes Dymelor at home, 500 mg QD; follows haphazard diet at home; weighs 200 lbs and is 6'0"; underwent cholecystectomy 12 years prior to admission; appetite is usually good, even with diabetic diet; prefers to eat 9-2-7—hospital serves 8-12-5; appears anxious concerning hospitalization; seems to have limited understanding of diabetes—possibly does not want to be concerned with it, since he states he has no problems; dislikes food served and times it is served—occasionally refuses to eat; drinks alcohol rarely—only socially; record intake, output; OOB with commode privileges; on 2000 caloric diabetic diet—3 eggs per week, no added salt, no coffee, tea, soda, may have decaffeinated coffee; Colace 100 mg QD; urines for clinitest and

Table **5-1**   (continued)

Areas of Nursing Responsibility	Applicable Data	Data Summary
		acetone-AC and HS; S/A urine coverage (with regular insulin-U-100)—4+ = 10 units, 3+ = 5 units; 2+ or 1+ = no insulin; daily FBS and 3 pm blood sugar; admission urine analysis—4+ sugar and small amount of acetone; FBS 286 on 7/1; cholesterol 270 on 7/1; blood sugar and cholesterol levels elevated
Exercise	1, 2, 4, 5, 6, 7, 8, 9, 10, 11, 16, 17, 21, 23, 24, 32, 35, 36, 37, 43, 44, 50, 51, 52, 53, 54, 63, 71, 88, 89, 90	Male, 52 years old; admitted with chest pain, nonrecurrent; low, substernal pain without radiation on admission; pain described as "dull" with "a feeling of fullness"; history of intermittent dyspnea with stress; no respiratory distress noted; normal color—circulation appears normal; warm, dry skin; denies nausea or dizziness; controlled, mild diabetes for five years; seems muscular and robust, but states he tires easily; weighs 200 lbs and is 6'0"; prefers to eat 9-2-7—hospital serves 8-12-5; CCU standing order places all patients on "danger list"; vital signs all within normal limits; no PVCs; appears anxious concerning hospitalization; seems outgoing, pleasant; has good sense of humor; seems sensitive to the feelings of others, especially family; appears extremely independent and questioning; does not like being in private room; wanders out to visit other patients often; occasionally sits at nurse's station; states that he dislikes being inactive; avid sportsman—sailing, water skiing, scuba diving, and tennis; captain of bowling league, meets twice a week; plays golf frequently; takes flying lessons—expects to be licensed in about one year; is karate instructor—holds black belt; record intake, output; OOB with commode privileges; Valium 5 mg PO QID; ECG changes consistent with subendocardial ischemia—6/30; ECG comparison shows continued STT wave changes in inferolateral leads consistent with ischemia—7/1; ECG shows continued STT wave changes over inferolateral leads consistent with subendocardial ischemia—7/2
Personal hygiene	1, 22, 37, 38, 39, 63, 72, 74, 81	Male, 52 years old; on cardiac monitor; appears extremely independent and questioning; maintains neat appearance; demonstrates good hygiene; insists on caring for self; record intake, output; OOB with commode privileges; S/A urine coverage (with regular insulin-U-100)—4+ = 10 units, 3+ = 5 units, 2+ or 1+ = no insulin; ECGs QD; admission urine analysis—4+ sugar and small amount of acetone
Sleep, rest patterns	1, 16, 32, 33, 43, 58, 64, 70, 71	Male, 52 years old; seems muscular and robust, but states he tires easily; appears anxious concerning hospitalization; sleeps well at home on one pillow with exception of last month prior to hospitalization, when he noted mild

Table **5-1**   (continued)

Areas of Nursing Responsibility	Applicable Data	Data Summary
		chest pain during night and occasionally used two pillows; does not seem to like being in private room; wanders out to visit other patients often; occasionally sits at nurse's station; visiting hours restricted to ten minutes every hour; vital signs as per CCU routine; Dalmane 30 mg PO QHS PRN; Valium 5 mg PO QID
Diversional activity	1, 2, 6, 7, 8, 9, 16, 22, 26, 27, 28, 29, 32, 34, 35, 36, 37, 40, 43, 44, 46, 50, 51, 52, 53, 54, 63, 64, 88, 89, 90	Male, 52 years old; admitted with chest pain, nonrecurrent; history of intermittent dyspnea with stress; no respiratory distress noted; normal color—circulation appears normal; warm, dry skin; seems muscular and robust, but states he tires easily; on cardiac monitor; wife appears extremely concerned, nervous, and protective; left school after eighth grade because of father's death; at 15, sought employment in order to support family; has worked full time since 15; appears anxious concerning hospitalization; verbalizes desire to be at home with family since they are separated only rarely; seems outgoing, pleasant; has good sense of humor; seems sensitive to feelings of others, especially family; appears extremely independent and questioning; questions why he is in coronary-care unit; does not seem to like being in private room; wanders out to visit other patients often; occasionally sits at nurse's station; states that he dislikes being inactive; unaware of purpose of coronary-care unit or why he is in it; avid sportsman—sailing, water skiing, scuba diving, and tennis; captain of bowling league which meets twice a week; plays golf frequently; takes flying lessons—expects to be licensed in about one year; karate instructor—holds black belt; record intake, output; OOB with commode privileges; vital signs as per CCU routine; ECG changes consistent with sub-endocardial ischemia—6/30; ECG comparison shows continued STT wave changes in inferolateral leads consistent with ischemia—7/1; ECG shows continued STT wave changes over the inferolateral leads consistent with subendocardial ischemia—7/2
Socializing and privacy	1, 16, 22, 32, 34, 35, 36, 43, 44, 50, 51, 52, 53, 54, 58, 71	Male, 52 years old; seems muscular and robust, but states he tires easily; on cardiac monitor; appears anxious concerning hospitalization; verbalizes desire to be home with family since they are separated only rarely; seems outgoing, pleasant; has good sense of humor; seems sensitive to feelings of others, especially family; does not seem to like being in private room; wanders out to visit other patients often; occasionally sits at nurse's station; states that he dislikes being inactive; avid sportsman—sailing, water skiing, scuba diving, and tennis; captain of bowling league which meets twice a week; plays golf frequently; takes flying lessons—expects to be licensed in about one

Table **5-1**   (continued)

Areas of Nursing Responsibility	Applicable Data	Data Summary
		year; karate instructor—holds black belt; visiting hours restricted to ten minutes every hour; Valium 5 mg PO QID
Elimination	11, 12, 15, 20, 37, 39, 42, 63, 65, 67, 68, 72, 81, 88, 89, 90	Controlled, mild diabetes for five years; takes Dymelor at home, 500 mg QD; follows haphazard diet at home; states his appetite is usually good, even with diabetic diet; appears extremely independent and questioning; demonstrates good hygiene; insists on caring for self; dislikes food served and times it is served; occasionally refuses to eat; record intake, output; OOB with commode privileges; on 2000 calorie diabetic diet—3 eggs per week, no added salt, no coffee, tea, soda, may have decaffeinated coffee; peripheral IV, keep vein open, D_5W—Lidocaine 2 Gm 500 D_5W at 2 mg/minute × 24 hours then DC; Colace 100 mg QD; S/A urine coverage (with regular insulin-U-100)—4+ = 10 units, 3+ = 5 units, 2+ or 1+ = no insulin; admission urine analysis—4+ sugar and small amount of acetone; ECG changes consistent with subendocardial ischemia 6/30, confirmed on 7/1 and 7/2
Safety	10, 17, 37, 39, 40, 43, 44, 46, 71	Denies nausea or dizziness; weighs 200 lbs and is 6'0"; appears extremely independent and questioning; demonstrates good hygiene; insists on caring for self; questions why he is in coronary unit; does not seem to like being in private room; wanders out to visit other patients often; occasionally sits at nurse's station; states that he dislikes being inactive; unaware of purpose of coronary-care unit or why he is in it; Valium 5 mg PO QID
Environmental considerations	3, 21, 22, 23, 34, 35, 37, 40, 42, 43, 44, 45, 63	Admitted through emergency room; prefers to eat 9-2-7—hospital serves 8-12-5; on cardiac monitor; CCU standing order places all patients on "danger list"; verbalizes desire to be at home with family since they are separated only rarely; seems outgoing, pleasant; has good sense of humor; appears extremely independent and questioning; questions why he is in coronary-care unit; dislikes food served and times it is served—occasionally refuses to eat; does not seem to like being in a private room; wanders out to visit other patients often; occasionally sits at nurse's station; states that he dislikes being inactive; one previous hospitalization for gall bladder surgery; record intake, output; OOB with commode privileges
Teaching	1, 6, 13, 14, 15, 16, 25, 26, 27, 28, 33, 35, 36, 37, 38, 39, 40, 41, 42, 44, 46, 50, 51, 52, 53, 54, 55, 65, 69, 71, 87	Male, 52 years old; history of intermittent dyspnea with stress; history of smoking 2 to 3 packs of cigarettes a day for 23 years; quit smoking three months prior to admission; states he follows haphazard diet at home; seems muscular and robust, but states he tires easily; desires definite diagnosis—MI currently not confirmed; wife appears extremely concerned, nervous, and protective; left school

Table **5-1**   (continued)

Areas of Nursing Responsibility	Applicable Data	Data Summary
		after completing eighth grade because of father's death; at 15, sought employment in order to support family; sleeps well at home on one pillow with exception of last month prior to hospitalization, when he noted mild chest pain during night and occasionally used two pillows; seems outgoing, pleasant; has good sense of humor; seems sensitive to feelings of others, especially family; appears extremely independent and questioning; maintains neat appearance; demonstrates good hygiene; insists on caring for self; questions why he is in coronary unit; seems to have limited understanding of diabetes or possibly does not want to be concerned with it since he states he has no problems; dislikes food served and times it is served—occasionally refuses to eat; states that he dislikes being inactive; unaware of purpose of coronary-care unit or why he is in it; avid sportsman—sailing, water skiing, scuba diving, and tennis; captain of bowling league which meets twice a week; plays golf frequently; takes flying lessons—expects to be licensed in about one year; karate instructor—holds black belt; drinks alcohol rarely and only socially; on 2000 calorie diabetic diet—3 eggs per week, no added salt, no coffee, tea, soda, may have decaffeinated coffee; urines for clinitest and acetone-AC and HS; Valium 5 mg PO QID; blood sugar and cholesterol levels elevated
Spiritual comfort and/or assistance	26, 34, 36, 37, 43	Wife appears extremely concerned, nervous, and protective; verbalizes desire to be home with family since they are separated only rarely; seems sensitive to feelings of others, especially family; appears extremely independent and questioning; does not seem to like being in private room; wanders out to visit other patients often; occasionally sits at nurse's station
Prevention of complications	2, 3, 4, 5, 6, 7, 8, 9, 10, 11, 12, 14, 15, 16, 22, 25, 32, 37, 40, 42, 44, 50, 51, 52, 53, 54, 55, and all data in the medical regimen and laboratory reports (see Box 5-3)	Admitted with chest pain, nonrecurrent; admitted through emergency room; low, substernal pain without radiation on admission; pain described as "dull" with "a feeling of fullness"; history of intermittent dyspnea with stress; no respiratory distress noted; normal color—circulation appears normal; warm, dry skin; denies nausea or dizziness; controlled, mild diabetes for five years; takes Dymelor at home, 500 mg QD; quit smoking three months prior to admission; states he follows haphazard diet at home; seems muscular and robust, but states he tires easily; on cardiac monitor; desires definite diagnosis—MI currently not confirmed; appears anxious concerning hospitalization; appears extremely independent and ques-

Table **5-1** (continued)

Areas of Nursing Responsibility	Applicable Data	Data Summary
		tioning; questions why he is in coronary unit; dislikes food served and times it is served—occasionally refuses to eat; states that he dislikes being inactive; avid sportsman—sailing, water skiing, scuba diving, and tennis; captain of bowling league which meets twice a week; plays golf frequently; takes flying lessons—expects to be licensed in about one year; karate instructor—holds black belt; drinks alcohol rarely and only socially; refer to all data in medical regimen and laboratory reports (see Box 5-3)
Assurance of physiologic status—health maintenance and promotion	6, 11, 12, 14, 15, 16, 17, 20, 25, 26, 29, 32, 33, 34, 41, 44, 47, 50, 51, 52, 53, 54, 55, 56, 57, 65, 67, 68, 69, 72, 73, 74, 75, 76, 77, 88, 89, 90	History of intermittent dyspnea with stress; controlled, mild diabetes for five years; takes Dymelor at home, 500 mg QD; quit smoking three months prior to admission; states he follows haphazard diet at home; seems muscular and robust, but states he tires easily; weighs 200 lbs and is 6'0"; states his appetite is usually good, even with diabetic diet; desires definite diagnosis—MI currently not confirmed; wife appears extremely concerned, nervous, and protective; has worked full time since he was 15; appears anxious concerning hospitalization; sleeps well at home on one pillow with exception of last month prior to hospitalization, when he noted mild chest pain during night and occasionally used two pillows; verbalizes desire to be home with family since they are separated only rarely; seems to have limited understanding of diabetes or possibly does not want to be concerned with it, since he states he has no problems; states he dislikes being inactive; married 30 years; wife works as dietary aid in hospital; avid sportsman—sailing, water skiing, scuba diving, and tennis; captain of bowling league which meets twice a week; plays golf frequently; takes flying lessons—expects to be licensed in about one year; karate instructor—holds black belt; drinks alcohol rarely and only socially; works as foreman at Smith & Wesson in quality control; believes that job is secure; on 2000 calorie diabetic diet—3 eggs per week, no added salt, no coffee, tea, soda, may have decaffeinated coffee; peripheral IV, keep vein open, D_5W—Lidocaine 2 Gm 500 D_5W at 2 mg/min × 24 hours then DC; Colace 100 mg QD; urines for clinitest and acetone-AC and HS; S/A urine coverage (with regular insulin-U-100)—4+ = 10 units, 3+ = 5 units, 2+ or 1+ = no insulin; daily FBS and 3 pm blood sugar; ECGs QD; cardiac enzymes Q8h × 3 then QD until normal; Electrolyte Profile QD; baseline CBC and clotting studies; ECG changes consistent with subendocardial ischemia—6/30, confirmed on 7/1 and 7/2

Table **5-1**   (continued)

Areas of Nursing Responsibility	Applicable Data	Data Summary
Emotional support, counseling	2, 3, 4, 5, 6, 7, 15, 22, 23, 24, 25, 26, 27, 29, 31, 32, 34, 35, 36, 37, 40, 41, 42, 43, 44, 46, 47, 48, 49, 57, 58, 71	Admitted with chest pain, nonrecurrent; admitted through emergency room; low, substernal pain without radiation on admission; pain described as "dull" with "a feeling of fullness"; history of intermittent dyspnea with stress; no respiratory distress noted; states he follows a haphazard diet at home; on cardiac monitor; CCU standing order places all patients on "danger list"; vital signs are all within normal limits—no PVCs; desires definite diagnosis—MI currently not confirmed; wife appears extremely concerned, nervous, and protective; left school after completing eighth grade because of father's death; has worked full time since he was 15; mother died at young age following what client calls "thyroid problem"; appears anxious concerning hospitalization; verbalizes desire to be home with family since they are separated only rarely; seems outgoing, pleasant; has good sense of humor; seems sensitive to feelings of others, especially family; appears extremely independent and questioning; questions why he is in coronary unit; seems to have limited understanding of diabetes or possibly does not want to be concerned with it, since he states he has no problems; dislikes food served and times it is served—occasionally refuses to eat; does not seem to like being in private room; wanders out to visit other patients often; occasionally sits at nurse's station; states that he dislikes being inactive; unaware of purpose of coronary-care unit or why he is in it; married 30 years; wife works as dietary aid in hospital; three children—two sons, one daughter; elder son and daughter married, one son in college; believes that his job is secure; visiting hours restricted to ten minutes every hour; Valium 5 mg PO QID

SUMMARY

This chapter discussed the data-processing segment of nursing. It was presented as a bridge connecting rote nursing responsibilities with individualized client considerations. A case example was used to illustrate the concept and will be followed through the later steps of the nursing process.

Chapter 6 discusses the nursing diagnoses emerging from data processing. Each diagnosis will be arranged into a priority format.

REFERENCES

Bower, F. (1982). *The process of planning nursing care* (3rd ed.). St. Louis: Mosby.

Gordon, M. (1982). *Nursing diagnosis: Process and application*. New York: McGraw-Hill.

Hall, L. (1964). Nursing: What is it? *The Canadian Nurse, 60*, 150–154.

Harrison, C. (1966). Deliberative nursing process versus automatic nurse action—The care of a chronically ill man. *Nursing Clinics of North America, 1*, 387–397.

Henderson, F. (1966). *The nature of nursing.* New York: Macmillan.

Hornstein, H. (1976). *Cruelty and kindness.* Englewood Cliffs, NJ: Prentice-Hall.

Lewis, E. (1968). This I believe . . . about the nursing process—Key to care. *Nursing Outlook, 16,* 26–29.

Marriner, A. (1983). *The nursing process: A scientific approach to nursing care* (3rd ed.). St. Louis: Mosby.

National Council of State Boards of Nursing. (1982). *Test Plan for the National Council Licensure Examination for Registered Nurses.* Chicago: Author.

Nightingale, F. (1969). *Notes on nursing: What it is and what it is not.* New York: Dover. (Original work published 1860).

Simms, L., & Lindberg, J. (1978). *The nurse person: Developing perspectives for contemporary nursing.* New York: Harper and Row.

Sundeen, S., Stuart, G., Rankin, E., & Cohen, S. (1981). *Nurse-client interaction: Implementing the nursing process* (2nd ed.). St. Louis: Mosby.

Watson, J. (1979). *Nursing: The philosophy and science of caring.* Boston: Little, Brown.

SELECTED READING

The classic selected reading for this chapter follows a case example through the nursing process to show individualized nursing care in action. It focuses on the uniqueness of the client and on ways in which the nurse respects such individuality in planning care. Data processing as developed in this chapter provides a framework for beginning practitioners to accomplish the same personalization of nursing-care plans. Since the case in the selected reading is more complex than the one used as an example in this chapter, it should be used as a review by the more advanced learner.

Deliberative Nursing Process versus Automatic Nurse Action— The Care of a Chronically Ill Man

Cherie Harrison, M.A.

A PROBLEM PATIENT

Mr. C. was first observed by the present writer sitting up in bed, leaning forward slightly, breathing forcefully and rapidly through his mouth. He was very thin, unshaven, slightly cyanotic, and he talked with difficulty. He stated that he had been nauseated earlier and that he could not shake a "sick feeling"; he had been unable to eat or to get out of bed to use the Bennett machine. He declined my offer to bring the Bennett machine to his bedside by stating that the machine would not help him feel better. He used his hand nebulizer twice during the interview. The patient's apprehension and despair were evident in his manner, and he stated, "No use fooling myself, it's the way it is."

Mr. C., a patient in a large metropolitan general hospital, was considered by the ward staff as an "uncooperative patient." Conversations with the ward personnel revealed that the two staff physicians viewed him as a "typical emphysema personality" with "neurotic dependency patterns" who was "not motivated to conscientiously cooperate with the prescribed treatment." The doctor who was directly responsible for Mr. C.'s medical care stated that the patient would have to be hospitalized for the rest of his life since he required "constant medical supervision." The head nurse felt that "Mr. C. just doesn't want to do anything for himself and wants to be left alone."

Reprinted with permission from *Nursing Clinics of North America*, 1966, Vol. 1, No. 3, pp. 387-397.

She had recently moved him into a room with another emphysematous patient in an attempt to gain Mr. C.'s cooperation in his medical regimen. The nurses' notes reflect Mr. C.'s behavior at this time: "——[patient] does not use Bennett machine full amount of time ——. [He is] refusing aminophylline suppositories for dyspnea as he views this [medication] as causing stomach distress and substernal pain." The chart further revealed that Mr. C. required "nerve pills" (Compazine and placebos) for "tension" and Darvon capsules for chest pain several times each night. Groceries and cigarettes were found in his bedside table.

Mr. C., 56 years old, had lived and worked in a city most of his life. He had never married; he left school after the eighth grade to support his parents until their death. He had lived with his sister since 1961. Mr. C. was a member of the Episcopal Church and had been an active member of Alcoholics Anonymous since 1948 (the ward staff did not know that Mr. C. belonged to A.A.). Until three years ago he had smoked approximately three packs of cigarettes a day. He had a steady employment record; he worked in the engineering department of a large medical center from 1937 to 1961.

The patient had been hospitalized nine times at the medical center where he worked. In 1940 he was diagnosed as suffering from chronic bronchitis. He developed asthma and was hospitalized for pneumonia in 1944. In 1957 chest x-rays revealed diffuse bullous emphysema. The increased dyspnea forced Mr. C. to retire from his work in 1961. The Personnel

Clinic provided the patient with a Bennett intermittent positive pressure breathing machine and a hand-bulb nebulizer for home use. Later that same year he was digitalized with Digoxin; this medication had been continued to date. It was necessary for Mr. C. to be hospitalized twice during 1963. The last admission to the medical center was in January, 1964, for breathing difficulties and somnolence. Early in 1964, Mr. C. was transferred from the medical center to the present hospital for chronic care of pulmonary emphysema with cor pulmonale.

On admission to this hospital, Mr. C. was 5 feet 10 inches tall and weighed 103 pounds. He had lost 65 pounds over the last three years. The progress note stated that on admission Mr. C. was "very apprehensive, frightened, exhausted, depressed." In January, April, and again in August, Mr. C. required treatment in the Drinker respirator in the intensive care unit for impending CO_2 narcosis. In September, 1964, Mr. C. was transferred to a convalescent ward, where this investigation took place.

PATHOPHYSIOLOGY OF EMPHYSEMA

Emphysema is a disease known to result in the impairment of pulmonary ventilation and in resulting disturbance of gas exchange.[5] Its development in most instances is characterized by a repetitive history of bronchial and pneumonic infections. These inflammatory processes result in the gradual and irreversible destruction of the small bronchioles, pulmonary blood vessels, and alveoli, and in a consequent loss of lung elasticity. The loss of lung elasticity significantly interferes with the mechanics of breathing.

In Mr. C.'s case alveolar ventilation, the amount of gas exhaled from the surface of the lung that takes part in gas exchange, was decreased greatly. Because of a loss in elasticity, there is an ever increasing accumulation of residual air in the lungs. The intrapleural pressure becomes less negative and during expiration the patient must expend great effort to force the air from his chest. The diaphragm, most important in maintaining normal negative intrapleural pressure, is pushed downward and works inefficiently. The rib cage becomes fixed in the inspirational pattern and expiration is chronically embarrassed.[5,9]

Elwood[4] states that there are three distinguishing features of this disability: marked arterial hypoxia, hypercapnea, and chronic cor pulmonale with recurring episodes of right heart failure. Mr. C. suffered from all three complications. Hypoxia, the depressed intake of oxygen into the alveoli, was evidenced by the decreased O_2 saturation level in arterial blood of 80 to 84% (normal 97%). Hypercapnea, the excess amount of carbon dioxide in body fluids, was seen in the elevated pCO_2 of the arterial blood of 54 to 58 mm. Hg (normal 40). The hypercapnea results in respiratory difficulties in the tissue cells and causes varying degrees of respiratory acidosis. Mr. C.'s compensated respiratory acidosis was reflected by the blood pH of 7.35 to 7.45 (normal 7.4).

In chronic cor pulmonale the heart is subjected to a greater effort by the necessity to pump blood through a restricted vascular pulmonary bed. This increase of work by the heart causes right ventricular heart failure with hypertrophy of the ventricle and hypertension in the pulmonary artery.[4,5,9] Mr. C.'s electrocardiograms had indicated sinus arrhythmia but not right ventricular hypertrophy.

The chronic hypoxia causes polycythemia to develop because in the presence of an arterial O_2 saturation of less than 80%, more red blood cells are produced. This compensating mechanism has physiological limitations and the resulting polycythemia becomes a disease secondary to pulmonary emphysema. This condition increases the viscosity of the blood, not only adding to the burden of the right ventricle but decreasing the renal blood flow rate.[5,9] Phlebotomies were performed on Mr. C. at the beginning of the study to decrease the blood viscosity; his hematocrit stayed within normal range following the phlebotomies.

The hypoxia, the hypercapnea, and the kidney compensating mechanism present a paradox in treatment. Treatment of the hypoxia with conventional oxygen therapy increases the severity of the hypercapnea by removing the lack of O_2 as the stimulus to the respiratory center, and increasing CO_2 retention. The rising pCO_2 level is accompanied by a proportionate rise in sodium bicarbonate, i.e., the kidney compensating mechanism. However, the compensating sodium ion reabsorption by the kidney tubules, with subsequent fluid retention, adds a burden to the heart in patients with cor pulmonale.[2,4] Diuretics were given daily to the patient to regulate this compensatory kidney mechanism by medical means to prevent acid-base imbalance, pulmonary edema, and heart failure.

When the compensating kidney mechanism fails, CO_2 narcosis threatens. This is a common cause of death in these patients and it is important that it be recognized at the onset. The patient begins to get drowsy and shows some mental vagueness; he has a slight cyanosis at rest. As the CO_2 retention increases he becomes sleepier, more confused, and more deeply cyanotic. One sign may be twitching of the fingers at rest which disappears on movement. Intermittent positive pressure breathing must be carefully supervised when early signs of impending CO_2 narcosis are present.[4]

I became aware that Mr. C. did not use the I.P.P.B. machine correctly. When Mr.C. demonstrated how he used the machine, it was obvious that he did not expire the compressed room air properly. He stated, "after six or seven minutes I become sleepy and sometimes fall asleep." Upon further investigation the surprisingly limited knowledge and understanding he had of his disease, except in the area of prognosis, became apparent.

Mr. C.'s complications (chronic cor pulmonale with mild episodes of right heart failure, chronic compensated respiratory acidosis, chronic arterial hypoxia, and hypercapnea) have required close medical supervision and intervention. Four primary medical objectives were identified: (1) To facilitate more effective breathing by decreasing the bronchiolar obstruction using bronchodilators, expectorants, and the Bennett intermittent positive pressure breathing machine in order to decrease arterial hypoxia and hypercapnea. (2) To maintain electrolyte and fluid balance by medication and diet in order to prevent CO_2 narcosis. (3) To decrease the burden of the right ventricle by medication, phlebotomies, and the previous two objectives. (4) To keep the patient hospitalized for the rest of his life in order to provide close medical supervision and "symptomatic relief."

THE DELIBERATIVE NURSING PROCESS

It is my firm belief that a patient must work through his problems in his own way. The patient should be supported by an environment that allows him to do this: an environment that provides the skills, the knowledge, and the assistance the patient requires in solving his individual problems. The problems of the patient and the challenges involved were the central reason for further investigation of Mr. C. and his needs. The problem-solving process was used in an effort to help Mr. C. cope more effectively with the difficulties which beset him and to assist him in strengthening his resources and his problem-solving capacities.

Basic to this problem-solving process was the establishment of a working relationship between Mr. C. and myself. This was effectively accomplished by using Orlando's[8] deliberative nursing process. Orlando presented a conceptual framework from which a nursing care model might evolve. The basic concept underlying her theoretical model involves the "nursing situation" which is comprised of three elements: the patient's behavior, the responses of the nurse, and the nursing action. The interaction of these three elements, when in action and moving through time and space, is the "nursing process." The nursing process is based on the nurse's knowledge (principles that underlie health, environment, and people). This knowledge allows the nurse to attach specific meanings to her observations of the patient's behavior and to plan for the nursing action needed. Orlando believes that nursing action offers whatever the patient may require in order for his needs to be met.

Specific steps in this deliberative nursing process are: (1) The nurse observes the patient's behavior and explores with him its meaning. She pursues the subject until she knows the meaning of the patient's behavior and the specific activity that is required to meet his need(s). (2) The nursing action is carried out in such a way that the patient is helped to inform the nurse as to how the action affects him (an element of basic trust is involved). (3) The nurse follows through on her action to see if the need was relieved. The meaning of the behavior and the nurse action is reevaluated until the need is met and the nurse's purpose in having helped the patient is achieved. (4) The nurse is available to respond to the patient's need and she conveys this to him. (5) The nurse knows how the nursing process affects the patient.

If the nursing process is carried out without exploration for the patient's need or consideration of how the process affects the patient, it constitutes what Orlando calls an "automatic process of activity." Automatic nurse action is usually ineffective in meeting the patient's need except in an emergency situation. This type of "situational" need may be defined as a requirement of the patient which (if and when supplied) diminishes his immediate distress or improves his immediate sense of well-being.

Employing the deliberative process the nurse proceeds to fulfill her independent role as a professional, as described by McManus.[7] Via the problem-solving approach she identifies the nursing problem of the patient and makes a nursing diagnosis. She further determines the objectives of nursing for the patient and his capacity for self-direction, and decides on a course of action. An individual program of nursing care is thus developed, incorporating psychological support and guidance as needed.

The nurse then sees to it that the nursing care program is carried out, either by herself when the patient's need dictates this, or by other members of the health team. She gives continuous direction and supervision of those who assist her, and evaluates and modifies the plan of nursing care as needed. She coordinates the nursing care program with the services of the medical and allied professional practitioners.

ILLUSTRATION OF THE PROBLEM-SOLVING APPROACH USING THE DELIBERATIVE NURSING PROCESS AS A GUIDE TO ACTION

Nursing objectives for Mr. C. were formulated at the beginning of the investigation; deliberate activity toward these objectives was initiated during weekly contacts with him for nine weeks. An evaluation of the nursing process used in meeting Mr. C.'s needs was continually validated by the patient's reactions and behavior.

Nursing Diagnosis

Mr. C.'s behavior suggested that he was depressed, anxious, unaccepting of assistance offered, and that he was not employing any spiritual, social, or intellectual resources. He had little knowledge or understanding of his disease entity except in the area of prognosis. His functional level was inconsistent with his physiological capabilities.

Nursing Objectives

Three primary objectives were identified: (1) To apply the deliberative nursing process with Mr. C. in order to assist him in changing this negative behavior to more positive interdependent behavior; to validate with Mr. C. his needs and his response to the nursing action, and to assist him in maintaining his capabilities, inner strengths, and interest in living. (2) To provide the acceptance, reality-support, and assistance required to help Mr. C. work through his problems with alveolar hypoventilation, thereby enhancing his participation in maintaining the maximum ventilation possible. (3) To support and assist the patient with the designated medical care, teaching the patient the scientific facts about his disability (within the limits of his understanding) and the reasons for the medical measures used.

Examples of Nursing Therapy

1. Problem Identified   The ward staff felt Mr. C. was "uncooperative." His need was to promote the development of productive interpersonal relationships.[1]

Approach used. The concept of Orlando's deliberative nursing process was used to ascertain and validate with Mr. C. his needs and problems.

NEED

- To be dealt with as an individual rather than a case, type, or category

- To express feelings, both negative and positive

- To be accepted as a person of worth, regardless of dependency, weakness, faults, or failures

- Understanding of and response to feelings expressed

- To be neither judged nor condemned for the difficulty in which he finds himself

- To make his own choice concerning his life

- To keep confidential information about himself as secret as possible

Evaluation of approach. The patient responded to the deliberative nursing process and began to participate actively in his medical regimen. With the aid of the Bennett machine, he was able to

Reason for approach. "Ineffective patient behavior is used to mean any behavior which prevents the nurse from carrying out her concern for the patient's care or from maintaining a satisfactory relationship to the patient. . . . The nurse must view it as a possible signal of distress or a manifestation of an unmet need."[8] Hildegard Peplau states, "The purpose of nursing has never been merely to help cure. Rather, it has been to offer a warmly human relationship through which people could develop and use their assets and external resources toward the solution of their health problems. The mission of nursing must continue to be creative interpersonal relationships through which patients will achieve self-actualization."[11]

Seven psychosocial needs that are directly related to therapeutic relationships with patients were identified by Biestek[3]:

PRINCIPLE

- Treatment as an individual

- Purposeful expression of feelings

- Acceptance as he is, not as you would want him to be

- Controlled emotional involvement of the nurse, relating to the patient's needs only

- Nonjudgmental attitude

- Patient self-determination; the environment provides the reality

- Confidentiality

get out of bed more often and do things for himself. He began to feel better, to be concerned about other patients near him, and to take an interest in his personal appearance. "I've felt well enough to go in and see Mr. W. next door; he is getting breathing exercises with me and does them better."

2. Problems Identified   Three related problems were: alveolar hypoventilation, moderate to severe dyspnea, and drowsiness when using the Bennett machine. His need was "to facilitate the maintenance of a supply of oxygen to all body cells."[1]

Approach used. I explored with Mr. C. why the I.P.P.B. machine and hand nebulizer were not helping him breathe better and why he was refusing the aminophylline suppositories.

Reason for approach. I could not understand why the Bennett machine was not assisting him in improving his ventilation. Slow, forced expiration should have improved his vital capacity and lowered the residual capacity, which should have improved the ventilation to the lung tissue. Aminophylline suppositories act chiefly on the smooth muscle of the bronchi, decreasing the hypertonicity.

Evaluation of approach. The patient was not expiring properly when using the Bennett machine and was exhibiting symptoms of CO_2 narcosis. Explanation of the physiological reasons for this and instructions on how to expire more adequately helped Mr. C. breathe out slowly and forcibly. He practiced forced expiration with and without using the Bennett machine. I taught Mr. C. to exhale forcibly before using the hand nebulizer so that the medication would be inhaled deeply into the bronchial tree.

The patient improved his technique in using the Bennett and began to use it at the prescribed times. Drowsiness did not recur and some relief of dyspnea was maintained, especially at rest. Mr. C. asked the doctor if breathing exercises might help him and these were ordered. He conscientiously tried to learn the breathing exercises, taught to him by a physical therapist, but was limited in abdominal inspirational breathing and tried too hard to establish the abdominal breathing rhythm.

It was suggested to the patient that he use the breathing exercises and the hand nebulizer for relief of his dyspnea so that he would not become entirely dependent on the Bennett machine. Mr. C. refused aminophylline suppositories because he felt they caused his "stomach distress"; but after an explanation of the bronchial action of the medication, he started using them to assist in breathing.

3. Problem Identified   Mr. C.'s fatigue threshold was low; therefore, he had a decreased capacity for activities. His need was "to promote optimal activity; exercise, rest and sleep."[1]

Approach used. The doctor ordered assistance in dressing activities and instructions in cane walking. These activities were begun cautiously, with progressive increase in activity level as pulmonary ventilation improved.

Reason for approach. Mr. C.'s hematocrit was within normal limits and the potential for thrombus formation did not seem to be a factor. Caution against overstepping his fatigue threshold was stressed because activity may cause an increase in metabolic lactates and increased acidosis. Hypercapnea greatly affects metabolic activity and oxidating processes within the cells, thereby causing a low fatigue threshold and a limit on the patient's activity. Activities therefore were limited to what Mr. C. felt he was capable of doing. We worked together on increasing his activities progressively, stopping when he became tired or more dyspneic.

Evaluation of approach. At times Mr. C. walked in his room holding onto a wheel chair. He was able to dress himself but he tired easily and became dyspneic when he used his arms above shoulder height. He continued to become fatigued while attempting to eat or ambulate, but felt that he had improved since starting the breathing exercises and since using the Bennett machine. During our last visit, he stated that he could sit up longer each day and that he was sleeping better without any need for his "nerve pills."

4. Problem Identified   Mr. C. appeared distressed, apprehensive, and complained of "nervous tension," "jitters," and chest pain (burning pain under the sternal notch). His need was for information and support to enable him to identify and accept his illness emotionally.

Approach used. The deliberative nursing process: The questions that he asked were answered and he was supported during the times he explored his illness emotionally. He was not reprimanded when he did not follow the medical regimen, e.g., when he was observed smoking.

Reason for approach. "Conquest of anxiety implies the acceptance of reality, the acceptance of divinity in ourselves . . . . Knowledge alone is not enough, for with knowledge alone we cannot vanquish anxiety. . . . We must strengthen our confidence in life."[10] Improving the nurse-patient relationship and the patient's ventilation should reduce his restlessness and apprehension. Mr. C. suffered burning chest pain each night for months. The pain was sometimes relieved by Darvon, a synthetic non-narcotic analgesic. The patient requested "nerve pills" several times each night, and placebo capsules were given to replace the Compazine that had been given for months previous to this study.

Evaluation of approach. Mr. C. stopped asking for "nerve pills" after the deliberative process was begun. He began to decrease his requests for medication whereas previously he had required several p.r.n. medications, especially during the night. He spoke at length about himself and his family and of the three years after his discharge from the service. He could not "settle down" and he drank too much. Mr. C. cried during this part of the interview. He related how active he had been in A.A. "It became my life, and I miss working with those guys." He said that the doctor had caught him smoking the other day; "I was so sure I could give it up when they told me to, especially after being able to give up drinking. . . . Maybe tomorrow I can resist smoking that cig when I wake up." During our last interview Mr. C. stated that he had not smoked a cigarette in five days. "Mr. Y. and Mrs. W. [patients] have the same problem and I am trying to help them."

Near the end of the interview Mr. C. thanked the writer for coming to see him every week: "You know, I would rather know what's wrong than to have someone shoot the bull with me."

Outcome

Although all of the nursing care objectives were not achieved, Mr. C.'s behavior did change from negative dependence to a more positive interdependent approach to therapy and activities of living in general. Of course this behavior change, whether real or apparent, will be fully evidenced only by time, for as Orlando[8] warns: "The improvement is always relative to what the nurse and patient start with, to the length of their contact and to what they are able to accomplish."

CONCLUSIONS

Patients and nurses do not always communicate with one another. Sometimes the patient may not be able to communicate effectively and his nonverbal behavior may be the only clue to his plea for help. The behavior becomes meaningful to the nurse if she is aware of the interactions between herself and the patient. We need to look at our communications, verbal and nonverbal, and ascertain how effective they are.

Automatic nurse action tends to stereotype a patient or place him in a fixed category. All emphysematous patients are not alike, any more than any of us are alike; stereotyping is a poor foundation for an effective nurse-patient relationship.

The deliberative nursing process stems from a theoretical model that seems to lend itself to a consistent, meaningful, and productive relationship with the individual patient. When the patient and his family are active participants in the planned program of care the basic purpose of nursing is more likely to be achieved and the planned care is successful: the nurse helps the patient meet his need(s). Inherent in the deliberative nursing process is the problem-solving approach which guides the nursing process.

A vital component of the problem-solving approach is the nurse's *acceptance of the patient as he is* when he enters the hospital. Many times we expect the patient to behave at or progress to a level which he never has achieved and is incapable of achieving. The nurse should consider the patient's resources (his personality, his family, and his community) and then keep in mind that he achieves his self-actualization level from these resources; they are the foundation upon which realistic individual planning for patient care can be achieved. The deliberative nursing process provides for effective nursing care because the nursing care goals are in harmony with the patient's goals, his capabilities, and his resources.

REFERENCES

1. Abdellah, F. G., et al. *Patient-Centered Approaches to Nursing.* New York, The Macmillan Co., 1960, p. 16.

2. *Basic Respiratory Physiology Taken from Standard Texts.* Bird Institute Lecture Series, Publication No. 9262. Palm Springs, California.

3. Biestek, F. P. *The Casework Relationship.* Chicago, Loyola University Press, 1957.

4. Elwood, E. *The Battle of Breathlessness. Nursing Care of the Disoriented Patient.* Monograph No. 13. New York, American Nurses' Association, 1962, pp. 5–15.

5. Guyton, A. C. *Textbook of Medical Physiology.* 3rd Ed. Philadelphia, W. B. Saunders Co., 1966.

6. Haas, A., and Luczak, A. *The Application of Physical Medicine and Rehabilitation to Emphysema Patients.* Monograph No. 21. New York, Institute of Physical Medicine and Rehabilitation, 1963.

7. McManus, R. L. Nurses want a chance to be professional. *Modern Hospital,* 64:89, October, 1958.

8. Orlando, I. J. *The Dynamic Nurse-Patient Relationship.* New York, G. P. Putnam's Sons, 1961.

9. Peplau, H. E. Automation: Will It Change Nurses, Nursing, or Both? *Technical Innovations in Health Care: Nursing Implications.* Monograph No. 5. New York, American Nurses' Association, 1962, p. 37.

10. Sodeman, W. A. *Pathologic Physiology.* Philadelphia, W. B. Saunders Co., 1956.

11. Steiner, H., and Gebser, J. *Anxiety: A Condition of Modern Man.* New York, Dell Publishing Co., Inc., 1962, pp. 11, 105.

Chapter 6

Nursing Diagnosis

After collecting data and processing information according to the areas of responsibility of nurses, it becomes necessary to make a decision—*a nursing diagnosis*—on the actual or potential health problems with which the client needs the nurse's assistance. Once made, the diagnoses must be ranked in priority according to the health status of the client within a given time, space, and recovery framework.

Bower (1982) stated that, as a client, one is free to make decisions about oneself and to be involved in one's own care. This coincides with the writings of May (1961), an existential psychologist who emphasized the dimensions of will, decision, and choice in one's life. Therefore, the nurse must recognize the client as an important contributor to decision making.

This chapter will discuss the cognitive dimensions of establishing a nursing diagnosis and the importance of responding to priorities. The case presented in Chapter 5 will then be used to demonstrate establishing diagnoses and setting priorities.

Referring back to the equation stated earlier, it can be seen readily that the nursing-care plan consisting of nursing diagnoses and orders results from a combination of various types of input: client data, system data, responsibilities, knowledge, and, of course, the nurse.

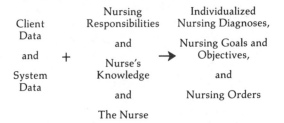

The third segment of the equation is the decision segment and is highly dependent on the first two parts. For strong, individualized nursing decisions to be made, sufficient data and knowledge are necessary.

Nursing literature is replete with discussions and definitions of the nursing diagnosis, so only a brief synthesis of these will be provided. McCain (1965) was early in stating that symptoms are grouped together and named. Rothberg (1967, p. 1040) defined the nursing diagnosis as "an evaluation by nurses of those factors affecting the patient which will influence his recovery." Thomas and Coombs (1966, p. 52) noted that it is a "statement of a conclusion resulting from a recognition of a pattern derived from a nursing investigation of the patient." They included two aspects: the process of diagnosis and the decision.

The nursing diagnosis also is viewed as a conclusive statement concerning an individual's nursing needs, based on scientific determination (Aspinall, Jambruno, & Phoenix, 1977; Komorita, 1963; Price, 1980) and incorporating every known and surmised factor within an individual that can have an effect on his dignity, rights, well-being, recovery, and pursuit of a meaningful lifestyle. It provides the basis for nursing orders (Yura & Walsh, 1983). Webster defined diagnosis as an investigation of the facts to determine the nature and cause of a condition, situation, or problem and the resultant decision based on such an examination.

Because nursing terms are not standardized, it is necessary to further mention the diversity in nursing language as it relates to the diagnostic function in nursing. There is controversy over the use of the term *nursing orders* versus *nursing approaches,* and many terms are used synonymously for *nursing diagnosis,* such as *patient problems, nursing problems, patient needs, nursing goals, the diagnostic process,* and so forth (Andruskiw & Battick, 1964; Blair, 1971; Price, 1980; Woods, 1966). The term *diagnosis* carries connotations that make it unacceptable to those who assume that only physicians can diagnose. However, the terminology used should not be a paramount issue as long as intent is clear, and *diagnosis* does convey professional accountability for a nurse's decisions. As far back as 1961, Abdellah emphasized establishing a nursing diagnosis as an independent function of the nurse.

Clear, simple, and specific statements should characterize nursing diagnoses. They should articulate succinctly an identified problem in the client's system. Furthermore, they should address problems and needs of the client and of all significant parts of the identified system. Problems include those factors considered potential problems as well as actual ones (Mayers, 1983).

The conceptual definition of the nursing diagnosis used in this and subsequent analyses in this book was presented first by Gordon (1976, p. 1299):

> Nursing diagnoses, or clinical diagnoses made by professional nurses, describe actual or potential health problems which nurses by virtue of their education and experience are capable and licensed to treat.

A problem exists when the client's actions in a specific area of nursing responsibility have not reached the level the nurse has established as optimal for that client. Figure 6-1 illustrates this point. A nursing diagnosis, then, is a *client problem* that needs to be solved—the actual condition that requires change. A statement of

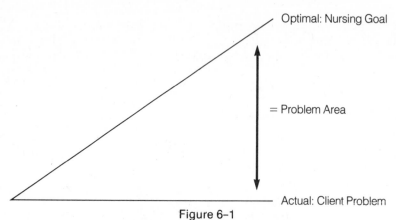

Optimal: Nursing Goal

= Problem Area

Actual: Client Problem

Figure 6–1
Problem of Disparity Between
Nursing Goals and Client Actions

the optimal condition is a *nursing goal.* Therefore, the problem (diagnosis) and the goal are two ends of the same continuum of desired change.

There has been tremendous energy devoted by our colleagues to developing a systematic classification of nursing diagnoses that represents the entire domain of nursing (Bircher, 1975; Campbell, 1978; Carpenito, 1983; Gebbie & Lavin, 1974; Gordon, 1982; Kim, McFarland, & McLane, 1984; Kim & Moritz, 1982; Roy, 1975). Roy (1975) underscored the need for such a classification to (a) organize the most relevant events nurses observe, (b) label phenomena so that prescribed actions are closely related to those data on which therapeutic judgments are made, and (c) further develop nursing science. To date, Carpenito (1983) and Kim, McFarland and McLane (1984) have reported on the list of approved nursing diagnoses that were accepted at the Fifth National Conference for Classification of Nursing Diagnoses by the group called the North American Nursing Diagnosis Association. Carpenito (1983) and Kim, McFarland, and McLane (1984) also provide the definition, etiology, and defining characteristics for each diagnosis. The following list contains these diagnoses.

NURSING DIAGNOSES ACCEPTED AT THE FIFTH NATIONAL CONFERENCE*

Activity intolerance

Airway clearance, ineffective

Anxiety

Bowel elimination, alterations in: Constipation
    Related to change in lifestyle
    Related to immobility
    Related to painful defecation

Bowel elimination, alterations in: Diarrhea
    Related to untoward side-effects

Bowel elimination, alterations in: Incontinence

Breathing patterns, ineffective
    Related to hyperpnea or hyperventilation

Cardiac output, alterations in: Decreased

Comfort, alterations in:
    Acute pain
    Chronic pain
    Pain in children

*SOURCE: *Classification of Nursing Diagnoses: Proceedings of the Fifth National Conference,* by M. J. Kim, G. McFarland, and A. McLane (Eds.). St. Louis: C. V. Mosby, 1984. Also published in Carpenito, L. *Nursing Diagnosis: Application to Clinical Practice.* Philadelphia: J. B. Lippincott, 1983. Specifications following the words "related to" are from Carpenito (1983).

Communication, impaired verbal
    Related to impaired ability to speak words
    Related to aphasia
    Related to foreign language barriers

Coping, ineffective individual
    Related to depression in response to
        identifiable stressors

Coping, ineffective family: Compromised

Coping, ineffective family: Disabling

Coping, family: Potential for growth

Diversional activity deficit
    Related to monotony of confinement
    Related to post-retirement inactivity
        (change in lifestyle)

Family processes, alterations in
    Related to an ill family member

Fear *(specify)*

Fluid volume deficit, actual

Fluid volume deficit, potential

Fluid volume excess
    Edema

Gas exchange, impaired
    Related to chronic tissue hypoxia

Grieving, anticipatory

Grieving, dysfunctional

Health maintenance, alterations in

Home maintenance management, impaired

Injury, potential for *(specify)*
    Poisoning
    Suffocation
    Trauma

Knowledge deficit *(specify)*

Mobility, impaired physical
    Related to alterations in lower limbs
    Related to alterations in upper limbs

Noncompliance *(specify)*
    Related to anxiety
    Related to negative side-effects of
        prescribed treatment

    Related to unsatisfactory relationship with
        caregiving environment or caregivers

Nutrition, alterations in:
    Less than body requirements
        Related to chewing or swallowing
            difficulties
        Related to anorexia
        Related to difficulty or inability
            to procure food

Nutrition, alterations in:
    More than body requirements
        Related to imbalance of intake vs.
            activity expenditures

Nutrition, alterations in:
    Potential for more than body requirements

Oral mucous membrane, alterations in
    Related to inadequate oral hygiene
    Related to stomatitis

Parenting, alterations in: Actual

Parenting, alterations in: Potential

Powerlessness
    Related to hospitalization

Rape trauma syndrome

Self-care deficit: Total
    Feeding
    Bathing/hygiene
    Dressing/grooming
    Toileting

Self-concept, disturbance in
    Sensory-perceptual alterations:
        Visual
        Auditory
        Kinesthetic
        Gustatory
        Tactile
        Olfactory

Sexual dysfunction
    Related to impotence
    Related to ineffective coping
    Related to lack of knowledge
    Related to change or loss of body part
    Related to physiological limitations

Skin integrity, impairment of: Actual

Skin integrity, impairment of: Potential

Sleep pattern disturbance

Social isolation

Spiritual distress
    Related to inability to practice
        spiritual rituals
    Related to conflict between religious or
        spiritual beliefs and prescribed
        health regimen

Thought processes, alterations in
    Related to inability to evaluate reality

Tissue perfusion, alteration in
    Cerebral
    Cardiopulmonary
    Renal
    Gastrointestinal
    Peripheral

Urinary elimination, alterations in patterns of
    Related to enuresis (maturational)
    Related to dysuria
    Related to incontinence

Violence, potential for
    Related to sensory-perceptual alterations
    Related to inability to control behavior

An inductive procedure is used to pinpoint a nursing diagnosis, and this procedure follows the equation at the beginning of this chapter. The information known about the client's system, the nursing responsibilities, knowledge, and the nurse is essential in writing individualized nursing orders, implementing nursing care, and evaluating nursing care. A deductive procedure is therefore employed after a nursing diagnosis has been established. Figure 6-2 is a diagram for these procedures.

Approved nursing diagnoses lend unity and clarification to nursing practice and scientific development. More than the diagnosis, however, is required to give individualized care. Mundinger and Jauron (1975) suggested that contributing factors must be identified in a

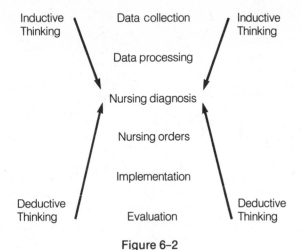

Figure 6-2

Deductive and Inductive Thinking in The Nursing Process (SOURCE: Adapted from *Nursing Leadership and Management: An Experiential Approach*, by E. L. La Monica. Copyright © 1983 by Wadsworth, Inc. Reprinted by permission of the publisher, Wadsworth Health Sciences Division, Monterey, California.)

two-part diagnosis, for example, "anxiety relating to impending hysterectomy." Approved nursing diagnoses do not currently exist for the plethora of phenomena nurses observe. The approved nursing diagnoses that do exist are just beginning to be understood and be used by practicing nurses. Since the process of arriving at a diagnosis is essential in order to plan and give comprehensive and individualized care, this chapter, by means of a case example, will examine the procedure of specifying a nursing diagnosis, identifying the approved nursing diagnosis wherever possible, stating the nursing goal(s) and objectives, and arranging them in order of priority.

The cognitive aspects of establishing nursing diagnoses have been discussed. Prior to continuing the case analysis begun in Chapter 5, the conceptual basis for recognizing and responding to diagnoses as priorities is presented.

CONCEPTUAL FRAMEWORK FOR ESTABLISHING DIAGNOSTIC PRIORITIES

The conceptual framework used in helping the nurse to arrange nursing diagnoses into priorities was developed by Abraham Maslow. He discussed a hierarchy into which classifications of human needs can be ordered (Maslow, 1970), as shown in Figure 6–3. In order of priority, these needs are: physiologic, safety, social, esteem, and self-actualization. The needs are vital parts of the client's system.

According to Maslow, the physiologic needs (shown at the bottom of the pyramid) are top priority when unsatisfied and remain as having the highest priority until satisfied. Once the physiologic needs become less important or are not threatened, safety needs take priority. This format follows through to self-actualization, which is a priority only when the other four areas in a person's need system are gratified. Hersey and Blanchard (1982)* diagram this movement as shown in Figure 6-4.

To understand Maslow's hierarchy of needs within a nursing framework more fully, a discussion of each need will follow.

Maslow's Hierarchy of Needs

Physiologic Needs. The physiologic needs are those that are basic to life: air, water, food, clothing, and shelter. According to Chapman and Chapman's advocacy helping model (1975), needs in this area of Maslow's hierarchy fall into two dimensions: lifesaving (prevention of imminent death) and life-sustaining (health maintenance and prevention of complications following bodily insult). At this level technologic input is high, and social/emotional support and client participation is low.

---

*Hersey and Blanchard write for a leadership perspective. Applications to nursing are this author's.

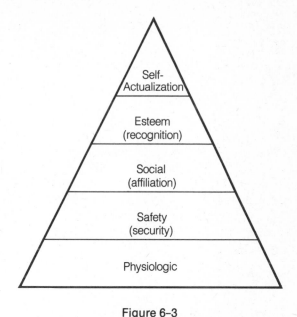

Figure 6–3

Maslow's Hierarchy of Needs (SOURCE: *Motivation and Personality*, 2nd Ed., by Abraham H. Maslow. Copyright © 1970 by Abraham H. Maslow. Reprinted by permission of Harper & Row Publishers, Inc.)

Sufficient operation of the body is a foremost priority. Until threat to life is removed, these needs are paramount (Hersey & Blanchard, 1982). It follows, therefore, that when a client is in physiologic crisis and must be monitored constantly, security needs—such as socio-economic issues—are not in priority; that is, when a client's life is in imminent danger, the client is not concerned about a possible change in work position because of the disease. When physiologic needs have been satisfied, however, other levels of needs become important.

Safety (Security). This is the second level of Maslow's hierarchy. Hersey and Blanchard (1982) defined these needs as involved with self-preservation. Included are freedom from

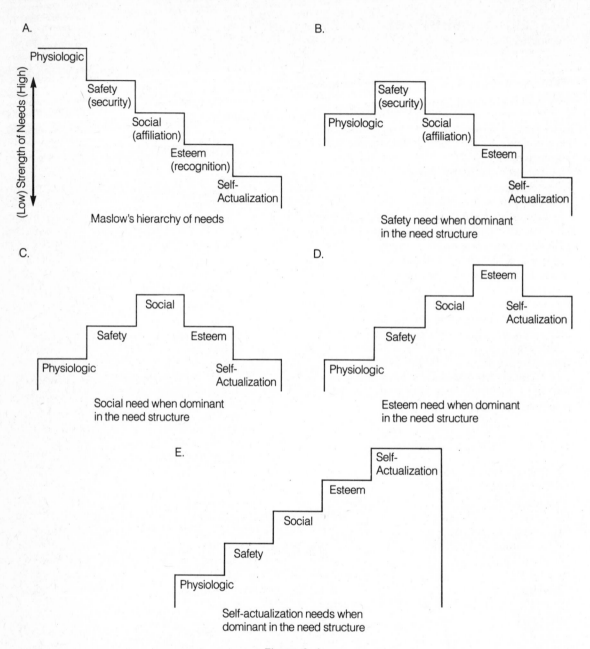

Figure 6–4

Movement of Maslow's Hierarchy of Needs

(SOURCE: *Management of Organizational Behavior: Utilizing Human Resources,* 4th Ed., by P. Hersey and K. H. Blanchard, pp. 27–29. Copyright © 1982 by Prentice-Hall, Inc., Englewood Cliffs, N.J. Reprinted by permission. Based on Maslow, 1970.)

physical danger and freedom from deprivation of basic physiologic needs. There is an awareness regarding one's own or one's family's safety and preservation. Hospital costs, medical fees, and job security are all examples of safety needs. Gellerman's (1978) research earmarked safety and security needs as appearing both overtly and covertly.

When basic life-threatening crises are past, safety needs emerge as priorities. Then, in order for a client to move to higher level needs, security needs must be somewhat satisfied.

Social (Affiliation).   Included in this need structure, cogently expressed by Hersey and Blanchard (1982), are meaningful interpersonal relationships, group acceptance, and belonging. When social needs are unsatisfied, a nurse may observe boredom in clients (Mayo, 1945), apathy, desire to have friends and family visit, and other signs. There may be expression of concern for other clients and employees in the environment. This is the movement from self to others. It parallels Chapman and Chapman's (1975) third dimension of their helping model, labeled "life-enhancing"—that is, one's relationship with the world.

Esteem.   When a client first seeks to belong, the positive values of belonging emerge as priorities and should be satisfied if a nurse desires the client to reach fullest potential. Instead of just feeling like a part of a system or group, the person who has esteem needs in focus will seek recognition and respect from others, prestige, and power. The client may want to be useful in some way, either by being personally involved in or by helping in another's case. For example, responsibility for helping a roommate may occur. It must be remembered that recognition involves another person. If one seeks esteem, this must be noticed and reinforced (Hersey & Blanchard, 1982). In other words, when a client tells you what she did to help herself or another, you should communicate to the client your awareness of the achievement.

Unfortunately, needs in this area are not always acted on in a positive framework (Hersey & Blanchard, 1982). The client, for example, who has a full leg cast and impaired mobility, yet consciously disobeys his order to stay in bed or call for help when using the bathroom facilities, may be exhibiting an unfulfilled esteem need. It becomes the nurse's responsibility to satisfy this need with measures that capitalize on the client's strengths. Once the need is satisfied by other means and in positive frameworks, maladaptive behavior will generally decrease.

Self-actualization.   This need structure is of the highest order, becoming prominent when all others are satisfied. It involves one's desire to reach fullest potential (Hersey & Blanchard, 1982). Moreover, this potential is founded on awareness of one's own strengths and weaknesses; it is reality based.

A nurse can perceive that clients are at this level when they strive to help themselves and their environment on their own—independently—yet, are dependent and interdependent according to their own direction, as is necessary.

Maslow's Hierarchy of Needs in Nursing Practice

Nurses must constantly strive to satisfy the needs of clients at the level implicitly and explicitly expressed by the person, and Maslow's structural framework provides a useful basis by which practitioners can determine priorities of client needs. This framework, however, should be considered only in response to the client's nursing diagnosis.

The levels of needs Maslow delineated should not be construed in nursing as absolute. They must be interpreted in light of the client's system and the nurse's goals. In other words, one can be predominantly at a social level regarding recovery, yet may in reality be at a self-actualizing level in the work position. Also, the levels of Maslow's hierarchy of needs must be visualized as overlapping when priorities are set.

Based on the areas of nursing responsibility delineated in Chapter 5, a general framework of use may be developed for these needs. Paralleling areas of nursing responsibility with Maslow's hierarchy can be a useful base in beginning to establish priorities of needs (see Table 6-1). The guidelines in Table 6-1 indicate where the need might emerge and also the progression through all levels of the hierarchy.

Thus far this chapter has discussed the cognitive dimensions of nursing diagnosis, in addition to Maslow's theory as the conceptual framework for determining priorities of diagnosed needs. The last portion of this chapter will use the case example begun in Chapter 5 to illustrate how to establish nursing diagnoses, as well as how to rank priorities.

CASE EXAMPLE ON NURSING DIAGNOSES AND PRIORITIES

Just as review, nursing diagnoses are decisive statements concerning a client's actual or potential health problem (Carpenito, 1983; Gordon, 1976; Kim, McFarland, & McLane, 1984); these should be framed by the uniqueness of the client. Nursing goals are statements of what the client needs to be assisted in achieving, given the nursing diagnoses; they are the optimal. Nursing diagnoses and goals should be arranged according to priorities.

One useful means for making diagnoses is to follow this formula:

The client needs _____

because _____

The first part of the formula becomes the statement of nursing goals. The latter part is the description of the actual situation from which the nursing diagnosis is deduced; this provides specific reasons behind an individual client's requirements. The rationale also becomes helpful in developing nursing orders (see Chapter 7).

It is possible to have more than one diagnosis from each area of responsibility. More-over, since there is overlap, it is important that the designer of nursing care gives comprehensive consideration to diagnosing, rather than worry about the proper place for diagnoses relative to the nurse's areas of responsibility. *The important goal is that all areas be considered.*

The specification of nursing diagnoses is illustrated in Table 6-2, based on the case of Mr. Munson, as begun in Chapter 5. (Refer back to Table 5-1 for the data summaries relative to each area of nursing responsibility.) According to this method, aspects of organizing the information needed to specify a nursing diagnosis include areas of nursing responsibility, a formula for stating the nursing goal (the client needs . . .) and its rationale (because . . .), and the resultant nursing diagnosis. Designating priorities and identifying approved nursing diagnoses will be discussed in the following paragraphs.

Once the nursing diagnoses are established, the next step is to apply Maslow's hierarchy to these diagnoses for Mr. Munson. Table 6-3 shows the nursing diagnoses, the goal(s) for each, and the type of need involved according to Maslow's theory.

After looking at the diagnoses in light of Maslow's hierarchy, the nurse decides which diagnoses are present-oriented and which diagnoses are future-oriented. Although it is possible for a diagnosis to be both present- and future-oriented, such a diagnosis is considered to be the former since it must be focused upon in the present. Indeed, nursing care should be progressive, beginning with what is absolutely essential to preserve life and continuing on thereafter to all other areas. The actions of putting the diagnoses into operation and of specifying nursing orders also reflect Maslow's need hierarchy. A diagnosis may be pertinent in a past framework, but its relevance may change with respect to the reality of here and now.

Table 6-4 divides the 18 diagnoses that have been specified into present-oriented and future-oriented diagnoses. It is underscored that physiologic and safety needs predominate in the present. As you study the diagnoses in totality, however, overlap can be observed.

Table **6-1**   Guidelines for Maslow's Hierarchy of Needs Paralleled with
Areas of Nursing Responsibility

Maslow's Hierarchy	Areas of Nursing Responsibility
Physiologic needs	nutrition sleep, rest patterns elimination prevention of complications assurance of physiologic status—health maintenance and promotion
Safety (security) needs	comfort exercise personal hygiene safety environmental considerations spiritual comfort and/or assistance emotional support, counseling teaching
Social (affiliation) needs	diversional activities socializing and privacy
Esteem (recognition) needs	an amplification of what has emerged before, but considering the client's need for achievement
Self-actualization needs	the client can take care of self—allow it

The next step of the procedure is to number the present-oriented diagnoses, moving from those needs that are absolutely essential to meet immediately (1) to those that can be put off for a while (11). There will be differences among practitioners in this area, but exact sequence is not an issue. Table 6-5 contains the priority list showing the nursing diagnoses arranged in order of priority; nursing goals also are stated.

This listing ranks the diagnoses in order of importance. You can see that there is more of a horizontal than a vertical priority among nursing diagnoses 1 through 7, as well as among 8 through 11. The client's needs should be met in this order. Also, future-oriented diagnoses must be kept in mind when designating orders, because they probably will emerge as priorities at a future point. It must be recognized, however, that there is a limit to what should be expected for accomplishment; it is impossible to encompass all needs, situations, and changes in one given time and space. Furthermore, it is stressful to overload a client or a nurse.

It is important to note that the nursing diagnoses resulting from data processing are not perceived specifically as pertinent only to the client in the case example; the essence of the diagnoses may be applicable to many clients. Yet, nursing goals are individualized. The process described ensures that you have knowledge of the individual client so that personalized care will be ordered and implemented as it relates to the diagnoses. By following the design in this chapter, the nurse should have at his or her fingertips the rationale for every action and the knowledge of what should be done to capitalize on the client's status and potential. Furthermore, the procedure for establishing nursing diagnoses has been reported to be successful in a variety of clinical practice areas and with patients in different stages of development in health and illness (Fredette & Gloriant, 1981; Gleit & Tatro, 1981; Gordon, Sweeney, & McKeehan, 1980; Leslie, 1981; Lunney, 1982).

Table **6-2** Specification of Nursing Diagnoses: Case Example

Areas of Nursing Responsibility	Nursing Goal	Rationale	Nursing Diagnosis
	Remember: This is a goal that the nurse wishes to achieve with the client.		*Remember: This should be a statement concerning the client's actual or potential health problem.*
Comfort	To continue to maintain his own personal comfort measures	He is not in any present distress; chest pain has not recurred and no respiratory distress is noted. Even though he is usually fairly active, it must be noted that he tires easily and has a history of intermittent dyspnea with stress. He sleeps with one to two pillows as he is comfortable. He is independent. It seems that he can care for this aspect himself.	Comfort: Self-maintenance*
Nutrition	To ingest balanced nutrients within a 2000 calorie diabetic diet	Client is not receiving proper nutrition; he does not like the food sent by the the kitchen and refuses meals since they are not in line with his usual eating patterns. This is contributing to a caloric deficit, and insulin regulation becomes difficult. At home he is controlled and has a good appetite. Neither behavior is evident in the hospital. Anxiety may be a causative factor in his lack of appetite. Teaching is needed, so the nutrition problem will be addressed in that section.	Nutrition, alterations in: Less than body requirements

Table **6-2**   (continued)

Areas of Nursing Responsibility	Nursing Goal	Rationale	Nursing Diagnosis
Exercise	To obtain knowledge of the disease process and its link with physical exercise To pace his physical activity schedule	He is a very active individual, engaging in many sports. Physically he looks muscular and robust, even though stating that he tires easily. With the presence of a possible MI, he may have to plan a more clearly paced schedule of physical activity and exercise. It is believed that he needs to become more receptive to changes through knowledge of his physical boundaries. When he accepts this—and because of his independent traits—he probably will be able to respond wisely to the exercise needs of his own body.	Knowledge deficit: MI and physical exercise
Hygiene	To be able to maintain his own hygienic measures	He is independent and seems totally capable of caring for himself. He can get OOB but, since he is on intake and output, he must be taught to chart himself. S/A coverage must be considered and care of monitor leads taught.	Hygiene: Self-maintenance*
Sleep, rest patterns	To be assured of adequate rest amid coronary-care procedures and environment	He tires easily and is anxious concerning hospitalization. At home he sleeps well with one or two pillows, whichever he desires. Monitoring of vital signs during the night is necessary. Medication for sleep is PRN, and he is on Valium for muscle relaxation, QID.	Sleep pattern disturbance

Table **6–2**   (continued)

Areas of Nursing Responsibility	Nursing Goal	Rationale	Nursing Diagnosis
Diversional activity	To select diversional activities in his present environment that reflect his likes and rest schedule	He is in the hospital because of a possible MI, even though no pain or respiratory difficulty is evident. Limited activity is important, with the diversion necessity. Tiring easily, he still seems to have difficulty accepting restrictions. He is anxious, wants a definite answer to his medical diagnosis, wants to go home, and enjoys visiting with other patients. His dislike of inactivity pervades all. Exercise as diversional activity was previously discussed in the Exercise area.	Diversional activity deficit related to monotony of confinement
Socializing and privacy	To have his needs for recognition, affiliation, and privacy met and maintained, as possible	He seems to be socially active and a leader in outside groups. Not being able to participate in a bowling competition—especially since he is captain of the team—makes him feel guilty. He maintains his independence but likes to talk with other patients. Commode privileges should be handled with finesse.	Self-concept, disturbance in: Self-esteem
Elimination	To continue to privately maintain elimination needs and report any signs of constipation	He is independent and able to care for himself. Urine must be tested for insulin coverage and, even though no bowel constipation is evident, the nurse must be alert for any dysfunction attributable to the nature of disease process.	Bowel and bladder elimination: Self-maintenance*

Table **6-2** (continued)

Areas of Nursing Responsibility	Nursing Goal	Rationale	Nursing Diagnosis
Safety	To plan and secure his own safety	He is an above-average-sized man who seems totally capable of ensuring his own safety. Since he is on Valium, he must be aware of its possible effects, even though no dizziness or nausea have been noted.	Knowledge deficit: Effects of drugs and therapeutic regimen
Environmental considerations	To adjust to the environmental limitations by understanding the rationale for the policies in existence	Setting is a coronary-care unit. He is on a monitor and has commode and OOB privileges. Visiting hours imposed by the hospital make the client unhappy since he feels excluded from his family and close friends. He wants to be with them for a longer period of time. Also, a dislike for being in a private room is obvious.	Knowledge deficit: Environment
Teaching	To accept and understand his diabetic condition	Despite the fact that the client seems to be an independent, responsible leader of others, he obviously has problems owning the diabetic process as part of himself. This is conclusive in his haphazard diet, in his high FBS and cholesterol readings, and in his statement that he has "no problems."	Coping, ineffective individual
	To plan and control his own balanced diet		Knowledge deficit: Nutrition for diabetes
	To regulate his own insulin needs		Knowledge deficit: Insulin administration
Spiritual comfort and/or assistance	To have a respectful and trusting relationship with the nurse so that needs can be discussed if they emerge as stressful	He seems to be sensitive and to be part of a close family structure. His need for spiritual support is not currently evident; however, the nurse must establish a close relationship in order to be available for guidance should	Anxiety

Table **6-2**   (continued)

Areas of Nursing Responsibility	Nursing Goal	Rationale	Nursing Diagnosis
		a need emerge in the client within this area. Having a possible MI is usually very frightening.	
Prevention of complications	To be free of signs and symptoms of cardiac complications	The client is in a critical period; the diagnosis of MI is not established. The nurse must be keenly alert for signs affirming the diagnosis. Also, recurrent MI symptoms can be lethal, and all fine discriminations pointing to that end must be observed, noted, and acted upon with haste. Awareness of arrhythmias evidenced on the cardiac monitor is especially important.	Cardiac output, alterations in: Decreased
Assurance of physiologic status—health maintenance and promotion	To understand his overall lifestyle and what is important to consider given his health status To establish a design for work, exercise, and the diabetic condition so that stressors are minimized and paced	He has diabetes and is extremely physically active. Being sensitive and bright, he constantly questions—verbally and nonverbally—and becomes anxious. As a foreman, he must look at his work responsibilities to ultimately design a pattern for his overall lifestyle that includes all activities, but with the activities evenly meshed and paced.	Knowledge deficit: Lifestyle alterations
	To have awareness of himself when stress mounts To control his own body-stress patterns		Coping, ineffective individual

Table **6-2**   (continued)

Areas of Nursing Responsibility	Nursing Goal	Rationale	Nursing Diagnosis
Emotional support, counseling	To have relief from the anxiety that pervades areas of the present situation and environment	He is pervasively anxious. He wants to control himself, and he must be aware of all that is going on regarding his care. Sometimes he hesitates to question, however, and the respectful, trusting, helping relationship diagnosed under spiritual needs comes into play here. *(Emotional support and counseling should be of concern in all the identified areas. Those aspects not covered, however, can be discussed here.)*	Anxiety

*Approved nursing diagnoses are not available for all the identified diagnoses; an asterisk next to the diagnosis denotes that it has not yet been approved.

SOURCE: *Classification of Nursing Diagnoses: Proceedings of the Fifth National Conference,* by M. J. Kim, G. McFarland, and A. McLane (Eds.). St. Louis: C. V. Mosby, 1984. Also published in Carpenito, L. *Nursing Diagnosis: Application to Clinical Practice.* Philadelphia: J. B. Lippincott, 1983.

Table **6-3**   Maslow's Hierarchy of Needs Applied to
Nursing Diagnoses and Nursing Goals: Case Example

Nursing Diagnosis	Nursing Goal	Type of Need
Comfort: Self-maintenance*	To continue to maintain his own personal comfort measures	Physiologic
Nutrition, alterations in: Less than body requirements	To ingest balanced nutrients within a 2000 calorie diabetic diet	Physiologic
Knowledge deficit: MI and physical exercise	To obtain knowledge of the process and its link with physical exercise	Safety
	To pace his physical activity schedule	
Hygiene: Self-maintenance*	To be able to maintain his own hygienic measures	Physiologic
Sleep pattern disturbance	To be assured of adequate rest amid coronary-care procedures and environment	Physiologic
Diversional activity deficit related to monotony of confinement	To select diversional activities in his present environment that reflect his likes and his rest schedule	Social
Self-concept, disturbance in: Self-esteem	To have his needs for recognition, affiliation, and privacy met and maintained, as possible	Esteem
Bowel and bladder elimination: Self-maintenance*	To continue to privately maintain elimination needs and report any signs of constipation	Physiologic
Knowledge deficit: Effects of drugs and therapeutic regimen	To plan and secure his own safety	Safety
Knowledge deficit: Environment	To adjust to the environmental limitations by understanding the rationale for the policies in existence	Safety/Social/Esteem
Coping, ineffective individual	To accept and understand his diabetic condition	Safety

Table **6-3** (continued)

Nursing Diagnosis	Nursing Goal	Type of Need
Knowledge deficit: Nutrition for diabetes	To plan and control his own balanced diet	Safety
Knowledge deficit: Insulin administration	To regulate his own insulin needs	Safety
Anxiety	To have a respectful and trusting relationship with the nurse so that needs can be discussed if they emerge as stressful	Social
Cardiac output, alterations in: Decreased	To be free of signs and symptoms of cardiac complications	Physiologic
Knowledge deficit: Lifestyle alterations	To understand his overall lifestyle and what is important to consider given his health status	All levels
	To establish a design for work, exercise, and the diabetic condition so that stressors are minimized and paced	
Coping, ineffective individual	To have awareness of himself when stress mounts	All levels
	To control his own body-stress patterns	
Anxiety	To have relief from the anxiety that pervades areas of the present situation and environment	All levels

*Approved nursing diagnoses are not available for all the identified diagnoses; an asterisk next to the diagnosis denotes that it has not yet been approved.

SOURCE: *Classification of Nursing Diagnoses: Proceedings of the Fifth National Conference,* by M. J. Kim, G. McFarland, and A. McLane (Eds.). St. Louis: C. V. Mosby, 1984. Also published in Carpenito, L. *Nursing Diagnosis: Application to Clinical Practice.* Philadelphia: J. B. Lippincott, 1983.

Table **6-4**   Present-Oriented and Future-Oriented
Nursing Diagnoses: Case Example

Present-Oriented Diagnoses	Future-Oriented Diagnoses
Comfort: Self-maintenance*	Knowledge deficit: MI and physical exercise
Nutrition, alterations in: Less than body requirements	Diversional activity deficit related to monotony of confinement
Hygiene: Self-maintenance*	Coping: Ineffective individual (diabetes)
Sleep pattern disturbance	Knowledge deficit: Nutrition for diabetes
Self-concept, disturbance in: Self-esteem	Knowledge deficit: Insulin administration
Bowel and bladder elimination: Self-maintenance*	Knowledge deficit: Lifestyle alterations
Knowledge deficit: Effects of drugs and therapeutic regimen	Coping, ineffective individual (body stress patterns)
Knowledge deficit: Environment	
Anxiety (nurse-patient relationship)	
Cardiac output, alterations in: Decreased	
Anxiety (environment)	

*Approved nursing diagnoses are not available for all the identified diagnoses; an asterisk next to the diagnosis denotes it has not yet been approved.

SOURCE: *Classification of Nursing Diagnoses: Proceedings of the Fifth National Conference,* by M. J. Kim, G. McFarland, and A. McLane (Eds.). St. Louis: C. V. Mosby, 1984. Also published in Carpenito, L. *Nursing Diagnosis: Application to Clinical Practice.* Philadelphia: J. B. Lippincott, 1983.

Table **6-5** Present-Oriented Nursing Diagnoses and Nursing Goals
Arranged According to Priorities: Case Example

Nursing Diagnosis (in order of priority, high to low)	Nursing Goal
1. Cardiac output, alterations in: Decreased	To be free of signs and symptoms of cardiac complications
2. Knowledge deficit: Effects of drugs and therapeutic regimen	To plan and secure his own safety
3. Bowel and bladder elimination: Self-maintenance*	To continue to privately maintain elimination needs and report any signs of constipation
4. Sleep pattern disturbance	To be assured of adequate rest amid coronary-care procedures and environment
5. Nutrition, alterations in: Less than body requirements	To ingest balanced nutrients within a 2000 calorie diabetic diet
6. Anxiety	To have a respectful and trusting relationship with the nurse so that needs can be discussed if they emerge as stressful
7. Anxiety	To have relief from the anxiety that pervades areas of the present situation and environment
8. Knowledge deficit: Environment	To adjust to the environmental limitations by understanding the rationale for the policies in existence
9. Hygiene: Self-maintenance*	To be able to maintain his own hygienic measures
10. Comfort: Self-maintenance*	To continue to maintain his own personal comfort measures
11. Self-concept, disturbance in: Self-esteem	To have his needs for recognition, affiliation, and privacy met and maintained, as possible

*Approved nursing diagnoses are not available for all the identified diagnoses; an asterisk next to the diagnosis denotes that it has not yet been approved.

SOURCE: *Classification of Nursing Diagnoses: Proceedings of the Fifth National Conference,* by M. J. Kim, G. McFarland, and A. McLane (Eds.). St. Louis: C. V. Mosby, 1984. Also published in Carpenito, L. *Nursing Diagnosis: Application to Clinical Practice.* Philadelphia: J. B. Lippincott, 1983.

SUMMARY

Chapter 6 has focused on nursing diagnoses, exploring the cognitive dimensions as well as a conceptual framework for establishing priorities. A case example constructed in Chapter 5 was used to exemplify these two processes.

The next chapter is concerned with writing nursing orders for each diagnosis. This is the planning step of the nursing process: designing a strategy to achieve goals. The content of Chapters 6 and 7, nursing diagnoses and nursing orders, generally makes up the nursing-care plan.

REFERENCES

Abdellah, F. (1961). *Meeting patient needs—an approach to teaching.* Paper presented at the biennial convention of the National League for Nursing. Cleveland, Ohio, April 10–14.

Andruskiw, O., & Battick, B. (1964). Identification of nursing problems. *Nursing Research, 13,* 75–78.

Aspinall, M. J., Jambruno, N., & Phoenix, B. (1977). The why and how of nursing diagnosis. *The American Journal of Maternal Child Nursing, 2,* 354–358.

Bircher, A. (1975). On the development and classification of diagnoses. *Nursing Forum, 14,* 10–29.

Blair, K. (1971). It's the patient's problem—and decision. *Nursing Outlook, 19,* 587–589.

Bower, F. (1982). *The process of planning nursing care* (3rd ed.). St. Louis: Mosby.

Campbell, C. (1978). *Nursing diagnosis and intervention in nursing practice.* New York: Wiley.

Carpenito, L. (1983). Nursing diagnosis: Application to clinical practice. Philadelphia: Lippincott.

Chapman, J., & Chapman, H. (1975). *Behavior and health care: A humanistic helping process.* St. Louis: Mosby.

Fredette, S., & Gloriant, F. (1981). Nursing diagnosis in cancer chemotherapy: In theory. *American Journal of Nursing, 81,* 2013–2022.

Gebbie, K., & Lavin, M. (1974). Classifying nursing diagnoses. *American Journal of Nursing, 74,* 250–253.

Gellerman, S. (1978). *Motivation and productivity.* New York: American Management Association.

Gleit, C., & Tatro, S. (1981). Nursing diagnoses for healthy individuals. *Nursing and Health Care, 11,* 456–457.

Gordon, M. (1976). Nursing diagnosis and the diagnostic process. *American Journal of Nursing, 76,* 1298–1300.

Gordon, M. (1982). *Nursing diagnosis: Process and application.* New York: McGraw-Hill.

Gordon, M., Sweeney, M. A., & McKeehan, K. (1980). Nursing diagnosis: Looking at its use in the clinical area. *American Journal of Nursing, 80,* 672–674.

Hersey, P., & Blanchard, K. (1982). *Management of organizational behavior: Utilizing human resources* (4th ed.). Englewood Cliffs, NJ: Prentice-Hall.

Kim, M. J., McFarland, G., & McLane, A. (Eds.). (1984). *Classification of nursing diagnoses: Proceedings of the fifth national conference.* St. Louis: Mosby.

Kim, M.J., & Moritz, D. (Eds.). (1982). *Classification of nursing diagnoses: Proceedings of the third and fourth national conferences.* New York: McGraw-Hill.

Komorita, N. (1963). Nursing diagnosis. *American Journal of Nursing, 63,* 83–86.

La Monica, E. (1983). *Nursing leadership and management: An experiential approach.* Monterey, CA: Wadsworth Health Sciences.

Leslie, F. (1981). Nursing diagnosis: Use in long-term care. *American Journal of Nursing, 81,* 1012–1014.

Lunney, M. (1982). Nursing diagnosis: Refining the system. *American Journal of Nursing, 82,* 456–459.

Maslow, A. (1970). *Motivation and personality* (2nd ed.). New York: Harper and Row.

May, R. (Ed.). (1961). *Existential psychology* (2nd ed.). New York: Random House.

Mayers, M. (1983). *A systematic approach to the nursing care plan* (3rd ed.). Norwalk, CT: Appleton-Century-Crofts.

Mayo, E. (1945). *The social problems of an industrial civilization.* Boston: Harvard Business School.

McCain, F. (1965). Nursing by assessment—not intuition. *American Journal of Nursing, 65,* 82–84.

Mundinger, M., & Jauron, G. (1975). Developing a nursing diagnosis. *Nursing Outlook, 23,* 94–98.

Price, M. (1980). Nursing diagnosis: Making a concept come alive. *American Journal of Nursing, 80,* 668–671.

Rothberg, J. (1967). Why nursing diagnosis? *American Journal of Nursing, 67,* 1040–1042.

Roy, Sr. C. (1975). A diagnostic classification system for nursing. *Nursing Outlook, 23,* 90–94.

Thomas, M., & Coombs, R. (1966). Nursing diagnosis: Process and decision. *Nursing Forum, 5,* 50–64.

Woods, N. (1966). Measuring a patient's need and progress. *Nursing Outlook, 14,* 38–41.

Yura, H., & Walsh, M. (1983). *The nursing process: Assessing, planning, implementing, evaluating* (4th ed.). Norwalk, CT: Appleton-Century-Crofts.

SELECTED READINGS

In the first of the two readings, Thomas and Coombs provide further discussion on the procedure for building a nursing diagnosis. They use an inductive approach to illustrate the thought processes used to arrive at the diagnosis. Rothberg, in the second article, gives a rationale for the need for nursing diagnoses in nursing practice. This is based on the diagnosis as a requisite for goal-directed care plans.

Nursing Diagnosis:
Process and Decision

Mary Durand Thomas, R.N., M.S.N.
Rosemary Prince Coombs, R.N., M.N.

The diagnostic process is not unique to any one occupation or profession. The medical history, the physical examination, and the laboratory tests which lead to the physician's diagnosis have been compared to the work of the police detective, who asks questions, examines clues, and submits material to a crime lab for the data he needs to identify a criminal accurately.[1] When a student is not achieving at the expected level, educators seek out the strengths and weaknesses of his performance so as to make an educational diagnosis.[2] A social worker gathers facts from the client and the client's family "to make as exact a definition as possible of the situation and personality of a human being in some social need."[3] In recent nursing literature, the term "nursing diagnosis" has occurred with increasing frequency.[4]

If everyone is diagnosing, how is nursing diagnosis similar to and different from the diagnoses made by other professions and occupations? There are similarities. Every diagnosis begins with the gathering of facts. The facts may be a hematocrit of 30 percent, the location of a stray bullet, the inability to add a column of figures, or the report that the father of a large family has lost his job. At some time during or at the completion of the fact-gathering, the practitioner in a given field recognizes a pattern. He then states his conclusion.

Differences in diagnoses arise from each

practitioner's view of his role behaviors and responsibilities and from the knowledge necessary for the practice of each profession. The nurse's definition of nursing determines both her view of nursing responsibilities and the knowledge those responsibilities require. Our definition of nursing is consistent with Hall's conception of nursing as a professional process involving three overlapping aspects: (1) *the nurturing aspect—a close interpersonal relationship concerned with the intimate bodily care of patients;* (2) *the medical aspect, shared with the medical profession and concerned with assisting the patient through his medical, surgical, and rehabilitative care;* and (3) *the helping aspect, shared with all professional persons and involving therapeutic interpersonal skills to assist the patient in self-actualization.*[5]

With a working definition of nursing in mind, a nurse can make a nursing diagnosis which specifies an aspect of the patient's condition that requires nursing care. How does a nurse make a nursing diagnosis? What is a nursing diagnosis?

We define a nursing diagnosis as *a statement of a conclusion resulting from a recognition of a pattern derived from a nursing investigation of the patient.* We visualize this definition as implying the two aspects of diagnosis—(1) *the process of diagnosing* and (2) *the decision, or actual diagnosis.* (Figure 1). We will explain this definition as we have used it to make nursing diagnoses. In practice, the process of diagnosing, including the nursing investigation and the thought process leading to the recognition of a pattern, precedes the actual diagnosis.

Reprinted with permission of Nursing Publications, Inc., 194-B Kinderkamack Road, Park Ridge, New Jersey, from *Nursing Forum,* 1966, Vol. 5, No. 4, pp. 50-64.

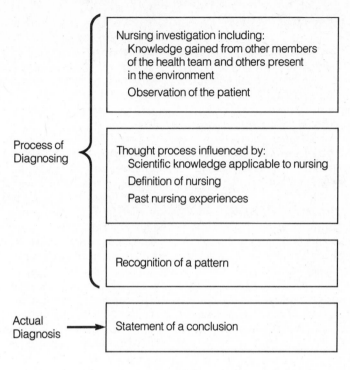

Figure 1

The Steps to Nursing Diagnosis

NURSING INVESTIGATION

The nursing investigation begins with a collection of facts. Some of these facts are gained from members of the health team through written and spoken communication.

The patient's chart is the major means of written communication. The admission, or face, sheet gives us facts regarding the patient's age, sex, marital status, occupation, religion, and place of residence. The medical history and physical examination provide us with the patient's past and present experiences of illness. In the physician's progress notes we find an overview of changes in the patient's condition since hospitalization. The physician's orders outline the plan for diagnostic studies and therapy. Reports of diagnostic studies add to our information about the patient's present illness. The nurses' notes are reviewed for nursing observations of the patient.

Spoken communication with nurses who have cared or are caring for the patient complement the information gained from the chart. These nurses may be asked such questions as: "Tell me about Mr. G. What is he like as a person?" and "What signs and symptoms did you observe?" Other health team members, such as the medical social worker, the physical therapist, the occupational therapist, and the inhalation therapist, may be asked questions relevant to their information about the patient.

Communication with the patient's family and friends may yield information regarding the patient's prehospitalization habits. A question such as "What was he like before he became ill?" may elicit facts not obtained from the health team members.

A major source of fact collection is our own observation of the patient. Observation, as we use it, implies the use of four of the five senses. We visually observe the patient to detect overt physical and psychological signs of illness. We talk to the patient and listen to his responses, and we may listen to sounds from the heart or chest or abdomen. We may touch the patient at the site of a subjective complaint, such as pain. We may smell discharges from body orifices or from a wound.

We make statements or ask questions in order to elicit further information from the patient regarding his expectations about hospitalization, his views of his illness, and his prehospital daily activities concerning food, exercise, elimination, and rest and sleep. We utilize information already obtained from other sources to guide our statements or questions and to prevent our subjecting the patient to repetitive questioning.

RECOGNITION OF A PATTERN

As we proceed in fact collection, we continually ask ourselves questions to determine the relatedness of facts and to structure our data collection. Mr. T mentions that his barium enema showed a "mass" in his abdomen. On his history it is noted that he had a cancerous lesion removed from his lip four years previously. Could he be concerned about a recurrence of cancer?

We ask ourselves how our present observations compare or contrast with those made previously by other health team members. A nurse observes that Mrs. E's newly applied cast is saturated with a blood stain measuring one inch in diameter. Fifteen minutes later we find the blood stain is two inches in diameter. Information concerning the possibility of hemorrhage may be sought by measurement of the blood pressure and heart beat, by inspection of skin color, and by consultation with the phy-

sician about his expectations regarding bleeding. Thus, one fact helps us to structure further observations.

The thought process through which the relatedness of facts is seen is influenced by our background of scientific knowledge, by past nursing experiences, and by our definition of nursing.

Scientific knowledge applicable to nursing may be drawn from such sciences as psychology, sociology, anthropology, anatomy, physiology, pathology, and bacteriology. Our education in these sciences forms our background working knowledge. Referral to new scientific findings keeps us informed about changing trends. Scientific knowledge is reinforced and expanded by our past nursing experiences with patients exhibiting similar signs and symptoms. Together, scientific knowledge and past experiences provide a mental card file of facts and principles to which we refer as we seek the significance of our observations.

Thus, as we seek the relationship of facts, we are influenced by these considerations: a certain scientific mechanism may be present; an observation from past experience is similar to that seen in this patient; a nurse has a responsibility in this area. Gradually or suddenly our thought process draws the facts into a pattern. The end result of this process we have named the recognition of a pattern.

STATEMENT OF A CONCLUSION

The actual nursing diagnosis is the statement of a conclusion. The diagnosis may be descriptive as "Communicates exclusively through gestures" or "Limited response to auditory and tactile stimuli." The diagnosis may be etiological as "Lessened intestinal peristalsis" or "Inadequate understanding of hospital environment because he does not speak English." As more facts are obtained through nursing investigation, a descriptive diagnosis may become an etiological diagnosis. Knowledge of the etiology may suggest more pertinent nursing care.

We have made diagnoses which are primarily physiological ("Lessened intestinal peristalsis") and others which are primarily psychological ("Feelings of powerlessness"). Some nursing diagnoses—for example, "Nausea"—imply both physiological and psychological aspects. "Nausea" is also an example of the use of a major medical symptom as suitable terminology for a nursing diagnosis.

A nursing diagnosis might be anticipated in a certain medical diagnosis; for example, "Pain" may be the nursing diagnosis in a patient with a myocardial infarction. Or, a nursing diagnosis may be distinct from the medical diagnosis; it may describe a condition due to hospitalization ("Lonesomeness") or to a complication of the primary illness ("Urinary retention" in a patient with benign prostatic hypertrophy).

We have made the same nursing diagnoses in patients with different medical diagnoses, since the same physiological or psychological processes may be present even when the total patterns as viewed by the physician are different. "Inadequate oxygenation" may be a nursing diagnosis in patients whose medical diagnosis is "asthma," "postoperative pneumonectomy," or "congestive heart failure."

The nursing diagnosis may be the same as the medical diagnosis. This occurrence is most likely in emergency situations when the nurse's therapeutic actions are the same as the physician's. An initial diagnosis of "Cardiac arrest" may be both a medical and a nursing diagnosis calling for immediate respiratory and cardiac resuscitation. Following emergency treatment the medical diagnosis may become "Ventricular fibrillation" or "Myocardial infarction," and the nursing diagnosis may become "Ineffective cardiac output" or "Fear of pain."

With the exception of such an emergency, a nursing diagnosis is not a medical diagnosis. A nursing diagnosis tends to be more individualized. Where a medical diagnosis serves to summarize a group of signs and symptoms, a nursing diagnosis may consist of one sign or symptom that focuses on the patient's particular response to his illness. A nursing diagnosis tends to reflect the progress of the patient. Whereas a medical diagnosis may remain the same until the patient has recovered or died, a nursing diagnosis indicates the significant responses the patient makes at the stages of his illness and therefore may change with daily changes in the patient. This individualization and reflection of patient progress make a nursing diagnosis useful in the round-the-clock performance of hospital nursing as well as in community nursing. Both are situations in which medical diagnosis is made but in which there are many hours of nursing responsibilities in the absence of the medical practitioner.

The process of diagnosing begins as soon as the patient comes under nursing care, and it continues until he no longer needs nursing care. As the nurse learns more about the patient, she may revise the nursing diagnosis. The diagnosis may become more specific; "Fear and anxiety concerning the surgical procedure" may become "Fear and anxiety concerning the possibility of cancer." Or the diagnosis may become more generalized; "Cyanosis" may become "Inadequate oxygenation."

In some instances, because of interruptions or masking of physiological or psychological cues, the nurse does not have sufficient facts to recognize a clear-cut pattern. The facts merely suggest a pattern. The decision, or diagnosis, then becomes what we call a rule-out, or tentative nursing diagnosis. This diagnosis is, in fact, a hypothesis which structures and stimulates the nurse's search for more information. We seek this information, usually by returning to the patient, to determine the accuracy or inaccuracy of the tentative nursing diagnosis.

At this point we do not believe that all nursing diagnoses can or should be of a given degree of specificity or generalization. It may be possible to organize nursing diagnoses into a classification system comparable to the classifications used by medicine. Such a system will not be possible until nurses are skilled in diagnosing and agree about the meaning and implications of the nursing diagnosis.

What is the value of a nursing diagnosis?

Examples of Nursing Diagnoses

Facts Obtained During Nursing Investigation	Major Points in the Thought Process Leading to Recognition of a Pattern	Nursing Diagnosis

Mr. A was a 55-year-old man hospitalized for a pneumonectomy complicated by a cerebral embolus, which in turn necessitated a tracheotomy and a gastrostomy.

Facts Obtained During Nursing Investigation	Major Points in the Thought Process Leading to Recognition of a Pattern	Nursing Diagnosis
Vocal cords bypassed by tracheotomy Had difficulty covering the opening of the tracheotomy tube with his finger Said "It hurts there (pointing to gastrostomy) when I talk." Had difficulty holding tablet while writing because of paresis of left arm	Physical discomfort and physical disability when attempting spoken or written communication	Limited ability to communicate 1) by vocal sounds 2) by writing
Nodded or shook head Exaggerated changes in facial expression Rubbed his stomach Pointed to his hip Shook his finger Held out hand to shake hands Waved When he does speak, he says only one or two words	He is trying to express himself in the way in which he experiences least frustration—usually through gestures or changes of facial expression	
At times shrugs shoulders or shakes head when nurse is unable to understand him	Repeated frustrations may lead to anxiety	Anxiety as a result of frustration at inability to communicate
Requested by wave of hand that tube feeding be stopped Held right hand over abdomen Lying very still	Signs indicative of mild stimulation of vomiting center	Nausea
Two days postoperative from hiatal hernia repair Nurse reported episodes of hiccoughs and indigestion	May have lessened gastric capacity from surgical trauma or lessened gastric motility	

Examples of Nursing Diagnoses (continued)

Facts Obtained During Nursing Investigation	Major Points in the Thought Process Leading to Recognition of a Pattern	Nursing Diagnosis
Feed Regurgitated	Excessive stimulation of oropharynx	Nausea
Coughing one ounce of mucus per hour		
Anxiety	Anxiety may stimulate the cerebral cortex to send afferent impulses to vomiting center	

Mrs. B was a 65-year-old woman hospitalized for polypectomy of the descending colon.

Facts Obtained During Nursing Investigation	Major Points in the Thought Process Leading to Recognition of a Pattern	Nursing Diagnosis
Stated "My stomach hurts."	Little evidence of gastro-intestinal activity	Lessened intestinal peristalsis
Abdomen distended.		
No flatus passed		
Few bowel tones		
Miller-Abbott tube in place	No peristalic stimuli	
Receiving continuous intravenous therapy		
Medical consultation suggested intestinal obstruction		
Face flushed, skin hot to touch	Signs of fever	Pathogenic bacteria infecting incision site
Oral temperature fluctuating between 100° and 102° F		
Moderate diaphoresis		
Leukocyte count elevated. Presurgical: 7000/cu. mm. One week postsurgical: 12,000/cu. mm.	Signs of infectious process	
Red, swollen, indurated area around lower half of midline incision site		
No evidence of healing in lower half of incisional wound		
Serosanguineous discharge from wound		
Talked of coming into hospital feeling well and now being sick	Expectations regarding hospitalization and treatment have not been met	Feelings of Powerlessness
Said she had expected that the polyps could be removed by way of the proctoscope and "now all this"		

Examples of Nursing Diagnoses (continued)

Facts Obtained During Nursing Investigation	Major Points in the Thought Process Leading to Recognition of a Pattern	Nursing Diagnosis
"I'm told it will take time to get well. But I don't know what they mean by time—a day, a week, a month."		Feelings of powerlessness
I don't understand why the doctor left the inhalator here. He knows. I don't know why he left it, but he knows."	Does not feel she can plan what is to come or what she can do	
I don't know why I have to have the intravenous tubes. The doctor probably knows best."	Does not understand or feel in control of her environment	
"All these tubes—I just want to get rid of them so I can be on my own."		
Gross jerky movements of limbs		
Picking at bed clothes	Signs of central nervous system disturbance	
Unable to stand without assistance		
Disoriented as to time, place, and family		R/O Electrolyte imbalance 1) hypocalcemia 2) hypopotassemia
Gastrointestinal decompression for one week		
Intravenous therapy with replacement of electrolytes KCl and NaCl	Loss of body electrolytes	
Five to six loose stools per 24-hour period for the last three days (Presurgery pattern of one stool per day)		

Mr. C was a 44-year-old man hospitalized for thrombophlebitis of the right leg and headaches in the left frontal region.

Had cerebral vascular accident one year ago which resulted in loss of vision in the left half of visual field		
Lost job because of impairment of vision	Has experienced losses	
His daughter was to be married in two months		Depressed; has thoughts of suicide

Examples of Nursing Diagnoses (continued)

Facts Obtained During Nursing Investigation	Major Points in the Thought Process Leading to Recognition of a Pattern	Nursing Diagnosis
Reported that he had had approximately four hours of "restless" sleep per night for the last two months	Symptoms of depression 1) Insomnia 2) Thoughts about death and suicide 3) Feelings of uselessness	Depressed; has thoughts of suicide
Talked of donating his body to the medical school		
Talked about his experiences with death in World War II		
"Everybody should die at 45" (three months away)		
Expresses concerns about suicide		
Said that he had thought of many ways of taking his own life but that he would not do so unless he became more disabled		
"You are useful only when you are rearing children."		
"If I become paralyzed, I'll take a gun and shoot myself."	Not comfortable being dependent upon others for some of his physical needs, although his physical condition necessitates this	
Said it would be more difficult for his family if he were disabled than if he committed suicide		
Repeatedly emphasized that he did not want to be a burden		Dependency longings
Up to the bathroom against the doctor's orders		
Unwraps leg against doctor's orders		
History of alcoholism	May be symptoms of dependency longings	
Smokes 2–3 packs of cigarettes per day		
Medical diagnosis of thrombophlebitis	Danger of emboli	
Veins in left thigh slightly engorged		

Examples of Nursing Diagnoses (continued)

Facts Obtained During Nursing Investigation	Major Points in the Thought Process Leading to Recognition of a Pattern	Nursing Diagnosis
Skin inflamed over the course of the vein	Danger of emboli	R/O Vascular insufficiency 1) cerebral 2) lower limbs
Medical order of bedrest		
History of cerebral vascular accident		
Reports frequent headaches over left temple	Possible vasoconstriction	
Smokes 2–3 packs of cigarettes a day		
Drinks coffee, 8–10 cups per day		

Nursing is seeking a scientific basis for practice. The process of diagnosing necessitates the use of scientific knowledge and requires the relation and application of this knowledge to nursing. The actual diagnosis establishes a point of departure, a basis for nursing care. George B. Shaw has been credited with saying "Diagnosis should mean the finding out of all there is wrong with a particular patient."[6] We believe a nursing diagnosis could mean the finding out of all that is necessary to know to begin a plan of nursing care.

REFERENCES

1. John A. Prior and Jack S. Silberstein, *Physical Diagnosis: The History and Examination of the Patient.* St. Louis: The C. V. Mosby Company. 1959. pp. 17–18.

2. Leo J. Brueckner, "Introduction" Educational Diagnosis. *Thirty-fourth Yearbook of the National Society for the Study of Education.* Guy Montrose Whipple (ed.). Bloomington, Ill. Public School Publishing Company. 1935. p. 2.

3. Mary E. Richmond, *Social Diagnosis.* New York: Russell Sage Foundation. 1917. p. 357.

4. Virginia Bonney and June Rothberg, *Nursing Diagnosis and Therapy.* New York: National League for Nursing. 1963.

5. Lydia E. Hall, "Nursing—What Is It?" Revised. Mimeographed. Loeb Center, New York, April 26, 1963, p. 1–5.

6. F. G. Crookshank, "The Importance of a Theory of Signs and a Critique of Language in the Study of Medicine" Supplement to C. K. Ogden and I. A. Richards, *The Meaning of Meaning.* 10th edition, London: Routledge and Kegan Paul, Inc. 1949. p. 343.

BIBLIOGRAPHY

Wilda Chambers, "Nursing Diagnosis," *American Journal of Nursing,* 62:102–104. November, 1962.

Nori I. Komorita, "Nursing Diagnosis," *American Journal of Nursing,* 63:83–86, December, 1963.

R. Faye McCain, "Nursing by Assessment—Not Intuition," *American Journal of Nursing,* 65: 82–84, April, 1965.

Catherine M. Norris, "Toward a Science of Nursing—A Method for Developing Unique Content in Nursing," *Nursing Forum,* 3: 22–24, Number 3, 1964.

Why Nursing Diagnosis?

June S. Rothberg

The author maintains that nursing diagnosis is essential to professional nursing. It ensures focus on the individual. It reveals the many factors which influence the patient's progress. And it results in a goal directed plan of nursing care that can be evaluated.

Nursing diagnosis is a term which, in recent years, has been used with ever increasing frequency and often with little accuracy. For various reasons, the term can be an emotion-laden or frightening concept to nurses and to other health personnel. Before discussing what a nursing diagnosis is, let us review what it is not. It is not a medical diagnosis made by nurses. It is not a psychiatric diagnosis made by nurses. It is not a socioeconomic diagnosis made by nurses.

In making a nursing diagnosis, the professional nurse may utilize specific information from the diagnoses which other qualified persons have made. However, she will add to this information her own independent observations to form an evaluation which is uniquely nursing.

In 1961, Abdellah stated, "We must face up to the responsibility that making a nursing diagnosis is an independent function of the professional nurse" (1). I believe that for far too long a time we in nursing have abdicated this responsibility.

As a starting point, in broad and very general terms, a nursing diagnosis may be thought of as an evaluation by nurses of those factors affecting the patient which will in-

fluence his recovery. These factors may include intrinsic dimensions such as physical condition or emotional state and, also, external influences such as economic problems. All nurses, I am certain, know of a patient whose physical progress was impeded because he was frantic over bills or who couldn't be discharged because he was unable to walk up three flights of stairs. Some of these factors will need to be referred to appropriate disciplines for action. Some are directly the responsibility of nursing.

It is precisely in the area of interdisciplinary functions and relations that difficulties in patient care arise. There is considerable overlap at the boundaries of each profession's practice. Instead of leading to increased cooperation and communication for the benefit of the individual and all society, this overlap has led to the reverse. The various disciplines are warily watching their own vested interests—guarding their particular prerogatives and preserves. Lest I be misunderstood, I mean nursing, too.

In the past 15 years, there has been a tremendous increase in the number of persons working in the health arena. The 1960 census indicated that in a 10-year span, the health field has risen from seventh to third place among major United States industries in terms of numbers of persons employed (2). This was six years ago! Not only are numbers increasing but as knowledge expands and is intensified, becoming more advanced and more highly technical, new specialties are proliferating. In my own field of rehabilitation, there are physical, occupational and recreational therapists, vocational and rehabilitation counselors, and prosthetists, to mention only a few of the occupational specialists. It is now possible for a person to obtain a professional degree (a bachelor of science) in orthotics, the newest specialty field.

With the impetus given by recent health and social legislation which is directed toward the preparation of health workers to meet the needs of our continually burgeoning and aging population, there will be an ever larger number of persons working in health fields.

We may expect ever greater fragmentation of services than current and anticipated growth warrants unless each and all of us become completely aware of a single overriding fact—the common denominator in health or disease is the individual man. It is not an institution—not a doctor—not a nurse—not any other health worker. It is the human being who needs to be kept well and treated when sick. Without awareness and understanding of this central fact, health care and particularly nursing care has neither direction nor meaning.

The challenge to us today is to furnish the kind of health care people need, when and where they need it. To do this, we must bring the patient into the foreground. There is no one idea having greater importance for nursing than that of viewing the patient as a person. It is only when the patient is so viewed, as a person, that care is provided to him according to his needs in an appropriate, continuous, and dynamic pattern which is sometimes described as comprehensive care. Nursing diagnosis makes it possible to provide such care.

One hears much today about meeting total needs of patients. This is a reaction to a practice which has concentrated primarily on two areas: routine physical care concerned with fundamental physiologic processes such as nutrition and elimination, and highly technical complex aspects of nursing. We have emphasized the physical and the technical while ignoring or not understanding the perceptions, the responses, the social, and the psychologic needs of people. To further complicate the picture, we have so fragmented our services that the basic physical care of patients has been relegated to increasingly less well-prepared personnel and we have taken to our professional bosom those highly

complex and often painful procedures which were formerly the province of the physician.

All too frequently, we have centered on the medical, the psychiatric, or other diagnosis. We have carried out medically prescribed orders, briskly and efficiently applied some highly routine or ritualized procedures, and considered the whole process nursing, while neatly ignoring the patients' perceptions, feelings, and individual problems.

As a reminder of the hazard, encountered when we concentrate on physical diagnosis as the sole determining factor in planning nursing care, consider the following. The patient in bed 13 has a gastric neoplasm, the one in bed 32 has a viral pneumonia, and the one in bed 20 has a cerebral aneurysm. What do we know about these three persons? Only their medical diagnoses! The person in each bed could be any combination of either half of the following: a man or a woman, 35 years old or 75, ill for years with a chronic disease or sick for the first time in his life, a valued and loved family member or a socially isolated person living without family or friends, destitute or financially secure.

It is the combination of such factors plus many others which will strongly influence the particular patient's progress and recovery. These characteristics exert this influence because they are the resources—physical, emotional, social, and economic—which the person can call upon to overcome his illness. Nursing diagnosis is the process which identifies the patient's resources and deficits, thus indicating his needs for nursing assistance.

Historically, patient care has been considered the core of all nursing activity regardless of the setting in which it was performed or the type of nursing function required. Modern nursing extends over the broad spectrum of health services and encompasses promotion of health, prevention of illness, as well as care of patients and their families. In order to administer patient care, the nurse must identify the individual's needs for nursing services. Ever since nursing was first performed, the nurse, by a process either wholly or partially conscious, looked at the patient and determined on the basis of intuition, experience, rote learning, knowledge, or in some cases ignorance, which nursing acts were needed to relieve his distress.

What must the nurse know about the patient? This is the central question in determining, in a professionally responsible manner, the patient's requirements for nursing services. What must she understand of the intrinsic processes (physical, physiologic, emotional), occurring within him? What must she know of the extrinsic factors (sociologic, economic) surrounding him, and the influence these exert upon him? How well does he manage himself in relation to the stresses he faces? What probable results can she expect from her nursing? When the nurse is able to answer these questions accurately, she is ready to provide appropriate comprehensive nursing.

Answering these questions in a clearly ordered, reasoned manner, based on scientific fact, requires the establishment of a nursing diagnosis and nursing therapy. Nursing diagnosis is an evaluation within the framework of current knowledge of the patient's condition as a person including physical, physiologic, and behavioral aspects.

Let us examine the key word of this definition: *evaluation*. An evaluation is a process, implying a continuing operation. There are many kinds of evaluations which go on all the time, continually influencing our choice of actions. Some are not conscious evaluations but are implicit or intuitive. At this moment, you are evaluating what you read. As I write, I am subconsciously evaluating your possible response to my words. But neither of us is sharply aware of this evaluation process as it goes on—it is almost automatic.

However, these kinds of evaluations—intuitive, implicit, and automatic—are not what is required in making a nursing diagnosis. It is definitive, clearly focused, and completely conscious evaluation which is necessary for our decision making about patients. In order to be of help to ourselves and especially to others, we must practice evaluation in an explicit manner

as a consciously planned activity. It may be practiced informally. However, it frequently is carried out within the framework of a formal evaluation instrument.

What is it we are evaluating? We are determining the patient's condition—the relative state of health or ill health in physical, functional (or physiologic), and behavioral areas. We are looking for both strengths and weaknesses in these areas and for both overt and covert problems.

How are we evaluating? We are consciously and systematically observing physical signs and activities, observing physiologic indications and reports, and observing social and interpersonal behavior. The interpretation of observations is based on principles from the biologic, physical, and social sciences which have been integrated into a nursing science.

Why are we evaluating? The purpose of such assessment is to determine the patient's (or the family's) need. We are trying to appraise the situation of the patient to learn what we as professionals can do for him.

Thus, the prime element in the process of evaluation or diagnosis is identification of individual needs. The second element is clear definition of goals for the patient's care. One such goal, in the physical realm, might be to obtain the maximum possible improvement in the patient's condition. Another goal might have to be more modest, such as the maintenance of his present condition without further deterioration. An even more modest but imperative goal must be the prevention of superimposed disabilities (3). A different kind of goal might be to increase the patient's verbal interaction with his roommates. Several categories of goals must be packaged together, since the patient being diagnosed is a person with a variety of responses, facets, and problems. Therefore, goals include desired physical, functional, and behavioral targets.

The nurse making a diagnosis determines which of the identified care needs are amenable to nursing. Once nursing problems have been defined clearly by the diagnosis, a course of nursing activities purposefully directed toward increasing the positive health of the patient can be initiated. The nurse selects the appropriate methods, resources, and personnel to meet the identified needs. Those needs which are beyond the scope of nursing are referred to the appropriate health workers. Thus, the unique function of the professional nurse is being performed—that of the diagnosis of the patient's need for nursing services and the decision upon a course of action to follow (4).

We have now moved into the realm of nursing therapy. Nursing therapy is defined as knowledgeable intervention in the form of nursing activities, based on the nursing diagnosis, and directed at moving the individual toward positive health (5). Nursing care plans are a step toward nursing therapy. There is absolutely no point in making a nursing diagnosis unless it leads directly to action in the form of nursing therapy. And, of course, appropriate comprehensive nursing therapy is impossible without a prior diagnosis of need. Nursing therapy is derived specifically from the diagnosis. Direction for the nursing intervention is given by the nursing diagnosis. The three elements of diagnosis—identification of individual need, establishment of goals, and selection of appropriate methods—together provide the knowledge required in order to act appropriately to move the individual toward more positive health.

New knowledge in the health sciences is expanding and pyramiding at a fantastic rate. Predictions about nursing practice of the future, made only five years ago, were considered by a majority of nurses to be science fiction, but today are reality. Nurses are working with patients treated in hyperbaric chambers, with bioelectric monitoring devices, with electronic

cardiac, bladder, and muscle pacemaker and implants. Microminiaturization techniques developed for outer space explorations have opened untold opportunities for the alleviation of man's physical ills.

In view of these technological changes, what happens to the fragility and importance of the individual? One way to meet the challenge is to consciously and clear-sightedly assess the patient's needs as an individual utilizing keen professional observation plus all the mechanical gadgets to obtain highly accurate information about his condition and to utilize skilled professional judgment to interpret and evaluate the information. Then, at all times remembering that all people have a diversity of needs, make a diagnosis and institute a plan of therapy to meet the individual problems of the person in our care.

REFERENCES

1. Abdellah, Faye. *Meeting Patients' Needs—An Approach to Teaching.* Paper presented at biennial convention of the National League for Nursing. Cleveland, Ohio, April 10–14, 1961.

2. Manpower in health. *Progressive Health Services* 10: May 1961.

3. Rothberg, June, ed. Foreword, [to the] Symposium on chronic disease and rehabilitation. *Nursing Clinics of North America* 1:352–354, Sept. 1966.

4. Abdellah, *op. cit.*

5. Bonney, Virginia, and Rothberg, June. *Nursing Diagnosis and Therapy; An Instrument for Evaluation and Measurement.* New York, National League for Nursing, 1963.

Humanistic Exercises

Exercise 7

Personalized Care Plan*

Purposes	1. To learn the steps of the nursing process.
	2. To explore all the personal aspects of self that make up one's existence.
	3. To develop an awareness of one's needs in relation to goal accomplishment.
	4. To isolate problem areas in individual goal accomplishment related to one's own life.
	5. To brainstorm about how one's needs can be met.
Facility	A large room with a table where participants will be able to sit in a circle and write.
Materials	Worksheet A: Data Base
	Worksheet B: Needs Schema
	Worksheet C: Personal Care Plan
	Worksheet D: Action Planning
	Paper, writing materials, posterboard, construction paper, or worksheets may be used, as well as blackboard or newsprint and magic markers.
Time Required	Three to four hours or more.
Group Size	Unlimited groups of four.

Needs Schema

1. comfort
2. nutrition
3. exercise
4. diversional activities
5. dependency
6. independency
7. socializing
8. security
9. esteem
10. self-actualization
11. to be appreciated
12. to be loved
13. safety
14. environmental considerations
15. teaching
16. prevention of complications

---

*This exercise, the PELLEM Pentagram (Chapter 17), and exercises contained in Part VI were jointly created and designed by Elaine L. La Monica and Eunice M. Parisi-Carew at the University of Massachusetts, 1975–1976.

Eunice Parisi-Carew received her doctorate from the University of Massachusetts in 1972 in the behavioral sciences. As a counseling psychologist, a member of Certified Consultants International, and a member of the National Training Laboratories, she has done extensive consulting in the areas of management, leadership, interpersonal and group dynamics, staff development, and organizational change. Currently, she is an independent consultant working with several large corporations and with government agencies.

17. skills and competencies
    a. organizational skills
    b. technical skills
    c. interpersonal skills
    d. decision-making skills
    e. communication skills
    f. teaching skills
18. others *(may be decided by individual members or groups)*

Design

1. The purposes of the exercise should be explained to the participants, expanding on the fact that nurses are involved with writing care plans for their clients every day. Since nurses are individuals, too, it might be helpful for participants to look at themselves, their needs, and their ways of meeting needs. Participants will actually be confronting and exploring their own selves, then receiving feedback on care plans with the intent of expanding the data and ideas. In a sense, each participant will both lead and be the subject of a team conference.

2. *Data base.* Each member should start with Worksheet A from this book and add sheets as necessary since this part may be lengthy. The sheet is divided into three columns entitled Psychologic, Physiologic, and Social. Under these headings, the participants place all the facts about themselves that come to mind. Examples of each would be the following:

Psychologic	*Physiologic*	*Social*
1. needs to be independent	3. small-framed	5. married
2. fears authority	4. blond	6. two children
		7. likes to have people near

3. After participants have filled in their data bases, they then share these in groups of four (for approximately 20 minutes).

4. After sharing, the participants are asked to go back and individually rethink and expand their data base by writing down any personal facts that were mentioned during the sharing but are not currently included. Following this, participants should number the data base consecutively as shown above.

5. Referring to the needs schema (Worksheet B), which may be listed on a blackboard, individuals should jot the needs down on paper and indicate what numbers from their data base apply or are important in considering those stated needs. An example would be the need for dependency. The following numbers might be placed after it from the data base information: 1, 2, 3, 5, 6, 7. There are no absolutes in this section; participants should just think about the data and, if it may be pertinent to the needs in some way, place the need number beside it. The purpose of this step is to provide an individualized picture of each person in relation to the stated needs.

6. From the needs schema, individuals should pick the ten top-priority needs that they think they have. Place a star next to them.

7. Numbering from 1 to 10, highest priority to lowest, members arrange in order these ten priority needs.

8. Going from the highest priority on down, personal diagnoses should be made concerning each need relevant to the pertinent data. Write these on Worksheet C. Leave a space between diagnoses:

Personal Diagnoses	Personal Goals	Personal Orders	Areas of Concern
1.			
2.			

(and so forth)

9. Use the following formula for writing each nursing diagnosis, filling in the blanks:

I feel that I need _____

because _____

The first blank becomes the goal; the second is the diagnosis. Emphasis at this point is on thoughts, rather than semantics. Members may have more than one diagnoses for each of the 10 priority items on the needs schema.

10. After individuals have written their diagnoses and recorded them, the next step is to individually brainstorm ways that the goals can be attained. Participants ask themselves, "If I could have everything the way I wanted it, what would be done to meet these needs?" Write these in the Personal Orders column and number them.

11. Members should now have ten diagnoses and goals and several personal orders under each. Participants regroup into fours and share these. Members should provide feedback for each other on each of the areas and offer additional suggestions for orders.

12. Following the sharing section, individuals next extrapolate from each diagnosis and its orders; they should note a maximum of four issues or areas of specific concern—that is, aggression, assertion, and so forth. They may ask themselves, "Of all this material, what are the central issues that I need to work on?"

13. Regrouping into fours, participants share these central issues and write them on Worksheet D, including everyone's individual issues and the number of times issues are mentioned by individuals.

14. Each small group of four should then decide on four issues or areas of concern that are highest priority in the group. This is usually based on the number of times it is mentioned by individuals and/or in discussion. These also should be recorded on Worksheet D.

15. A large group is formed and all of the issues are written on a blackboard or newsprint; rate priorities of needs according to the number of times issues are mentioned by groups. This list provides a lead-in for focusing on issues of concern to the group.

16. Discuss the experience.

Variations

This exercise may be done in part by homework assignments or may be divided into concurrent sessions as study of the nursing process progresses. An added dimension would be for individuals to look at the needs not in top priority and suggest when it is anticipated that these needs would emerge for action.

Discussion

The central issues obtained from the participants can form the basis for further work in the group. The nursing orders can be used in action steps. What is intended to be gained is a picture of one's life in relation to individual needs, followed by a plan for how needs can be met. Looking at oneself in such a manner often makes self-awareness possible and goal directed. The steps followed in this Personalized Care Plan are analogous to those in the nursing process.

Exercise 7
Data Base

Psychologic	Physiologic	Social

Exercise 7   Worksheet B
Needs Schema

1. comfort
2. nutrition
3. exercise
4. diversional activities
5. dependency
6. independency
7. socializing
8. security
9. esteem
10. self-actualization
11. to be appreciated
12. to be loved
13. safety
14. environmental considerations
15. teaching
16. prevention of complications
17. skills and competencies
    a. organizational skills
    b. technical skills
    c. interpersonal skills
    d. decision-making skills
    e. communication skills
    f. teaching skills
18. other _____
19. _____
20. _____

Exercise 7   Worksheet C

Personal Care Plan

Personal Diagnoses	Personal Goals	Personal Orders	Areas of Concern

Exercise 7 Worksheet D
Action Planning

Central Issues of Individuals in the Small Groups

Issue	Times Mentioned	Issue	Times Mentioned
_____	_____	_____	_____
_____	_____	_____	_____
_____	_____	_____	_____
_____	_____	_____	_____
_____	_____	_____	_____
_____	_____	_____	_____
_____	_____	_____	_____

Central Issues of the Small Group

_____

_____

_____

_____

Exercise 8

Term Paper—The Nursing Process*

Purposes
1. To carry out the steps of the nursing process with a patient in a clinical setting.
2. To formally report the results of the method.

Facility
A clinical setting in which each student can choose and work with a client family.

Materials
Paper, construction paper, poster boards, scrolls, or any other media desired by the learner on which the report can be made.

Time Required
Variable, but generally a long-range project or term assignment.

Group Size
Not applicable.

Design
Term/Course/Module Assignment
1. Use a client and/or family and/or community as the focus of the project.
2. The project is to include the following parts:
   a. Brief overview of client; include the time period covered by the paper relative to client's stage of illness/wellness and the reason(s) for care.
   b. Data—include sources for data collection.
   c. Data processing relevant to needs.
   d. Diagnosis.
      1) determination of nursing diagnoses, goals, and/or objectives.
      2) priority arrangement.
   e. Action.
   f. Responses (actual).
   g. Action(s) that would have been more effective.
3. Steps:
   a. Gather all available data—itemize and organize.
   b. For each of the needs listed below, indicate which combination(s) of data are relevant to determining the specifics of this patient's need

---

*This exercise is an adaptation of one used by Virginia Earles, University of Massachusetts, Division of Nursing, 1975.

    c. Write—data process nursing diagnoses for patient's actual or potential health problems.

    d. Pick the ten top-priority diagnoses of this patient or family and indicate order of priority.

    e. Write nursing orders for each of the ten priority needs.

    f. For each of the diagnoses not in the top ten, suggest when you anticipate that each would emerge for action.

    g. Indicate what was actually done relevant to each diagnosis.

    h. Evaluate each client/family response in relation to its effectiveness.

Needs Schema

1. comfort
2. nutrition
3. exercise
4. personal hygiene
5. sleep, rest patterns
6. diversional activity
7. socializing and privacy
8. elimination
9. safety
10. environmental considerations
11. teaching
12. spiritual comfort and assistance
13. prevention of complications
14. assurance of physiologic status—health maintenance and promotion
15. emotional support and counseling

Variations

Reports of the project can be made in class, thus giving the opportunity for teaching and learning experience to the reporter.

This exercise may be done in part by assignments as study of the nursing process progresses.

Part III

Planning: Designing a Strategy to Achieve Goals

Chapter 7

Nursing Orders

Part III contains two chapters—this one on nursing orders and Chapter 8 on problem-oriented records—both of which are necessary in planning. Planning involves taking the nursing diagnoses (a client's actual or potential health problem) and the nursing goals (what the client needs to be assisted in achieving—the optimal) and specifying the nursing orders (nursing behaviors) that are aimed at eradicating the nursing diagnoses and achieving the nursing goals for and with the client. Planning, according to the National Council of State Boards of Nursing (1982) further includes cooperating with other health-care personnel for delivering care and recording information.

Chapter 7 begins with the theoretic aspects of designating and writing nursing orders. This will be followed by a discussion of nursing-care plans and of the creative process for developing and writing nursing orders. Then the case study begun in Part II of this book will be used to illustrate *nursing orders*—that is, specific nursing behaviors that are developed for the nursing diagnoses and which parallel the nursing goals presented at the conclusion of Chapter 6.

Let us recall the equation we used to illustrate earlier chapters:

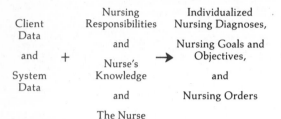

As the equation shows, nursing orders are a part of the results of data collection and processing. Together with the nursing diagnoses and the nursing goals and objectives, the nursing-care plan is formed.

COGNITIVE DIMENSIONS OF NURSING ORDERS

The nursing-care plans observed in charts, on the kardex, and in clinical-unit care-plan books generally denote the nursing diagnoses and orders for each client. Often, the nursing history also will be attached.

Care plans can be observed in a variety of forms, and nursing literature has devoted many pages to the need for a diversity of types from written formal plans to informal ones (Ciuca, 1972; Forman, 1979; Grey & Aldred, 1980; Harris, 1970; Kershaw, 1979; Mackie, 1979; Palisin, 1971; Vasey, 1979; Wagner, 1969). Considering the responsibility of the nurse to perceive and plan for an array of overt and covert patient needs for a group of patients and considering that the plans will be implemented by a variety of professional and technical care-givers, systematic and formal planning is essential. Little and Carnevali (1967) designated formal planning as absolutely necessary to incorporate all health-care efforts and to maintain a goal of providing quality, comprehensive care to consumers. Furthermore, care plans knit together the aspects of care required for a client—various data, histories, diagnoses, goals, orders—and communicate the essentials to every member of the nursing and health team. Progress can be noted and new data integrated constantly. Client transfer to other in-house units or to community-agency referrals can be made more efficiently when accompanied by a concise, systematic report of past and present client needs, as well as potential needs in the future.

Writing Nursing Orders

A nursing order should be a specific statement of what actions to take based on the goal(s) and objectives(s) a nurse wishes to achieve with and for a client, relative to an established diagnosis; hence, nursing orders are explicit statements of things needing to be done or actions that should be taken. Since the use of terms for the planning phase of the nursing process varies in nursing literature, a brief discussion of the terms used in this book follows.

The term *goal* suggests a broader area than *objectives*, and has been discussed in the previous chapter and at the beginning of this chapter. Objectives are more specific than goals, and they relate to the goals. It *may* be necessary to write one or more objectives for each goal to elucidate the process and content of the goal more clearly. For example, to move from the point of total unfamiliarity with diabetes, insulin administration, needed equipment, and self-injection to management of one's own diabetic needs, specific steps for accomplishment may best be delineated. These steps are useful in progressively evaluating where the client is in relation to objective fulfillment. Further, this can facilitate continuity of care. The case example used later in this chapter provides examples for this process.

Perhaps one of the clearest descriptions of a related term is Mager's (1975) definition of a *terminal behavior* as that which the learner should demonstrate when influence ends. There are two aspects of Mager's statement that are pertinent. First, "demonstrate" implies behavior that is visible and measurable to some degree (Mager, 1975). Logically speaking, therefore, objectives and orders must be as specific, succinct, and observable as possible. Clear objectives include statements on where the client is heading (Smith, 1971) relative to the diagnosis at hand. They should not portray general nursing behaviors such as "giving emotional support" (Smith, 1971), but should be action oriented, indicating specific, desirable client behaviors as well as those specific behaviors to be employed by the nurse in assisting the client to reach optimal health.

Second, Mager's (1975) statement that terminal behaviors refer to those that should be fulfilled by the time your influence ceases must be adapted to a nurse/client relationship. Specifically, the system of health care should be considered as "your influence." Short- and long-term nursing objectives and orders can then be developed and progress reports or evaluations written and communicated to the caregivers in various parts of the health system and in accordance with the client's presence within the structure. In other words, orders that may be begun in a coronary-care unit and might emerge as a number-one priority in a rehabilitation unit should be considered by the coronary-care nurse even though the nurse writing the order will not move with the client.

Nursing orders are nursing behaviors designed to meet the goals and objectives of nursing care. Three basic areas must be considered when writing nursing objectives and orders for each diagnosis. According to Bloom (1954), there are three types of objectives that can be used as a way of thinking about the nursing-orders system: cognitive, affective, and psychomotor. Cognitive aspects refer to the theoretic (or content) domain, such as knowledge of diabetes as a disease. The affective domain covers feelings and attitudinal processes: one's acceptance of an illness, relief of anxiety, and the like. Psychomotor aspects refer to necessary skills, such as competence in giving one's own insulin using aseptic technique. All three areas must be considered in writing objectives and orders for a given diagnosis. In addition, it is obvious that the nurse's overall order system should integrate medical orders.

Note that all nursing orders should be stated in a behavioral format, because the purpose for writing orders is to delineate the steps required to move a client's behavior toward a goal whose aim is relief of a designated diagnosis. Refer to Figure 7-1 for a visualization of this progression.

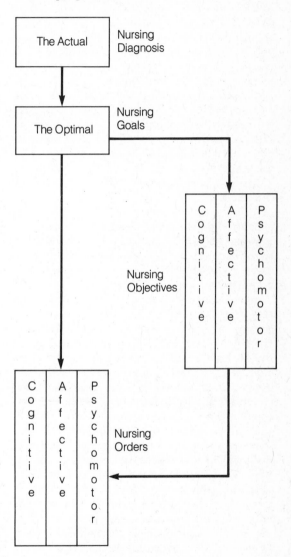

Figure 7–1

Steps in Moving from the Nursing Diagnosis to Nursing Orders

Creative Order Writing. Kelly (1966) noted the paucity of nursing orders in care plans in comparison to the great number of physician's orders. Moreover, even with the intent to practice *individualized* nursing care, it is easy to fall into a pattern of writing nursing orders that are nonspecific to the client. These tend to be bland and impotent, adhering to hospital policies and procedures much more than addressing specific client needs and the *best* way to fulfill those needs.

Following general procedure may become automatic. It becomes easy to do again what has been done before, and this process leads to preconceived notions, or mental sets, concerning what should be done with the client. As these automatic mental sets are formulated and reinforced, perceptual fields may narrow. This can result in routine orders and ways of implementing them. Instead, we need to foster expansion of perceptual fields through creative nursing orders that respond to the individuality of the client's system and that pinpoint the best ways to enable the client to reach fullest potential by using his own assets.

Eisenman (1970) conducted an investigation that unfortunately found student nurses becoming less creative during nursing education. He later researched whether or not student nurses high in creativity (as measured by perceptual preferences for complexity) would be accepting of clients labeled mentally ill or physically disabled (Eisenman, 1972). He contrasted these results with those of student nurses low in creativity. Results indicated that those who had a preference for complexity displayed increased acceptance of these clients, while those who preferred simplicity displayed decreased acceptance. These studies have important implications in nursing practice and education. First, creativity must specifically be developed, not dampened. Second, if a system (education or practice) dampens creativity to any degree, it becomes the responsibility of practitioners themselves to ensure that overt, conscious measures are taken to compensate for

the natural tendency to formulate mental sets, make care routine, or be blocked from thinking by the system's policies *before* one actually thinks of newer approaches in care and ways to implement them.

It becomes essential to look upon an individual, a disease, a strength, or a weakness and form opinions that are based on an expansive perceptual field and creative ways of setting decisions in motion. McNeil (1973), in discussing the aesthetic educational process, stated that a teacher with only one or two ways of teaching is limited in meeting the learners' differences in the way each learns best. If one relates this to nursing practice, routine orders very well may not be what is best for the client. Table 7-1 compares the nursing process with the components of the creative process.

The step that can be used first to foster creativity and develop orders that reflect the individuality of the client is exploration. Here— before nursing orders are designated—brainstorming takes place. This process involves freeing the mind of right/wrong and can-do/cannot-do. It is the process of expanding possibilities, and it answers the question, "If I could develop orders for this client, ideally doing anything I want, being as specific and personal to the client as possible and reflecting what I know about the client, what would I want done and how?" Any ideas are important, and no value judgments of good or bad are operative. After the ideas are listed, one chooses those that can be implemented with ease, picking out one or two that require minor alterations of agency or hospital norms. Then they are implemented according to the brainstormed "how." In this way creativity is fostered, rather than dampened. Moreover, care is not routine and guided by mental sets, because one is always considering and working on something new in relation to a unique person. It follows, of course, that new modes of client care have the ability to become part of the standard approach, with formal changes occurring as necesary and when documented as effective. It follows, also, that

Table **7-1**   The Nursing Process Compared with the Creative Process*

Nursing Process	Creative Process
Assessment	*Motivation*
Collection of data from many sources	Assuming that a person is creating because of internal and external forces
Classification, analysis, and summarization of data to determine nursing problems and/or needs	
Note: *At this point in the nursing process it is very easy to get caught in the routine, trite methods of problem-solving and to fail to study the individual needs of the unique patient*	*Exploration*
	Observing, surveying, and exploring all the possibilities that are available for use
	Improvisation
	Outgrowth of what is discovered through exploration
	Unplanned, impromptu manipulation of ideas, thoughts, concepts
	Working with the interrelatedness and movements that are suggested in the explored possibilities
Planning	*Experimentation*
Design for action	Combining and planning the structure of ideas, materials, and concepts in a certain area
Development of strategies or alternative approaches to meeting the needs of patients	Designing alternative methods and structures suitable for implementation
Implementation	*Application*
"Trying on" and carrying out of the proposed plan of care	Experimenting and applying strategies and designs that are then "tried on"
Evaluation	*Evaluation*
Based on available feedback, use of new information to revise the care plan as necessary	*Extension*
	Opening and experimenting with new avenues of ideas; repeating the process
	Extending or implying further areas of study

*SOURCE: The components of the creative process as herein described were developed by S. Brainerd. *A Curriculum for an Aesthetic Program for Teacher Education.* Doctoral dissertation, University of Massachusetts, School of Education, Amherst, 1971.

just because a procedure is standard, it is not necessarily ineffective or unsuitable for a particular client; the nurse must use judgment. Such application of creativity in the writing of nursing orders has been reported positively ("Instructor Teaches," 1981).

The cognitive aspects of nursing orders and the components of objective writing for nursing orders have been discussed, and brainstorming has been introduced as a method to facilitate individualization of nursing-care plans. Next, following the established diagnoses in Chapter 6, the same case study will be discussed in the next portion of this chapter. Developing nursing objectives and orders from the nursing diagnoses and goals set forth in Chapter 6 will be the focus.

CASE EXAMPLE ON NURSING ORDERS

The case example will be developed more completely by dealing with the nursing diagnoses that are presently essential in the client's system and by dealing with them in order of priority (see Table 6-5). Diagnoses of less than immediate priority will become a focus of emphasis in the rehabilitation phase of the client's progress—that is, when plans for discharge are in the picture. It is important to remember that medical orders are included in the nursing orders, since this is one aspect of nursing responsibility. Also, to personalize nursing orders, it is often necessary to refer back to the data-collection and processing stages and obtain and examine client data necessary to make the orders come alive in the client's system (see Boxes 5–1, 5–2, and 5–3 and Tables 5-1 and 6-2).

An example of nursing orders developed for the client, Mr. Munson, according to the priorities of his needs is given in Table 7-2. Nursing orders are developed for each diagnosis, including objectives and specific actions related to the objectives.

Table 7–2   Nursing Diagnoses, Goals, Objectives, and Orders: Case Example

Nursing Diagnosis	Nursing Goal	Nursing Objectives	Nursing Orders
1. Cardiac output, alterations in: Decreased	To be free of signs and symptoms of cardiac complications	To be free of complications relating to the disease states of MI and diabetes To be free of pain	a. Monitor constantly; be alert for arrhythmias. b. If arrhythmias occur, treat immediately as specified by standing orders and document by running a strip on the monitor; CALL FOR A PHYSICIAN STAT. c. Monitor vital signs QH; be alert for changes. d. Listen to lungs for signs of congestion, QID. e. Be alert for nonverbal signs of chest pain or related pain; check with client frequently. f. Be alert for signs of dyspnea and give oxygen at 4 liters/min PRN.

Table **7-2**   (continued)

Nursing Diagnosis	Nursing Goal	Nursing Objectives	Nursing Orders
			g. Observe skin color and body temperature frequently for flushing or pallor.
			h. Monitor lab reports for signs of abnormalities; if any exist, report them to the physician stat.
			i. Keep an accurate I & O sheet in client's room.
			j. Test urine for S/A AC and HS; give insulin as indicated.
			k. REPORT ALL CHANGES IN CLIENT'S CONDITION TO PROFESSIONAL NURSE IN CHARGE.
2. Knowledge deficit: Effects of drugs and therapeutic regimen	To plan and secure his own safety	To understand the reason for hospitalization in the coronary-care unit To be aware of the purposes of procedures To be aware of his diabetic condition	a. Explain concept of coronary-care unit to client; if feasible, give him a tour of the unit or show him pictures. b. Familiarize him with all the equipment in his room and with how it works, emphasizing the purposes of each piece; carry this out in small steps. c. Explain rationale for all care that he will receive: monitor, medications, treatments, I & O, S/A test, diabetic diet, visiting hours, and so on. d. Make sure he understands your explanations by encouraging him to respond to your statements.
3. Bowel and bladder elimination: Self-main-tenance*	To continue to privately maintain elimination needs and report any signs of constipation	Not required; goal is sufficient	a. Talk with him regarding the importance of charting I & O and testing urine. b. Find out whether he is interested in caring for these aspects himself.

Table **7-2**   (continued)

Nursing Diagnosis	Nursing Goal	Nursing Objectives	Nursing Orders
			c. If he is, then develop a plan for teaching that moves from your demonstration, to the client doing and being checked, and then to the client's assuming total responsibility himself.
			d. Keep chart of intake measures or equivalents on bedside table.
			e. Keep I & O sheet near client.
			f. Keep all equipment handy.
			g. Be alert for constipation—be sure to check for bowel elimination every day.
			h. Observe inconspicuously for any straining during bowel elimination.
4. Sleep pattern disturbance	To be assured of adequate rest amid coronary-care procedures and environment	Not required; goal is sufficient	a. Administer medications on time—Valium.
			b. Give sleeping medication if necessary.
			c. Since he is anxious about the hospital, sit and talk with him often—comfortably.
			d. Quietly monitor vital signs at night; try to discover his sleeping patterns, and do not disturb him when he is in deep sleep.
			e. Keep two pillows at bedside within easy reach; he can use these as necessary.
			f. Try to get a feeling for his cycle during the day; learn his periods of rest and activity. Then build treatments and procedures around these times, allowing him to rest when he can.

Table **7-2** (continued)

Nursing Diagnosis	Nursing Goal	Nursing Objectives	Nursing Orders
5. Nutrition, alterations in: Less than body requirements	To ingest balanced nutrients within 2000 calorie diabetic diet	To be free of anorexia To adapt to a special diet To adapt to hospital's food patterns, when necessary	a. Request that his meals be kept warm until he wants to eat or be sent up at 9–2–7; make special arrangements with department head in the kitchen. b. Explain diabetes and the importance of eating well-balanced meals. c. Tell client that you will help him in any way you can so that he receives foods that are in accordance with his likes. d. Obtain food-exchange lists from dietician, and plan meals with client. e. Be aware of whether this plan is working, and make changes accordingly.
6. Anxiety	To have a respectful and trusting relationship so that needs can be discussed with the nurse if they emerge as stressful To have relief from the anxiety that pervades areas of the present situation and environment	Not required; goals are sufficient	a. Spend time sitting down and talking with client. Do not ask questions; rather, respond to his feelings, letting him know that you have heard what he says. b. Let him know when you will be back to talk. c. Always be alert for signs of stress, anxiety, boredom. Note what you see by telling the client that he looks _____ . Listen to what he says in response to your statement. d. ALWAYS RESPOND TO WHAT THE CLIENT IS SAYING; PUT YOUR AGENDA IN THE BACKGROUND.

Table **7-2**   (continued)

Nursing Diagnosis	Nursing Goal	Nursing Objectives	Nursing Orders
7. Knowledge deficit: Environment	To adjust to the environmental limitations by understanding the rationale for the policies in existence	To socialize as much as possible	a. Explain rationale for visiting hours. b. If you do not think that visitors for a longer period of time will harm anyone else in the unit, allow client's visitors to remain as long as possible. Always observe client for signs of fatigue. c. If client is OOB, you might set up chairs in the hall and have the client visit with family and friends there. d. Move client's bed nearer to another client. e. During quiet hours, have client sit in nurse's station, monitored directly by the large receiver.
8. Hygiene: Self-main- tenance*	To be able to maintain his own hygienic measures	To care for himself independently whenever possible To have modesty and privacy respected	a. Allow client to care for his hygiene needs to the degree desired, respecting the exercise or activity level needed for recovery. b. Have all equipment handy for the client. c. Explain why limits are placed on his activity. d. Provide privacy while client is using the commode. e. Be alert for signs of embarrassment in client— blushing, nervousness, slow speech—and intervene by engaging client in conversation aside from what you are doing. Or, mention what you are doing and explain your reasons fully. Do what you feel most comfortable with, respecting the client's needs.

Table **7-2** (continued)

Nursing Diagnosis	Nursing Goal	Nursing Objectives	Nursing Orders
			f. Involve wife in his care if both he and she desire this.
			g. Be discreet in everything you do for the client.
9. Comfort: Self-maintenance*	To continue to maintain his own personal comfort measures	Not required; goal is sufficient	a. Continually be alert for what makes him comfortable and for his favorite manner of having things done; amplify these.
			b. Sit and talk with him concerning things at home that he might like to bring into his room; follow through by having family obtain these items.
			c. Always respond to his likes and dislikes; then respect them!
10. Self-concept, disturbance in: Self-esteem	To have his needs for recognition, affiliation, and privacy met and maintained, as possible	To have client feel self-satisfied by being recognized as needed by others	a. Always notice and verbally respond to what the client has accomplished.
			b. Reinforce positively all aspects of client's growth.
			c. Give client small things to do for himself, you, and other clients. Examples: talk or sit with another client who seems depressed; keep track of visiting hours for himself and others.
			d. Verbalize the positive aspects of the accomplishment of the client—for example, eating better, requiring no extra insulin. Use this also as a way to reinforce teaching areas.

*Approved nursing diagnoses are not available for all the identified diagnoses; an asterisk next to the diagnosis denotes that it has not yet been approved.

SOURCE: *Classification of Nursing Diagnoses: Proceedings of the Fifth National Conference,* by M. J. Kim, G. McFarland, and A. McLane (Eds.). St. Louis: C. V. Mosby, 1984. Also published in Carpenito, L. *Nursing diagnosis: Application to clinical practice.* Philadelphia: J. B. Lippincott, 1983.

Some readers may think that the amount of detail in the nursing diagnoses, goals, objectives, and orders shown in Chapters 6 and 7 is not feasible given the time constraints of nursing practice. Anxiety may increase when questioning the practicality of such an account. The specific purpose of such detail, however, *is to assist the learner* of nursing practice. Most of the orders are within the realm of practice for the experienced nurse, thereby making the orders automatic areas of response, which are then individualized for the client. For the practicing nurse, therefore, the detail shown can serve as a reinforcer and a review.

SUMMARY

Chapter 7 has focused on the cognitive aspects of nursing objectives and orders. This area forms the bulk of a nursing-care plan and should contain behavioral statements concerning what is needed to bring the client toward goal accomplishment and diagnosis eradication. The creative process was emphasized as a means for providing the nurse with a tool to develop nursing care that is truly individualized. The case example followed throughout Part II of the book was further developed to include objectives and orders for each diagnosis. Chapter 8 focuses on another procedure for recording nursing care.

REFERENCES

Bloom, B. (Ed.). (1954). *The taxonomy of objectives.* New York: Longmans, Green.

Brainerd, S. (1971). *A curriculum for an aesthetic program for teacher education.* Doctoral dissertation, University of Massachusetts, School of Education, Amherst.

Carpenito, L. (1983). *Nursing diagnosis: Application to clinical practice.* Philadelphia: Lippincott.

Ciuca, R. (1972). Over the years with the nursing care plan. *Nursing Outlook, 20,* 706–711.

Eisenman, R. (1970). Creativity in student nurses: A cross-sectional and longitudinal study. *Developmental Psychology, 3,* 320–325.

Eisenman, R. (1972). Creativity in student nurses and their attitudes toward mental illness and physical disability. *Journal of Clinical Psychology, 28,* 218–219.

Forman, M. (1979). Building a better nursing care plan. *American Journal of Nursing, 79,* 1086–1087.

Grey, J., & Aldred, H. (1980). Care plans in long-term facilities. *American Journal of Nursing, 80,* 2054–2057.

Harris, B. (1970). Who needs written care plans anyhow? *American Journal of Nursing, 70,* 2136–2138.

Instructor teaches students creativity in nursing care. (1981). *The American Nurse, 13,* 12.

Kelly, N. (1966). Nursing care plans. *Nursing Outlook, 14,* 61–64.

Kershaw, J. (1979). Teaching the nursing process: Standard care plans. *Nursing Times,* August 16, 75, 1413–1416.

Kim, M. J., McFarland, G., & McLane, A. (Eds.). (1984). *Classification of nursing diagnoses: Proceedings of the fifth national conference.* St. Louis: Mosby.

Little, D., & Carnevali, D. (1967). Nursing care plans: Let's be practical about them. *Nursing Forum, 6,* 61–67.

Mackie, L. (1979). Revitalizing the nursing care plan. *Nursing Times,* August 23, 75, 1440–1442.

Mager, R. (1975). *Preparing instructional objectives* (2nd ed.). Belmont, CA: Fearon.

McNeil, J. (1973). *The creative process.* Unpublished paper, University of Massachusetts, Center for the Study of Aesthetics in Education, Amherst.

National Council of State Boards of Nursing (1982). *Test Plan for the National Council Licensure Examination for Registered Nurses.* Chicago: Author.

Palisin, H. (1971). Nursing care plans are a snare and a delusion. *American Journal of Nursing, 71*, 63–66.

Smith, D. (1971). Writing objectives as a nursing practice skill. *American Journal of Nursing, 71*, 319–320.

Vasey, E. (1979). Writing your patient's care plan . . . efficiently. *Nursing '79, 9*, 67–71.

Wagner, B. (1969). Care plans: Right, reasonable, and reachable. *American Journal of Nursing, 69*, 986–990.

SELECTED READING

This article by Smith provides additional guidelines and discussion on writing nursing objectives. The emphasis is on specifically stating the objectives for client behaviors. Smith also talks about articulating what the nurse must do to assist the client to achieve the stated objectives.

Writing Objectives as a Nursing Practice Skill

Dorothy M. Smith

Objectives for patient care should be written as expected patient behaviors, "The patient will circle those foods that are not appropriate on his low sodium diet," and not as personnel behavior, "Encourage fluids," says this author. Such objectives can guide nurses to where they are going in patient care and let them know when and where they have arrived, she maintains.

In the preface to his book *Preparing Instructional Objectives*, Mager tells a story of a sea horse who set out to find his fortune. On the way, he met other sea creatures who promised him a speedier trip by selling him different methods of transportation and short cuts. His last short cut took him into the mouth of a shark, and he was devoured. Mager says the moral of the fable is that if you don't know where you are going, you are liable to end up somewhere else and not even know it (1).

Commonly used words to express "where are you going" are "goal," "objective," "end," "intention," "aim." In a previous article describing a tool for collecting data and planning care, I used the word "goal" (2). Subsequent work indicates that the word "objective" seems to be easier for staff and students to use. "Setting objectives" is a familiar phrase in education and there is much literature on the value of behavioral objectives.

Since the client of nursing is the patient, I believe the objectives of nursing must be stated in terms of patient behavior. Then evaluation

of practice (did you get to where you were going) consists of finding out whether the objectives were attained. Objectives of this kind can be narrow, concrete, specific, and unambiguous and clearly communicate intent to all members of the staff and to the patient and his family.

Such objectives are developed from data obtained from the patient as well as from nursing knowledge. They are developed with the patient and within the context of the patient's healthy and pathological states of body and mind. Thus, the objectives and the methods or strategies for achieving them are generally a series of compromises between ideal and real, known and unknown, and predictable and unpredictable (relatively sure and relatively unsure). This article will not deal with these compromises but rather with the skill that is needed to express "where you are going" in terms of patient behavior.

Writing objectives as expected patient behavior and in a way that makes evaluation possible is a difficult task. There is a tendency to write too broadly; for example, "The patient will accept his illness," or, "The patient will understand his diagnostic tests."

There is also a tendency to confuse objectives with standards. Standards are predetermined criteria for nursing care all patients have a right to expect. Standards are derived at best from research, although some may develop from long-standing unvalidated experience. Objectives are more individualized. Nevertheless, in the course of time, today's objectives may become tomorrow's standards.

Often objectives, regrettably, are expressed as personnel behavior—"to give emotional support to the patient," or "to encourage fluids," or "to teach the patient how to give his own insulin." We believe that the behavior (technical, interpersonal, and cognitive) of personnel reflects educational, professional, and institutional objectives and standards and cannot be used as a direct measure of nursing practice objectives.

The inability to reach a nursing practice objective with a patient may be traced back to human error, negligence, ignorance, an inadequate system or procedure, or to any number of factors. But evaluating any of these factors in and of themselves does not constitute measurement of nursing practice objectives for a patient.

Personnel may perform tasks superbly, but end up in the shark's interior. On the reverse side, the state of our science and art is such that we sometimes reach the objective in spite of potentially dangerous, intuitive efforts carried on in a seemingly disorganized and unsystematic fashion. We must learn to analyze why we got where we wanted to go or why we did not get there.

EXAMPLES

The following examples of objectives are stated as expected patient behavior. Since these are real objectives for real patients, we have evidence of rationale for the objectives (data and knowledge). However, here we are concerned not with the appropriateness of the objective but with the statement of the objectives: Is the intent of the journey clear, and can we tell if we got there?

- The patient will measure his own intake and output and record it as instructed.
- The patient will demonstrate three types of antepartal exercises and state the purpose of each during each clinic visit.
- The patient has moist mouth and lips as evidenced by absence of furring on the tongue and dryness and caking of the lips.

- The patient will sleep more comfortably at night as evidenced by a decrease in the number of episodes of shortness of breath from 2300 to 0700 hours.
- When requested, the patient will list in writing from memory those foods that are not appropriate on a low sodium diet.
- Each morning, the patient will circle, from a list of foods, those that are appropriate on his low calorie diet.
- The patient will discuss with his nurse the statement that he repeated several times during the initial interview, "The wife is living a lonely life while I am in the hospital."
- The patient will discuss her labor experience with the nurse at 1400 hours.

Some of our staff prefer, "The patient is able. . . ." I prefer the stark "will." Greenwood says:

> The scientist's prime aim is the description of the social world; the practitioner's prime aim is the control of that world (3).

FEELINGS ABOUT CONTROL

Nursing practitioners are seeking control. We apply knowledge for control; for the best, we hope. The word "control" may frighten some readers.

Principles of control, based on scientific knowledge, must be related to the patient, to his feelings, his perception, and his condition. Control is involved, and to deny this is to deny nursing practice itself.

Objectives are discussed with the patients (and families when appropriate), as are the methods to be employed. The patient's responsibilities and the nursing responsibilities are defined. Progress notes related to specific objectives are charted. When appropriate (with new data and knowledge), objectives are discontinued, or modified, and new ones added. It is interesting to note that the following kinds of comments were made when objectives, as described in this article, were discussed with nurses:

- We have objectives. We just cannot put them into words.

- Doing things and getting the work done is so important that there is no time for anything else.

- If I were to do this (that is, set objectives) my staff would feel that I was letting them down, because I was not out helping them.

- You cannot tell a patient what the objectives are. He will get too involved, and he needs all his energy to get well.

- There is only one objective—to care for the whole patient. More objectives will only fragment the patient.

- That stuff is for students—maybe—but it is not practical when you are dealing with life and death.

- It is not possible, because patients are individuals and you cannot have a system with individuals, only with things.

- It is real interesting, but we could not do anything like that in our agency because they would not let us.

- You will never measure nursing. It is too intangible and personal.

Such feelings and thoughts are not necessarily shared by all or even a majority of nurses. In answer to such comments I say both to these nurses and to myself, because we all have some of these feelings some of the time, that it is imperative that nursing find some way to show to ourselves and the public and our colleagues in the health field that our practice is socially useful, worthwhile, tangible, and measurable.

"Nurses are such wonderful people," is not enough. Education, in and of itself, is not enough. Hard work is not enough. We must begin to measure in a systematic way what we accomplish for and with patients, and we must put this into words that can be understood. Perhaps this way is not *the* way to do it. What suggestions do you have for keeping us out of the shark's stomach (and not even knowing we are there)?

REFERENCES

1. Mager, R. F. *Preparing Instructional Objectives.* Palo Alto, Calif., Fearon Publishers, 1962, p. vii.

2. Smith, Dorothy M. Clinical nursing tool. *American Journal of Nursing,* 68:2384–2388, Nov. 1968.

3. Greenwood, Ernest. Practice of science and the science of practice. In *Planning for Change,* ed. by Warren E. Bennis and others. New York, Holt, Rinehart and Winston, 1961, p. 74.

Chapter 8

Problem-Oriented Records

This chapter is devoted to the definition and description of problem-oriented records. The steps of the problem-oriented record (POR) system are parallel to the steps of the nursing process and the scientific method, underscoring the importance of this system in ensuring quality health care for the consumer. In using the POR, the methods discussed previously are essential; data collection, data processing, nursing diagnoses, and nursing orders all become elements of the POR. The nurse takes these methods, combines them with skills and competencies, and follows a specific format to yield a POR designed to enhance individualized, quality, client care. In this chapter, the protocol for the problem-oriented system is elaborated, followed by the advantages and disadvantages of its usage. The POR method presented in this chapter is used in many inpatient health facilities and is widely applied in outpatient community-health agencies (Mayers, 1983). Even if this specific method is not currently used in your facility, it is a valuable method to understand.

PROBLEM-ORIENTED RECORDS DEFINED

There is some debate about whether the problem-oriented approach is simply a standardized procedure for record keeping or whether it is a scientific and philosophic approach in health care. The term *problem-oriented records* seems to connote the former—a procedure for record keeping—but a careful study of the concept behind the system connotes the latter, a scientific and philosophic approach. In actuality, the POR system constitutes a combination of both schools of thought. Lawrence Weed (1970) developed a method of using the POR that captures the combination of record keeping and philosophy. Weed began with the scientific method, applied it to medical/health care, and delineated a standard, written format for communicating with colleagues. Of course, the POR is new neither in nursing nor in any other science; what is new, however, is the standardized procedure for communicating in writing and the instant recognition of POR as a formalized procedure. Anyone who is familiar with and committed to using Weed's method follows a specific protocol using proper language; it is designed for universal understanding. Perhaps this can be considered a milestone in health-care record keeping and, specifically, nursing record keeping.

Problem-oriented records involve both an application of the scientific method in health care and a logical, succinct system of record keeping. The POR incorporates a philosophic base mandating that clients be helped systematically and holistically. It defies fragmentation of care or the studying of patient problems as mutually exclusive. Built into the record-keeper system, moreover, is the means by which different professionals can concern themselves with select problems; the interaction of the many facets of client care is portrayed directly and clearly in the charting procedure. Further, POR aids in the documentation of both nursing and medical diagnoses (Fredette, 1984).

In addition to being a landmark in coordinating care for patients, POR is also revolutionizing the education of health practitioners and the evaluation of health services (Schell & Campbell, 1972). Properly used, the POR method permits a learner to visualize the inductive and deductive reasoning that leads a health practitioner to particular conclusions; to conceptualize the rationale for all actions; and to study a whole person. Thus, evaluation of care can be based on complete retrospective data as well as on the alleviation of client problems through specific actions. POR therefore encourages greater quality in client care as well as more thorough evaluation of care (Yura & Walsh, 1983).

Even though the term *problem-oriented records* is a descriptive phrase coined by Lawrence Weed for the medical profession, the procedural system has been applied to all health caregivers. The specific POR system developed by Weed has been adapted for use on nursing records in hospitals and other community agencies (Bloom, Dressler, Kenny, Molbo, & Pardee, 1971; Bonkowsky, 1972; Bower, 1982; Carnevali, 1983; Marriner, 1983; Sundeen, Stuart, Rankin, & Cohen, 1981) and is used in private and group professional offices and outpatient clinics, with all professionals writing on one record.

Parallels between the nursing process, the scientific method, and the POR can be drawn as shown in Figure 8-1. All these methods are dynamic, and the evaluative facets of each create new data that begin the process again.

PROTOCOL OF PROBLEM-ORIENTED RECORDS

The procedure used in POR, as developed by Weed (1970), has four essential parts: data base, problem list, initial plans, and progress notes. These four dimensions form the client's whole chart.

Figure 8–1

Parallels between the Nursing Process, the Scientific Method, and Problem-Oriented Records

Nursing Process	Scientific Method	Problem-Oriented Records
	Problem Finding	
Data collection ⟶	1. Gathering information ←	
	2. Examining information ←	Data base
Data processing ⟶	3. Interpreting information ←	
Nursing diagnosis ⟶	4. Identifying problem(s) ←	
	5. Stating the problem(s) ←	Problem list
	Problem Solving	
	1. Developing alternatives ←	
Nursing orders ⟶	2. Making a decision ←	
	3. Deciding on a plan of action ←	Plan of care
Implementation ⟶	4. Executing the plan of action ←	
Evaluation ⟶	5. Evaluating the results ←	
	6. Redefining problem and change ←	Progress notes

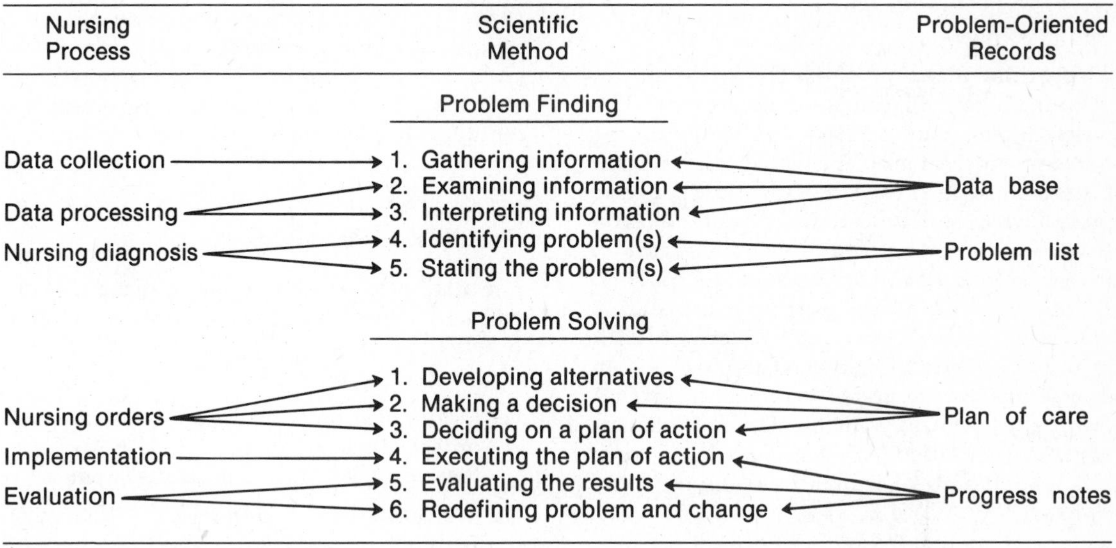

Data Base

The data base parallels the assessment phase of the nursing process. According to Weed (1970), the data base section includes the client's profile, history, physical, and laboratory reports. Usually, these four aspects of data are gathered on standardized forms. They are predefined as essential, and it is guaranteed that these data will be obtained for every client.

The nature of the nurse's input on this record varies, depending on the structure of the organization. If a nurse is a practitioner in a group practice, the nurse may have the responsibility for obtaining all aspects of data on the client's initial visit to the facility. Should POR be used in nursing units only by nurses, then the record is adapted to address only areas of nursing responsibility. The responsibilities of the professional nurse, therefore, reflect the purpose for which the POR is used and the structure of the group using it.

Problem List

The problem list corresponds to the nursing diagnoses, the result of analyzing and processing the data. The problem list is a numbered and titled list on which is included every problem the client has or ever has had. Weed (1970) defined the problem list as anything that requires management or diagnostic workup, including social and psychological problems. It is a dynamic list, with problems being resolved, added, or clarified. This part of the chart provides a quick reference on the client's overall health state. As can be seen, Weed's definition is interpreted to include nursing problems or diagnoses. Recalling the definition of nursing diagnoses—actual or potential health problems of clients—one can see a close parallel to the problem list.

Depending again on the purposes for which the POR is used, both medical and nursing diagnoses should be included in the problem list unless the record is only for nursing use; then, only nursing diagnoses are charted.

Initial Plans

The initial plans of the POR parallel the planning phase of the nursing process. The plans contain items corresponding in identifying number with the problems listed on the POR; plans include diagnostic, therapeutic (drugs and procedures), and educational aspects of care, relative to each problem. The plans are, in essence, the orders—both medical and nursing.

When medicine and nursing professionals are using the same chart, orders relative to each problem are listed together. This provides an easy guide to integrated care, assuring that comprehensiveness is maintained and relevant expertise is unified. All health workers' input follows this pattern, if they are using the same chart.

Progress Notes

The progress notes of the POR parallel the implementation and evaluation phases of the nursing process. These notes are written, as are the others, by everyone involved in the client's care and are identified by a number that corresponds to the problem and plan in focus. A specific format is followed, with the writer stating the date, time, problem name, and problem number in the chart. As physicians, nurses, or any other professional sees the client, he or she comments on the problem in focus in the progress notes. Obviously, all professionals do not comment on all of the problems; rather, they comment on those within their professional domain and areas of expertise. Thus, there is room for specialization in POR, and the specialists always can conceptualize the whole plan by perusing the chart. The specific format (SOAP) for writing progress notes is shown in Table 8-1; the example is a diagnosis from the case used in previous chapters.

This format—organizing by Subjective information, Objective information, Assessment,

and Projected course to follow (SOAP)—places emphasis on unresolved problems, with those already resolved being evaluated briefly (Weed, 1970). Progress notes provide the base for adding, altering, or deleting items from the problem list and orders (plan). Flow sheets and discharge notes relative to each problem are contained in the progress notes.

ADVANTAGES OF PROBLEM-ORIENTED RECORDS

The attributes of the POR system and method are many. Weed (1970) focused primarily on the benefits in medical dimensions; these are adapted here to nursing:

1. Different professional disciplines converge on specified outcomes of health care that focus on the entire client and system.

2. The POR is somewhat like a dictionary, with all individuals involved in the care having quick access to all aspects of the plan; all professionals involved use the same language and procedures for communicating.

3. Nurses, allied health workers, and physicians can see what they have done and learn from what others have done and observed; thus, education is underscored.

4. Clinical research is facilitated by the completeness of the records.

5. Quality of care is easily audited with deficiencies, if any, surfacing clearly.

6. All aspects of the client and system are respected and given attention.

7. The interactions of problems may become more apparent.

8. Satisfaction regarding outcomes is increased because of the visibility of progress.

9. Health-team members are able to work truly as a team—collaboratively.

10. Client data are shared by all involved health workers.

Table **8–1**   Problem-Oriented Records: Procedure for Writing Progress Notes

Nursing Diagnosis: Nutrition, alterations in: Less than body requirements	
Step	Examples of Each Step
(S) *Subjective Information*	
Description of symptoms by client	Client does not like the food sent by kitchen; he refuses to eat meals since they are not in line with his usual eating patterns. Client states that he feels anxious.
Feelings of client	
Concerns of client	
(O) *Objective Information*	
Observations of nurse, physician, others	Client has a daily caloric deficit. Insulin administration is not regulated; urine sugar and acetone levels fluctuate considerably.
What was done for client	
Results of tests and objective parameters	
(A) *Assessment*	
Record the professional's judgment, thinking, and opinion on the problem	Client is not eating a balanced diet, given diabetic condition; unregulated insulin needs.
(P) *Projected course to follow*	
Determine whether consultation is necessary	1. Request that his meals be kept warm until he wants to eat or be sent up at 9–2–7; make special arrangements with the department head in food services.
	2. Explain diabetes and the importance of eating well-balanced meals.
	3. Tell client that you will help in any way you can so that he receives foods that are in accordance with his likes.
	4. Obtain food-exchange lists from dietician, and plan meals with client.
	5. Be aware of whether this plan is working and make changes accordingly.

DISADVANTAGES OF PROBLEM-ORIENTED RECORDS

Although the disadvantages are few in comparison to the advantages, they are worthy of mention:

1. Education of all involved health-care workers regarding the procedures of POR can be lengthy.

2. The record system, if done inadequately, may expose practitioners to criticism from colleagues (Schell & Campbell, 1972). Even though the nursing audit is educational, it can also be threatening.

3. The system is only as good as the practitioners; if the client is viewed as merely a "problem" or a "disease," the POR system will do nothing to change this fragmentation of a person.

Careful use of the POR, as well as careful respect and attention paid to all involved persons, can minimize or eliminate these disadvantages, however.

SUMMARY

Chapter 8 looked at the problem-oriented record, both as a scientific method of health care and as a standard procedure for record keeping. The protocol of the POR was delineated, followed by discussion of the advantages and disadvantages of the system. The next Part of the book focuses on implementing nursing care according to the level of maturity of the client and the nurse and according to the skills necessary to accomplish each facet of care.

REFERENCES

Bloom, J., Dressler, J., Kenny, M., Molbo, D., & Pardee, G. (1971). Problem oriented charting. *American Journal of Nursing, 71,* 2144–2148.

Bonkowsky, M. (1972). Adapting the POMR to community child health care. *Nursing Outlook, 20,* 515–518.

Bower, F. (1982). *The process of planning nursing care: Nursing practice models* (3rd. ed.). St. Louis: Mosby.

Carnevali, D. (1983). *Nursing care planning: Diagnosis and management* (3rd ed.). Philadelphia: Lippincott.

Fredette, S. (1984). When the liver fails. *American Journal of Nursing, 84,* 64–67.

Marriner, A. (1983). *The nursing process: A scientific approach to nursing care* (3rd ed.). St. Louis: Mosby.

Mayers, M. (1983). *A systematic approach to the nursing care plan* (3rd. ed.). Norwalk, CT: Appleton-Century-Crofts.

Schell, P., & Campbell, A. (1972). POMR—Not just another way to chart. *Nursing Outlook, 8,* 510–514.

Sundeen, S., Stuart, G., Rankin, E., & Cohen, S. (1981). *Nurse-client interaction: Implementing the nursing process* (2nd ed.). St. Louis: Mosby.

Weed, L. (1970). *Medical records, medical education, and patient care.* Cleveland: Press of Case Western Reserve University.

Yura, H., & Walsh, M. (1983). *The nursing process: Assessing, planning, implementing, evaluating* (4th ed.). Norwalk, CT: Appleton-Century-Crofts.

SELECTED READING

This article by Fredette provides an excellent example of nursing care and its documentation using the SOAP procedure.

When the Liver Fails

Sheila La Fortune Fredette

Liver failure can mean anything from the discomfort of ascites to the crisis of hemorrhage. Knowledge of underlying pathophysiology is the key to effective nursing diagnosis.

Understanding how the liver works—or fails to work—is basic to anticipating problems associated with acute liver dysfunction. Understanding those problems in terms of treatable nursing diagnoses can enhance your ability to care for patients effectively.

Various personal, environmental and health factors are responsible for liver destruction. Alcoholism, for example, is a major cause of liver failure, as is drug abuse. Most prescription, nonprescription, and illicit drugs are detoxified in the liver, and long-term unmonitored use can destroy cells. Furthermore, it has been suggested that some environmental pollutants and chemicals adversely affect liver cells.

Liver damage, frequently masked until 80 percent of the organ is destroyed, has many implications for both medical and nursing regimens. For example, the patient with congestion of the liver associated with chronic congestive heart failure is prone to digitalis toxicity because destroyed liver cells fail to detoxify daily doses of digitalis. A liver that improperly metabolizes anesthetic or analgesic agents can cause death if too much of these unmetabolized central nervous system depressants accumulate.

Nursing diagnoses are based on manifestations of underlying pathophysiology. Usually, several pathophysiological factors act together to cause one or more clinical problems. Likewise, more than one nursing diagnosis can be derived from one set of clinical data. Nursing diagnoses in liver dysfunction can include any of the following:

- alterations in nutrition,
- risk of infection,*
- alterations in tissue perfusion,
- potential for injury with bleeding tendency,
- impaired skin integrity,
- alterations in cardiac output,
- alterations in comfort,
- alterations in thought processes, specifically cognitive impairment.

The problem-oriented approach—recording subjective (S) and objective (O) client data, the nurse's assessment (A) or interpretation of the data, and the intervention plan (P)—aids in documenting nursing diagnoses.

Alterations in Nutrition. When liver cells fail, deficiencies can occur in carbohydrate, fat, and protein metabolism. Deficiencies in the liver's ability to convert amino acids into glucose (glyconeogenesis), to store excess glucose (glycogenesis), and to release stored glucose as needed (gluconeolysis) result in erratic serum glucose levels. The inability of dysfunctional liver cells to carry on the many

*This diagnosis is not among those accepted for clinical testing by the National Task Force on the Classification of Nursing Diagnoses.

fat interconversions, plus the lack of sufficient bile to emulsify fats so they can be absorbed, cause a fat deficiency. Protein deficiency can result in anemia that will be exaggerated by bleeding and by the liver's inability to store iron and vitamin B_{12}.

Further, anorexia is a major problem for the patient with liver dysfunction. Decreased food intake couples with impaired absorption and storage of nutrients (including fat-soluble vitamins A, D, E and K) to deprive body cells of nutrients. Once begun, the cycle of anorexia is difficult to break.

The SOAP Approach

- Subjective data: Complaint of weakness and fatigue.
- Objective data: Weight loss of 20 lb in 6 months; loss of muscle mass, evidenced by emaciation and flabby skin; dull hair; pallor; low hemoglobin; macrocytosis.
- Assessment (nursing diagnosis): Nutritional deficit related to anorexia and to faulty absorption, metabolism, and storage of nutrients.
- Plan (nursing): Maintain nutrient intake at or above body requirements, using the following strategies:

Take a diet history to determine food preferences.

Accurately count calories (including intravenous calories).

Make sure calorie intake is at least 1,200 per day to prevent breakdown of tissue protein. Suggest tube feedings if patient cannot eat enough.

Offer mouth care prior to meals.

Encourage small, frequent feedings.

Provide emotional support; e.g., stay with client during meals or have your meal at bedside with client.

Request vitamin and mineral supplements.

- Plan (medical): Diet prescribed depends on clinical state; usually high carbohydrate, moderate fat, and high protein—unless ammonia levels rise, indicating a need for protein restriction.

Risk for Infection. * The liver plays an important role in preventing infection. Phagocytic functions are carried out by the Kupffer's cells that line venous channels of the liver. These cells remove up to 99 percent of the bacteria in venous blood (1). When one considers the colon bacilli and other debris in intestinal blood, this phagocytic function assumes added significance.

Any impairment in the ability of the Kupffer's cell to filter the venous blood places the client in danger of infection.

The SOAP Approach

- Subjective data: History of many or chronic and slow-healing infections.
- Objective data: Negative for signs of current new infection.
- Assessment (nursing diagnosis): Risk for infection* related to compromised state induced by deficient immunological system.
- Plan (nursing): To prevent the development of infection by such measures as reverse isolation and control of patient's contact with others during acute illness; meticulous attention to handwashing and other medical asepsis.

To detect any signs of infection (skin, urinary, respiratory) early through careful observation, such as chest auscultation every shift to evaluate respiratory status.
- Plan (medical): Antibiotics and respiratory therapy may be prescribed.

Alteration in Tissue Perfusion and Potential Impairment of Skin Integrity. Four factors—ascites, generalized edema, nutritional deficits, and blood loss—work together to cause inadequate tissue perfusion.

The clinical symptoms of ascites and gen-

---

*This diagnosis is not among those accepted for clinical testing by the National Task Force on the Classification of Nursing Diagnoses.

eralized edema have three separate, yet related, causes: portal hypertension, faulty protein metabolism, and inadequate detoxification of chemicals. Portal hypertension results from obstruction of the normal flow of blood and lymph. This increase of hydrostatic pressure within the blood vessels forces fluid out through blood vessel walls. As cells within the liver become engorged, fluid transudes through the liver surface into the abdominal cavity. Also, as hepatic venous pressure rises, fluid and protein solutes are forced into the lymphatic system, and lymph flow can increase greatly. This fluid is nearly pure plasma with a colloid osmotic pressure greater than extracellular fluid, thus drawing even more fluid into the abdominal cavity.

Leakage of fluid through blood vessel walls is further exaggerated because the liver is less able to synthesize the protein, albumin. When serum albumin levels fall, the colloidal osmotic pressure of plasma falls, and fluid exits through blood vessel walls. Any fall in protein intake further reduces albumin levels and exacerbates fluid leakage.

A sick liver that cannot detoxify aldosterone and antidiuretic hormone—the body's normal water regulators—further adds to the problem of water retention throughout the body. Normal perfusion of gases through the waterlogged cells is inefficient, resulting in hypoxia (which may be complicated further by impaired breathing due to the ascites or by impaired gas exchange related to pulmonary edema). Tissue hypoxia can also lead to impaired skin integrity.

The SOAP Approach

• Subjective data: complaints of feeling bloated, being unable to find a comfortable position, having difficulty breathing.
• Objective data: Increased abdominal girth; weight gain; pitting edema in feet and ankles; redness over sacral and hip areas; moist rales, labored breathing; slowed capillary refill time; hemoptysis; positive guaiac stool test; reduced hematocrit and hemoglobin.

• Assessment (nursing diagnosis): Inadequate tissue perfusion and potential impairment in skin integrity related to ascites, edema, bleeding, nutritional deficits, albumin deficiency.
• Plan (nursing): To relieve discomfort of ascites, position on side with head elevated and pillow supporting intercostals.

To assess ascites, measure abdominal girth and weight daily, and measure intake and output.

To prevent skin breakdown, use alternating pressure mattress; turn patient, inspect and care for pressure areas q2h; at least once each shift, check all skin surfaces.

During hemorrhage, use the usual interventions to monitor and control bleeding, plus energy-conserving measures, including complete bed rest and physical care.

For pulmonary edema, follow usual respiratory interventions.
• Plan (medical): Usually includes prescription for oxygen, blood, diuretics, salt-poor albumin, electrolyte replacement.

Bleeding Tendency* and Potential Alteration in Cardiac Output.   Diseases of the liver can so depress the formation of prothrombin, fibrinogen, and other clotting factors that the patient develops a tendency to bleed. A superimposed deficiency of fat-soluble vitamin K, common in liver disease, only contributes to the problem.

Existing portal hypertension associated with liver disease can lead first to venous distention, then to varices, and eventually to ruptured vessels. The rupture can be of small collateral venous channels established to disperse the excess fluid, or major blood vessels in the esophagus, stomach, or intestines may rupture.

Blood loss, either cumulative (in the case of slow bleeding) or spontaneous with massive hemorrhage, will of course alter cardiac output.

---

*This diagnosis is not among those accepted for clinical testing by the National Task Force on the Classification of Nursing Diagnoses.

The SOAP Approach

• Subjective data: Complaints of weakness, hemoptysis, bloody stools.

• Objective data: Pallor, dyspnea, petechiae, prolonged prothrombin time, drop in hemoglobin and hematocrit, bleeding from any body orifice or injection site, tachycardia, hypotension.

Assessment (nursing diagnosis): Bleeding tendency* related to reduced synthesis of prothrombin, portal hypertension, or both.

• Plan (nursing): Reduce the risk of bleeding by such measures as the following:

Observe for bleeding, including guaiac tests of stool and emesis.

Request stool softener.

Avoid giving coarse foods.

Insert rectal thermometer and suction tube gently, if they become necessary because of a decrease in level of consciousness.

Use measures to prevent skin breakdown.

Administer oxygen as needed for dyspnea and during any massive bleeding; reduce metabolic demands for oxygen by bed rest.

• Plan (medical): Prescriptions will usually include blood, antacids, vitamin K, gentle cathartic, bland diet, oxygen.

Alteration in Thought Processes. The liver's inability to metabolize protein has implications beyond nutritional deficits. Because the liver cannot convert ammonia (the end product of amino acid metabolism) into urea, blood ammonia rises. Ammonia is extremely toxic, especially to the brain, often leading to hepatic coma (2).

The rise in blood ammonia will be further aggravated when portal hypertension causes GI bleeding. When GI bleeding has occurred, intestinal bacteria will hydrolyze the patient's own blood proteins into amino acids and then deaminize them. As this ammonia is absorbed, the blood ammonia levels rise further.

In addition, when a fibrotic liver blocks the flow of blood, much of the ammonia never reaches the liver cells for deamination to urea. In some patients these factors—portal hypertension leading to gastrointestinal bleeding and faulty protein deamination—can combine to cause extremely high ammonia levels that severely alter thought processes. In addition, any hypoxia from blood loss can further impair mental function.

The SOAP Approach

• Subjective data: Speech or behavior that indicates loss of memory, confabulation, hallucinations, disorientation, confusion.

• Objective data: Variation on a mental assessment scale; disorientation to time, person, or place; aimless wandering, combative behavior; liver flap, elevation of blood ammonia, elevation of blood urea nitrogen.

• Assessment (nursing diagnosis): Alteration in thought processes related to faulty protein metabolism, bleeding in the gastrointestinal tract, or hypoxia.

• Plan (nursing): Assess level of consciousness or degree of coma.

Try to raise level of consciousness in the semiconscious or comatose patient; for example, if you get a reflex response, repeat it, trying to elicit a stronger response.

Protective devices as necessary.

• Plan (medical): Prescriptions may include enemas to remove blood in gastrointestinal tract, antibiotics to reduce intestinal flora, and dietary protein restriction.

Alteration in Comfort and Impairment of Skin Integrity. Liver enzymes usually convert bilirubin (an end product of normal red blood cell destruction) into a water-soluble form that is excreted. Faulty processing of bilirubin results in an accumulation of serum bilirubin that spills over into the extra-cellular fluid, tissues, and urine. Pruritus from bile salt deposits can lead to skin breakdown.

The SOAP Approach

• Subjective data: Complaints of persistent itchiness.
• Objective data: Restlessness, scratching, rubbing arms and legs on bed linen, jaundice, dark urine, elevated bilirubin, clay-colored stool.
• Assessment (nursing diagnosis): Discomfort and impairment of skin integrity related to jaundice and pruritus.
• Plan (nursing): Keep skin moist by using tepid water or emollient baths; avoid soap; frequently apply emollient lotions.

To reduce risk of skin damage, cut patient's nails short; wrap comatose patient's hands.

Treat any skin lesion promptly to prevent infection.

Assess need for PRN antihistamines.
• Plan (medical): Antihistamines and tranquilizers may be prescribed, but with caution and in lowered doses as they are metabolized by the liver.

OTHER DIAGNOSES

Any number of nursing diagnoses may apply for a patient with a dysfunctional liver, and each diagnosis can be worked through in the manner presented above. Among those commonly recognized are:

Sexual dysfunction related to retention of estrogens (in the male)

Anxiety related to the stress of illness and hospitalization

Fluid and electrolyte disturbances* related to edema and to nutritional deficiency

Disturbance in self-concept related to ascites and jaundice

Impaired physical mobility related to weakness or confusion

Self-care deficit related to hypoxia or cognitive impairment

Ineffective individual or family coping related to alcoholism

Knowledge deficit about recovery and prevention of exacerbation related to lack of information.

Nursing diagnoses are a method of documenting nursing practice based on sound theoretical knowledge. Such diagnostic nursing judgments lead to a logical plan of care that can be followed by all nurses.

REFERENCES

1. Dappas, Attallah, and Alvares, Alvito. How the liver metabolizes foreign substances. *Sci. Am.* 232:22, June 1975.
2. Guyton, A. C. *Textbook of Medical Physiology.* 6th ed. Philadelphia, W. B. Saunders Co., 1981.

---

*This diagnosis is not among those accepted for clinical testing by the National Task Force on the Classification of Nursing Diagnoses.

Humanistic Exercises

Exercise 9
The Nursing-Care Plan

Purposes

1. To practice developing rationally based nursing diagnoses and orders using case material.
2. To develop succinctness and clarity in writing comprehensive nursing-care plans.

Facility

Writing space and areas where groups of four can share.

Materials

Worksheet A: Nursing-Care Plan
Paper and pencils.

Time Required

One hour.

Group Size

Unlimited groups of four.

Physiologic Data
42 years old
male
c/o occipital lobe headaches
dizziness
excess thirst
frequent urination
malaise—symptoms of 6 months' duration
gained 20 lbs
5'6", 200 lbs
tonsillectomy at age 12 in South Carolina
allergic to Penicillin
tetanus booster, 1972
polio booster, 1968
regular diet

Psychologic Data
feels he has blood pressure problems
feels healthy
pressure on job (auto assembly-line foreman)
difficulty sleeping
feels anxious (smoking 1 to 3 packs/day; liquor intake is moderate)
eats and smokes when "uptight"
has no hobbies except keeping up house and yard
feels pressured to get better and go back to work

Sociologic Data
married
no previous hospitalizations
five children (ages 16, 12, 10, 8, 6—3 boys, 2 girls)
bills all over—unable to pay
Protestant
served four years in the army

Sociologic Data (continued)

works 40 hours/week

owns home—1 bath, 3 bedrooms

lives in suburbia

high school education

income $8500/year

oldest child of four siblings

brother—age 40, L & W, S. Carolina

sister—38, diabetes since age 12

brother—30, OK

father—died of heart disease and hypertension at 68

mother—64, L & W

wife prepares food

gets up at 5:30 A.M. and has four cups of coffee

eats no breakfast or lunch

has two cups of coffee for lunch

eats large supper at 6:30 P.M.

Doctor's Admission Orders

admit to Ward B

height and weight

TPR BID for 3 days

x-ray of chest

CBC

urinalysis

fasting blood sugar

BUN

VDRL serology test

consultation with podiatrist

routine recreational-outing privileges—accompanied

FBS

BRP

1800 cal low-salt diet

Dalmane 30 mg PO, HS PRN for sleep

BP Q4h when awake

Design

1. Using the data base above, learners should individually develop a nursing-care plan using Worksheet A.

2. Have each participant share his or her care plan with the other members of the group of four. Each person should have this opportunity.

3. Participants should pay particular attention to the differences and similarities of the care plans. Since everyone started with the same data base, similarities increase the reliability of perceptions, and differences underscore the individuality of perceptual fields. The latter especially should be looked at.

4. If time permits, the group can devise a nursing-care plan that reflects their combined beliefs—the results of a team conference.

Variations

This exercise can be a homework assignment. It can also be assigned in steps as study of the nursing process progresses.

Exercise 9
Nursing-Care Plan

Worksheet A

Nursing Diagnoses	Nursing Goals	Nursing Orders

Exercise 10

Problem-Oriented Nursing Records

Purpose	To gain experience in using the problem-oriented system of charting.
Facility	Access to traditionally charted client records.
Materials	Worksheet A: Data Base
	Worksheet B: Patient/Family Problem Index
	Worksheet C: Patient-Care Plan—Flow Sheet
	Worksheet D: Progress Notes
	Pen or pencil.
Time Required	Two hours.
Group Size	This is a homework assignment.
Design	1. Students should choose a client in a health-care setting where problem-oriented nursing records are not routinely used.
	2. Using Worksheets A, B, C, and D, the regular patient chart should be adapted to the problem-oriented system. Nursing care should be the focus, of course.
Variations	1. The instructor can prepare a case data base, and groups of four to six students can adapt the case to the problem-oriented method in class. In a large (total class) group, each smaller group can then report to each other. Differences should be discussed.
	2. This exercise can be a class-report assignment for several students. The teaching experience will then also be an objective.
	3. The data base from Part III, Exercise 9, can be used to develop the problem-oriented records.
	4. The worksheets can be used as a basis for the structure of POR and nursing-care planning on a continual basis.
	5. The records can be used to include total health-care planning (physician's diagnoses and orders and so forth).

Exercise 10
Data Base

Worksheet A*

Family Name

Family Roster

Family/Household Member	Sex	Birth Date	Comments: Relationship, Occupation, and So Forth
1.			
2.			
3.			
4.			
5.			

History (Sign and date entries): physical, functional, nutritional, and so forth

Environment: housing, sanitation, transportation, and so forth

Adjustments: social, emotional, cultural, vocational, religious, and so forth

---

*Guidelines for Worksheets A, B, C, and D have been adapted from those published by the National League for Nursing, New York, 1974.

Exercise 10   Worksheet B
Patient/Family Problem Index

Date	Problem Number	Problems (Current and Potential)	Date of Onset	Date Resolved	Past Problems (Inactive)

Exercise 10   Worksheet C
Patient-Care Plan—Flow Sheet

Date	Problem Number	Plan: Actions to Be Taken	Flow Sheet					
			Date					

Exercise 10   Worksheet D
Progress Notes

Date	Problem Number	Progress Notes			
		Subjective (S)	Objective (O)	Assessment (A)	Plans (P)

Part IV

Implementing: Initiating and Completing Actions

Chapter 9

Implementation

Implementation, the fourth phase of the nursing process, is the act of putting the nursing-care plan (nursing interventions) into operation; it is taking action to meet objectives and goals. Marriner (1983, p. 170) described it as "the actual giving of nursing care." Implementation involves carrying out nursing orders and physicians' orders (Marriner, 1983) within the unique learning framework of the client. Since the nurse is considered the person responsible for comprehensively coordinating the care of the client, the work of staff responsible for various aspects of care must be supervised. Information must be charted and exchanged (National Council of State Boards of Nursing, 1982).

The client is always the primary participant in the care plan and in the individualization process. The nurse, because of expertise, is co-leader. The nurse is responsible for discovering the best method for involving the client in the individual care plan and for delegating responsibility to other professional and technical caregivers as necessary. This involves four steps, three of which are covered in this chapter. The nurse's role is to

1. Designate the parts of the health-care system that will implement the care plan,

2. State the skills and competencies necessary to carry out the plan,

3. Diagnose the level of maturity (relative to each task) of the client in order to discover the leadership style needed by the nurse to implement the care plan, and

4. Diagnose the level of maturity (relative to each task) of the others in the health-care system who may be delegated portions of the client's care; this involves leadership and management skills applied in the administration of nursing care.[1]

The case begun in Chapter 5 and continued in Chapters 6 and 7 will form the foundation for amplifying the aforementioned steps. The following sections discuss the first three steps of the nurse's role.

PARTS OF THE SYSTEM

As previously discussed in Chapter 1, the most direct means for identifying a system is to state its purpose (Banathy, 1968), but system purposes evolve and change. In the implementation phase of the nursing process, the system's purpose is to deliver individualized, comprehensive nursing care with, to, and for the client (individual or family). The system includes, therefore, those persons who will deliver the care and those who will receive the care. Figure 9-1 shows a hypothetical example of system components that may be important, based on the case study.

Those people directly and indirectly involved in any care must be designated as part of the network. All persons must be considered, since it is the interaction of the parts, as well as

the individual entities, that produces and affects outcome.

The next step is to consider the skills necessary in order to implement the nursing orders relative to each nursing diagnosis.

SKILLS AND COMPETENCIES NECESSARY IN IMPLEMENTATION

The skills and competencies necessary to actualize the nursing orders and deal with the diagnoses must be determined. Certain skills are required of each part of the system and can be derived by answering and re-answering this simple question: What particular skills and competencies are needed by this particular person to carry out this specific nursing order? Referring to Figure 9-1, it is logical to deduce that the segments of the system involve two classifications of persons: nursing caregivers and nursing care-receivers. An operational definition of skills and competencies for caregivers and care-receivers may provide further clarity. Webster defined *skill* as "the ability that comes from knowledge, practice, aptitude, and experience to accomplish a task." *Competency* is "the quality of being adequate and qualified to carry out a responsibility."

Referring to the nursing diagnoses (Chapter 6) and orders (Chapter 7) of the case example used in this book, skills and competencies are listed in Table 9-1 for caregivers and care-receivers as they directly relate to fulfillment of nursing care.

It becomes evident the care-receiver's skills are relatively smaller in number than those of the providers when an acute phase of illness is involved. This is explained in Chapman and Chapman's (1975) advocacy helping model in which the degree of client participation decreases as severity of illness increases. Therefore, as the seriousness of illness decreases, the level of client participation increases. This factor provides further evidence of the dynamic processes in nursing care and of the need for a systems approach to plan individualized care.

---

[1]Refer to *Nursing Leadership and Management: An Experiential Approach* by Elaine L. La Monica. Wadsworth Health Sciences Division, Monterey, Ca., 1983.

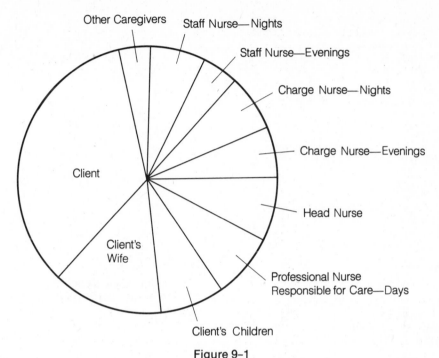

Figure 9-1

Care-Receiver/Giver's System in
the Coronary-Care Unit

LEVELS OF MATURITY OF CAREGIVERS AND CARE-RECEIVERS

After delineating the skills and competencies necessary to set nursing orders in motion, it is imperative to determine whether caregivers and care-receivers have the necessary level of maturity relative to each task. Simply stated, is the giver/receiver capable of adequately performing the task? Maturity refers to ability and willingness to accomplish specific tasks (Hersey & Blanchard, 1982), and levels of maturity move from low to moderate to high. This section focuses on using a leadership model for diagnosing the level of maturity of the client and of the primary caregiver. (Refer to La Monica, 1983, for a thorough discussion of leadership and management.)

The Situational Leadership Theory, developed by Hersey and Blanchard (1982), is the model that will be helpful in discovering how it is most appropriate to actualize the nursing-care plan—that is, how to intervene most effectively to develop those skills necessary for both the caregivers and the care-receivers. (Hersey and Blanchard's model is designed for leadership training; the integration into nursing is done by this author.) It is necessary for the nurse to view herself as the leader in her own learning, as well as co-leader with the client in client recovery. It is assumed that the client needs help in some areas, and the nurse is expected to have the expertise to provide the needed assistance. Furthermore, it is necessary to discern the degree and form of nurse intervention in relation to each task involved in the client's care. Thus, the nurse must be alert to tasks the client

Table **9-1**   Nursing-Care Plan with Skills and
Competencies of Caregivers and Care-Receivers

Nursing-Care Plan	Skills and Competencies

Nursing Diagnosis

Cardiac output, alterations in: Decreased

Nursing Goal

To be free of signs and symptoms of cardiac
  complications

Nursing Objectives

To be free of complications relating to the
  disease states of MI and diabetes

To be free of pain

Nursing Orders	*Care-Receivers*
1. Monitor constantly; be alert for arrythmias.	1. Willingness to permit the nurse to carry out this area of care
2. If serious arrythmias occur, treat immediately as specified by standing orders and document by running a strip on the monitor; CALL FOR A PHYSICIAN STAT.	*Caregivers*
3. Monitor vital signs QH; be alert for changes.	1. Knowledge of and experience with the process of this illness
4. Listen to lungs for signs of congestion, QID.	2. Observation
5. Be alert for nonverbal signs of chest pain or related pain; check with patient frequently.	3. Listening
6. Be alert for signs of dyspnea and give oxygen at 4 liters/min PRN.	4. Recording I & O
7. Observe skin color and body temperature frequently for flushing or pallor.	5. Testing urine for S/A
8. Monitor lab reports for signs of abnormalities; if any exist, report them to the physician stat.	6. Physical assessment
9. Keep an accurate I & O sheet in patient's room.	7. Interpreting ECG readings
10. Test urine for S/A AC and HS; give insulin as indicated.	8. Decision making
11. REPORT ALL CHANGES IN CLIENT'S CONDITION TO PROFESSIONAL NURSE IN CHARGE.	

****

Nursing Diagnosis	*Care-Receivers*
Knowledge deficit: Effects of drugs and therapeutic regimen	1. Awareness of environment
	2. Awareness and understanding of nursing care and medical regimen

Table **9-1**   (continued)

Nursing-Care Plan	Skills and Competencies

Nursing Goal

To plan and secure his own safety

Nursing Objectives

To understand the reason for hospitalization
   in the coronary-care unit

To be aware of the purposes of procedures

To be aware of his diabetic condition

Nursing Orders

1. Explain concept of coronary-care unit to client; if feasible, give him a tour of the unit or show him pictures.
2. Familiarize him with all the equipment in his room and with how it works, emphasizing the purposes of each piece; carry this out in small steps.
3. Explain rationale for all care that he will receive: monitor, medications, treatments, I & O, S/A test, diabetic diet, visiting hours, and so on.
4. Make sure he understands your explanations by encouraging him to respond to your statements.

Caregivers

1. Effective interpersonal skills—empathy
2. Teaching
3. Expertise with environment
4. Knowledge of and experience with nursing and medical treatment

* *

Nursing Diagnosis

Bowel and bladder elimination:
   Self-maintenance*

Nursing Goal

To continue to privately maintain elimination needs and report any signs of constipation

Nursing Objectives

Not required; goal is sufficient

Nursing Orders

1. Talk with him regarding the importance of charting I & O and testing urine.
2. Find out whether he is interested in caring for these aspects himself.

Care-Receivers

1. Recording I & O
2. Care of monitor leads
3. Testing urine for S/A
4. Familiarity with equipment
5. Knowledge of disease process
6. Awareness of the importance of maintaining comfortable elimination patterns

Caregivers

1. Recording I & O
2. Observation
3. Knowledge of the importance of elimination practices in relation to the disease process

Table **9-1**   (continued)

Nursing-Care Plan	Skills and Competencies
3. If he is, then develop a plan for teaching him that moves from your demonstration, to the client doing and being checked, and then to the client's assuming responsibility himself.	4. Teaching 5. Listening
4. Keep chart of intake measures or equivalents on bedside table.	
5. Keep I & O sheet near client.	
6. Keep all equipment handy.	
7. Be alert for constipation—be sure to check for bowel elimination every day.	
8. Observe inconspicuously any straining during bowel elimination.	

****

Nursing Diagnosis

Sleep pattern disturbance

Nursing Goal

To be assured of adequate rest amid coronary-care procedures and environment

Nursing Objectives

Not required; goal is sufficient

Nursing Orders

1. Administer medication on time—Valium.

2. Give sleeping medication if necessary.

3. Since he is anxious about the hospital, sit and talk with him often—comfortably.

4. Quietly monitor vital signs at night; try to discover his sleeping patterns, and do not disturb him when he is in deep sleep.

5. Keep two pillows at bedside within easy reach; he can use these as necessary.

6. Try to get a feeling for his cycle during the day; learn his periods of rest and activity. Then build treatments and procedures around these times, allowing him to rest when he can.

Care-Receivers

1. Awareness of the need for rest and of the resources available

2. Freedom to request rest measures

Caregivers

1. Administering medications safely and with knowledge of their effects

2. Physical-assessment skills

3. Observation

4. Listening

5. Effective interpersonal relationships

Table **9-1**   (continued)

Nursing-Care Plan	Skills and Competencies

Nursing Diagnosis

Nutrition, alterations in:
  Less than body requirements

Nursing Goal

To ingest balanced nutrients within a 2000
  calorie diabetic diet

Nursing Objectives

To be free of anorexia

To adapt to a special diet

To adapt to hospital's food patterns,
  when necessary

Nursing Orders

1. Request that his meals be kept warm until
    he wants to eat or be sent up at 9-2-7; make
    special arrangements with department head
    in the kitchen.

2. Explain diabetes and the importance of
    eating well-balanced meals.

3. Tell client that you will help him in any way
    you can so that he receives foods that are in
    accordance with his likes.

4. Obtain food-exchange lists from dietician,
    and plan meals with client.

5. Be aware of whether this plan is working,
    and make changes accordingly.

Care-Receivers

1. Knowledge of the importance of diet
    maintenance

2. Awareness of unique dietary needs

Caregivers

1. Knowledge and experience with dietary
    needs of diabetic clients

2. Collaboration

3. Observation

4. Listening

5. Interviewing

6. Teaching

****

Nursing Diagnosis

Anxiety

Nursing Goals

To have a respectful and trusting relationship
  so that needs can be discussed with the nurse
  if they emerge as stressful

To have relief from the anxiety that pervades
  areas of the present situation and environment

Nursing Objectives

Not required; goals are sufficient

Care-Receivers

1. Trusting relationship with caregivers

2. Perception of nurse's empathy

Caregivers

1. Effective interpersonal relationships

2. Counseling

3. Empathy

4. Listening

5. Observing

6. Interviewing

Table **9-1** (continued)

Nursing-Care Plan	Skills and Competencies

Nursing Orders

1. Spend time sitting and talking with client. Do not ask questions; rather, respond to his feelings, letting him know that you have heard what he says.

2. Let him know when you will be back to talk.

3. Always be alert for signs of stress, anxiety, boredom. Note what you see by telling the client that he looks _____ . Listen to what he says in response to your statement.

4. ALWAYS RESPOND TO WHAT THE CLIENT IS SAYING; PUT YOUR AGENDA IN THE BACKGROUND.

****

Nursing Diagnosis

Knowledge deficit: Environment

Nursing Goal

To adjust to the environmental limitations by understanding the rationale for the policies in existence

Nursing Objective

To socialize as much as possible

Nursing Orders

In addition to orders listed under safety,

1. Explain rationale for visiting hours.

2. If you do not think that visitors for a longer period of time will harm anyone else in the unit, allow client's visitors to remain as long as possible. Always observe client for signs of fatigue.

3. If client is OOB, you might set up chairs in the hall and have client visit with family and friends there.

4. Move client's bed nearer another client.

5. During quiet hours, have client sit in nurse's station, monitored directly by the large receiver.

Care-Receivers

1. Awareness and understanding of environment and its constraints

Caregivers

1. Teaching

2. Expertise with environment

3. Observation

4. Empathy

Table **9-1**   (continued)

Nursing-Care Plan	Skills and Competencies

Nursing Diagnosis

Hygiene: Self-maintenance*

Nursing Goal

To be able to maintain his own
hygienic measures

Nursing Objectives

To care for himself independently
whenever possible

To have modesty and privacy respected

Nursing Orders

1. Allow client to care for his hygiene needs to
the degree desired, respecting the exercise
or activity level needed for recovery.

2. Have all equipment handy for client.

3. Explain why limits are placed on his activity.

4. Provide privacy while client is using
commode.

5. Be alert for signs of embarrassment in
client—blushing, nervousness, slow
speech—and intervene by engaging client in
conversation aside from what you are doing.
Mention what you are doing and explain
your reasons fully. Do what you feel most
comfortable with, respecting the client's
needs.

6. Involve wife in his care if both he and she
desire this.

7. Be discreet in everything you do for the
client.

Care-Receivers

1. Knowledge of environment

2. Awareness that he is respected—physically
and emotionally

3. Awareness of what he is able to do

4. Awareness of procedures that must be
accomplished

5. Familiarity with use of equipment

Caregivers

1. Teaching

2. Collaboration

3. Decision making

4. Observation

5. Respect for client's integrity

6. Empathy

7. Effective interpersonal behaviors

****

Nursing Diagnosis

Comfort: Self-maintenance*

Nursing Goal

To continue to maintain his own personal
comfort measures

Care-Receivers

1. Trusting relationship with caregivers

2. Perception of nurse's empathy

3. Knowledge of environment

4. Awareness of what makes him comfortable

5. Ability to communicate comfort

Table **9-1**   (continued)

Nursing-Care Plan	Skills and Competencies
Nursing Objectives Not required; goal is sufficient *Nursing Orders* 1. Continually be alert for what makes him comfortable and for his favorite manner of having things done; amplify these. 2. Sit and talk with him concerning things at home that he might like to bring into his room; follow through by having family obtain these items. 3. Always respond to his likes and dislikes; then respect them!	*Caregivers* 1. Observation 2. Listening 3. Interviewing 4. Advocacy 5. Effective interpersonal communications

****

Nursing-Care Plan	Skills and Competencies
Nursing Diagnosis Self-concept, disturbance in: Self-esteem *Nursing Goal* To have his needs for recognition, affiliation, and privacy met and maintained, as possible *Nursing Objective* To have client feel self-satisfied by being recognized as needed by others *Nursing Orders* 1. Always notice and verbally respond to what the client has accomplished. 2. Reinforce positively all aspects of client's growth. 3. Give client small things to do for himself, you, and other clients. For example: Talk or sit with another client who seems depressed; keep track of visiting hours for himself and others. 4. Verbalize the positive aspects of the accomplishments of the client—for example, eating better, requiring no extra insulin. Use this also as a way to reinforce teaching areas.	*Care-Receivers* 1. Awareness of his accomplishments 2. Listening 3. Awareness of environment *Caregivers* 1. Effective interpersonal skills 2. Positive-reinforcement behaviors 3. Creativity 4. Teaching 5. Listening

*Note: Approved nursing diagnoses are not available for all the identified diagnoses; an asterisk next to the diagnosis denotes that it has not yet been approved.

SOURCE: *Classification of Nursing Diagnoses: Proceedings of the Fifth National Conference,* by M. J. Kim, G. McFarland, and A. McLane (Eds.). St. Louis: C. V. Mosby, 1984. Also published in Carpenito, L. Nursing diagnosis: Application to clinical practice. Philadelphia: J. B. Lippincott, 1983.

can accomplish independently, as well as to those requiring assistance.

There is a gap, however, between expertly planning individualized nursing care and implementing individualized interventions. Even though care can be tailored to the needs of the individual client, the communication processes, if not synchronized with the maturity level of the client in relation to the task, can be highly ineffective with the client. By diagnosing the level of maturity of the client and implementing nursing orders accordingly, the hope is that the effectiveness of any nursing intervention can be maximized. This means that the intervention must be received and accepted by the client to be useful. Furthermore, those areas in which the client can carry on independently should be allowed and encouraged, with support given only when needed.

The nurse's level of maturity in relation to a task plays just as important a role in implementing a nursing order as does the client's level of maturity. The nurse must engage in a self-study of maturity in relation to a task; this self-diagnosis will raise the nurse's consciousness and will illuminate areas for further study and experience. It will also designate the type of learning essential to facilitate growth.

SITUATIONAL LEADERSHIP THEORY[2]

Because a nurse should assist the client to reach fullest health potential, a leadership model is applied to the implementation of nursing care in order to determine what *assist* means. In theory, as a client's ability in a task moves from low to moderate to high, the nurse's style of intervention, or behavior, must change. For

example, a client who is unwilling and unable to plan his unique diet needs should be treated differently from one who is able but unwilling, even though both may need to be taught. Furthermore, a client who is both able and willing in this same situation needs no nursing intervention, and such intervention could be perceived as interference.

Application of Situational Leadership Theory (Hersey & Blanchard, 1982), which is based on research, provides the caregiver with leadership behaviors that have the highest probability for successfully motivating the client to learn. It guides the nurse in how to accomplish nursing orders in reference to identified, specific skills and competencies.

At this point, it is necessary to remember what is meant by *behavior*. First of all, behavior consists of actions and reactions perceived by others. This is different from *attitudes*, which are emotion-based values, beliefs, and opinions. As will be discussed in Part VI, attitudes and behaviors function best when integrated with each other. To think that "everyone knows what I really mean" is to be deluded. People truly know what a person means only by what behaviors they observe. Therefore, a nurse's behavior should reflect the nurse's attitude. *Task behavior* is the nurse's action of designating what needs to be done or learned, how it must be done or learned, when, where, and why. It involves mostly one-way communication. *Relationship behavior* is the nurse's socioemotional support, positive reinforcement, psychological strokes, ability to listen, and maintenance of a warm personal relationship with the receiver. It involves two-way communication patterns (Hersey & Blanchard, 1982).

There are four areas of behavior involved in implementing nursing care: (1) diagnosing the level of maturity of the client relative to individual skills and competencies, (2) designating the appropriate behavior style on which to base interventions, (3) diagnosing one's own level of maturity relative to the necessary skills and competencies, and (4) carrying out the order.

[2]Situational Leadership Theory is a model designed by Hersey and Blanchard (1982). It is applied to nursing leadership and management by La Monica (1983) and is also applied in the nursing process in this chapter.

Care-Receiver's Level of Maturity

The first aspect of Situational Leadership Theory to be considered is that of diagnosing the client's *ability* and *willingness* to accomplish the task. Decide on a maturity level based on the following four bench marks (Hersey & Blanchard, 1982, p. 154):

Maturity Level	Client Status
M1—Low Maturity	Unable and unwilling or insecure
M2—Low to Moderate Maturity	Unable but willing or confident
M3—Moderate to High Maturity	Able but unwilling or insecure
M4—High Maturity	Able, willing, and confident

It follows that, if a client needs to maintain a strict 2,000 calorie diabetic diet, does not have any knowledge on the subject, and is not interested in learning, the client would be diagnosed as M1 in relationship to the task. If the client shows interest but has no knowledge, then the client would be at the M2 level. Further, if the client has the knowledge but pays no attention to diet, M3 is indicated. The M4 level reflects a person with knowledge and ability, in that the diet is followed independently and without any intervention.

Once the maturity level is decided for a specific skill or competency (and this procedure should be used on individual skills, since the maturity levels may vary), then the level must be applied in the leadership model.

Appropriate Behavior Style

Figure 9–2 is a diagram of Situational Leadership Theory. Noted in the figure are two sections; the bottom refers to the maturity of the client, while the top indicates the appropriate leadership style of the nurse. The curvilinear line running through the uppermost segment reflects the way people grow from immaturity to maturity and the appropriate leadership style necessary in facilitating learning. Four quadrants are contained in the model, reflecting different balances of task behavior and relationship behavior. S1, S2, S3, and S4 refer to the style numbers.

It may be helpful to imagine yourself learning a skill—for example, skiing. At the onset, what is probably needed is a high degree of teacher explanation of exactly what is needed to get down the mountain alive—things such as "stand up," "bend knees," "relax," and "keep the skis straight." This is task behavior. As the act of descending the hill becomes easier, relationship behavior is indicated along with task behavior. This includes positive reinforcement, such as "You are looking better—not quite as stiff," "How does it feel to fly through the air?," and "You are getting it, but remember to keep your knees bent!" Gradually, as one moves from immaturity to maturity in skiing, neither task nor relationship behavior is necessary. The skier engages in the sport because it is now a part of the skier's personal life. The curvilinear line represents this growth process. It moves in the fashion described because of the learning theories that support this growth process; if your skiing teacher left you completely on your own after you successfully descended the mountain once, learning would not be completely or effectively fulfilled. Appropriate behavior should be reinforced positively.

Figure 9–3 shows how the nurse can decide on the appropriate leadership style after diagnosing the maturity level of the client. If a client is diagnosed at the M1 level, as shown in the figure, simply draw a right angle from the client's point on the immaturity–maturity continuum up to where your line intersects the curvilinear function (Hersey & Blanchard, 1982). It is in the quadrant of the intersection that the nursing intervention must be based *in relationship to the skill or competency*.

As an example, let us refer to the client who is unwilling and unable to follow the diabetic diet. An S1 quadrant—high task and

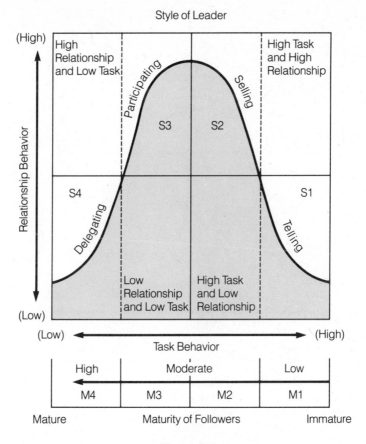

Style of Leader

Figure 9–2.

Situational Leadership (SOURCE: *Management of Organizational Behavior:*
Utilizing Human Resources, 4th Ed., by P. Hersey and K. H. Blanchard, p. 152.
Copyright © 1982 by Prentice-Hall, Inc., Englewood Cliffs, N.J. Reprinted by permission.)

low relationship—is indicated according to Situational Leadership Theory. This means that the nurse must begin by telling the client what to do (that is, that the diet must be followed), how it should be followed, and the need for accuracy in following it. Since the purpose is to move the client to maturity on this task, as soon as the nurse observes willingness, adaptation, or receptiveness, the original diagnosis changes from M1 to M2 and the style of leadership from S1 to S2. At this point, the nurse should continue to engage in task-relevant behavior and slowly begin to involve the client in two-way communication, providing positive support, giving feedback, asking and answering questions, and so forth. It becomes obvious that no matter where one starts, movement should always be toward maturity because the nurse desires that clients eventually become able to direct and intervene totally on their own behalf. A nursing diagnosis is eradicated when the client is able and willing to care for that area

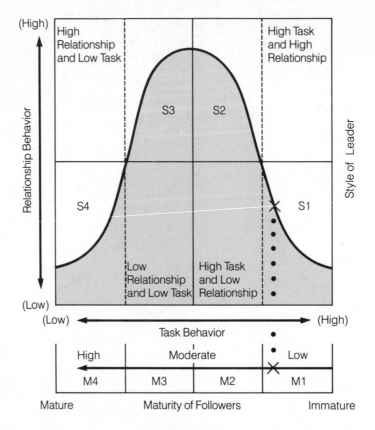

Figure 9-3

**Situational Leadership: Determining an Appropriate
Leadership Style** (SOURCE: *Management of Organizational Behavior:
Utilizing Human Resources*, 4th Ed., by P. Hersey and K. H. Blanchard, p. 200.
Copyright © 1982 by Prentice-Hall, Inc., Englewood Cliffs, N.J. Reprinted with permission.)

himself. The push, therefore, is always to move from S1 to S2, S2 to S3, and S3 to S4, one quadrant at a time—slowly. If a client regresses, then move backward one quadrant at a time.

Hersey and Blanchard (1982) delineated four verbs that clarify the leadership styles. (These can be seen in Figure 9-2.)

S1 = High Task, Low
     Relationship   = "Telling"

S2 = High Task, High
     Relationship   = "Selling"

S3 = High Relationship,
     Low Task   = "Participating"

S4 = Low Task, Low
     Relationship   = "Delegating"

Telling is reflective of one-way communication whereby the nurse must be explicit concerning what needs to be accomplished and how it must be accomplished to safeguard the health of the client. *Selling* is a leadership style in which the nurse must still be responsible for carrying out the task but at the same time engage in two-way communication to attempt to move the client into involvement. *Participating* is a collaborative effort between client and nurse, with the nurse moving toward a supportive role, since the client is able to accomplish the task. *Delegating* involves letting the client have full control, since the client is both able and willing (Hersey & Blanchard, 1982, with nursing adaptations by this author).

Caregiver's Level of Maturity

The same leadership model may be used as a consciousness-raising exercise to determine the nurse's own needs in relation to implementing a specified task. To do this, simply diagnose your own maturity on the scale, and then determine the appropriate leadership style needed. Quadrants S1, S2, and S3 indicate that outside help is necessary; ask for it, find it, and receive it. S4 signifies that one can carry on alone; implement.

Referring back to the example of teaching a client about a diabetic diet, suppose in this case it is the nurse who has the desire but does not have knowledge. An M2 level is indicated with an S2 leadership style required. High task and relationship means the nurse must be directed to the knowledge, must be taught, and also must be involved in two-way communication processes with the teacher, as well as with the client. From that point, the growth processes remain the same, moving through each quadrant as maturity increases. As another example, suppose a nurse has knowledge but is not highly motivated to work through this process with the client; this is an M3 level. What is necessary is to seek someone who can support, listen to, and help the nurse in accomplishing this task; this is high relationship, low task. Finally, to mesh attitudes with behaviors, all feelings must be worked through, recognizing that all nurses and others have both positive and negative feelings at different times, reflecting various circumstances.

Carrying Out the Orders

Going back to the skills and competencies delineated earlier in this chapter, one must consider each as a separate entity. A diagnosis of the level of maturity of the caregiver and the care-receiver relative to individual skills and competencies must be made and followed through to the implementation of individualized nursing care. It should be noted, too, that maturity levels are not consistent; any person has evidence of all facets of the continuum in his or her behavioral system. Moreover inasmuch as maturity flows in relation to many circumstances, especially in response to environmental changes and illness, people can be expected to move back and forth in maturity as situations change. It is the nurse's major responsibility to respond to any changes in self as well as in clients, rediagnosing and intervening as required.

Implementation of nursing care and the appropriateness of leadership styles can be effective or ineffective; this requires evaluation, which will conclude the steps of the nursing process and which will be presented in Part V. Chapter 10 is a discussion of teaching and learning, a major skill required for implementing nursing care.

SUMMARY

Chapter 9 focused on implementation of the nursing-care plan. Designation of the system involved in this implementation process and delineation of the skills and competencies of the caregivers and care-receivers was shown according to the case example begun in Chapter 5. These skills are necessary in carrying out nursing diagnoses and orders. Situational Leadership Theory was used as the theoretic framework for determining the manner of appropriate intervention, with both the nurse and client being considered.

REFERENCES

Banathy, B. (1968). *Instructional systems.* Palo Alto: Fearon.

Carpenito, L. (1983). *Nursing diagnosis: Application to clinical practice.* Philadelphia: Lippincott.

Chapman, J., & Chapman, H. (1975). *Behavior and health care: A humanistic helping process.* St. Louis: Mosby.

Hersey, P., & Blanchard, K. (1982). *Management of organizational behavior: Utilizing human resources* (4th ed.). Englewood Cliffs, NJ: Prentice-Hall.

Kim, M. J., McFarland, G., & McLane, A. (Eds.). (1984). *Classification of nursing diagnoses: Proceedings of the fifth national conference.* St. Louis: Mosby.

La Monica, E. (1983). *Nursing leadership and management: An experiential approach.* Monterey, CA: Wadsworth Health Sciences.

Marriner, A. (1983). *The nursing process: A scientific approach to nursing care* (3rd ed.). St. Louis: Mosby.

National Council of State Boards of Nursing. (1982). *Test Plan for the National Council Licensure Examination for Registered Nurses.* Chicago: Author.

SELECTED READING

For further reading on the leadership and management concepts presented in this chapter, the learner is referred to La Monica (1983), Chapter 4, "Diagnosing the System," and Chapter 5, "Leader Behavior Theory."

Chapter 10

Teaching/Learning

The focus of this chapter is the teaching/learning process, an essential skill during the implementation phase of the nursing process. Discussion revolves around diagnosing the learning needs of caregivers and care-receivers in order to carry out the nursing-process methods to their fullest potential. Learning principles and teaching strategies are discussed, and these form the foundation for teaching and learning in nursing practice.

TEACHING/LEARNING AND THE NURSING PROCESS

Teaching is a behavioral method for facilitating another person's learning. Learning is an internal experience for the receiver. It denotes an integration of thoughts, ideas, theory, and experience—past and present. The areas of self included in the PELLEM Pentagram (Chapter 17) are guides through which one can understand the integration of teaching behaviors into a person's cognitive, affective, and psychomotor processes, resulting in learning. Furthermore, learning is change, since new matter added within a system (specifically a person) produces an added mind dimension that makes a person different from before the process began.

In keeping the focus of teaching and learning in mind while using the nursing process and interacting with a client and the client's system, two functions are involved. First, the nurse assesses the learning needs of the client; these become the teaching responsibilities of the nurse. Second, to carry out teaching responsibilities, the nurse must assess the learning needs of himself or herself relative to teaching the client: Does the nurse have the background to know what should be taught and the best method for doing so? The teaching/learning process can therefore be conceptualized as a two-way interaction between learner and teacher, each dimension being dependent on the other with both parties learning.

It follows that the nurse becomes involved in two diagnostic steps, which are an extension of the identification of caregivers' and care-receivers' needed skills and competencies, discussed in Chapter 9:

1. Assessing the learning needs of the client,

2. Assessing the nurse's own learning needs to carry out teaching responsibilities—self-diagnosis

It is deemed essential that the professional nurse consider both steps in order to provide comprehensive nursing care. The experience of this author has been that learning needs always exist, although they must be satisfied within the limits of priority, time, and space, reflective of a given purpose. Further, this author admonishes continual consideration of these steps so as not to close doors before you realize what you're shutting out. Finally, learning needs should be considered in light of both past and present educational theory.

LEARNING-THEORY PRINCIPLES

Conley (1973, pp. 212–214) explicated eight generalizations from the literature on learning theories by synthesizing a wealth of theory and research. Each principle will be discussed separately and applied in the framework of this chapter:

1. *"Learning requires perceiving"* (Conley). Dewey (1963, 1966) interpreted learning as a sociologic phenomenon between an organism and the organism's environment. He noted, however, that learners must perceive a situation or subject as important for themselves and relevant or needed in order for learning to occur. Bruner (1960) called this "learning readiness."

2. *"Unique characteristics of the learner govern the extent of what is integrated"* (Conley). Differences among learners have been noted by many theorists in education. Piaget, for example, underscored intellectual variations based on the developmental maturation of a human being (Ginsburg & Opper, 1979; Wadsworth, 1979). Thorndike noted individual differences while developing "connectism" as a theory (cited in Hilgard, 1956), and Wertheimer (1945), a *Gestalt* psychologist, earmarked the importance of past experience in learning. Research has consistently proven that learning differences exist among individuals, and this disparity can be attributed to a variety of factors.

3. *"The degree of learning is influenced by one's environment"* (Conley). Again coming from a sociologic framework, behaviorists such as Watson (1916, 1972), Dewey (cited in Hilgard, 1956) in his functionalist perspective, and von Bertalanffy (1969) in general system theory have shown that the environment is an important variable affecting learning.

4. *"Learning is dependent upon the activity of the learner"* (Conley). This principle involves problem solving and behavior toward goal accomplishment by the learner. Hull (1942) discussed this in terms of his drive-reduction theory: When one has a need or drive to learn, problem-solve, or accomplish, one is motivated to satisfy this need.

5. *"Motivation of the learner influences what is learned"* (Conley). Internal motives such as

achievement, esteem, and self-actualization (Maslow, 1970), as well as external drives and incentives, must be considered. Both play a key role in determining what one learns.

6. *"Reinforcement of desired behavior increases the probability that the behavior will reoccur in another situation"* (Conley). Behaviorist theories have long documented this principle: positive reinforcement of those behaviors that one desires is effective.

7. *"Transfer of learning occurs when similar conditions are present in old and new situations"* (Conley). Thorndike (cited in Hilgard, 1956) was very early in documenting this principle. Guthrie (1952) later reaffirmed that a stimulus pattern that produces a certain response will tend to replicate the response if it or a similar pattern is repeated. Bruner (1960) underscored the importance of transfer in learning through this principle.

8. *"Practice determines the effectiveness and efficiency in learning"* (Conley). Repetition is of primary importance in learning. Thorndike (cited in Hilgard, 1956) was early in noting this effect. Furthermore, research has shown that time between practice periods and evaluation between intervals facilitates learning.[1]

According to Rogers (1969), learning has a quality of personal involvement—it is self-initiated and self-reliant. These beliefs are reflected in his learning principles, which are as follows:

1. Human beings have a natural potential to learn.

2. Learning is greatly enhanced when learners perceive relevance in the content being taught.

3. Learning that threatens one's self-image tends to be resisted; reduction of external threats eases this effect and facilitates experience.

4. Learning is facilitated when the learner is involved in the process.

5. Self-initiated learning is most powerful; it is lasting and pervasive.

6. Learning the process of learning is most important because it allows one to be continually open to experience.

Understanding and use of general principles developed by learning theorists must ground a nurse's teaching processes. Within this framework, there is a variety of instructional modes and media that the nurse can employ to meet the learning needs of client and self.

TEACHING STRATEGIES

The use of teaching strategies must be based on principles of learning, as well as dimensions of the learner and the teacher. The term *strategy* implies a means or method for achievement of a goal. It is not the aim of teaching; rather, it is the vehicle through which teaching occurs. This vehicle should reflect the best way to accomplish teaching objectives, synchronized with the perceived best means by which the learner will integrate new knowledge and the experience and ability of the teacher in using the strategy.

There are no absolutes in choosing a teaching strategy, and the instructor is limited only by personal ingenuity and creativity in composing a variety of modes and media around teaching objectives and what is known about the client and self. It is with this background that this portion of the chapter broadly discusses teaching strategies—modes and media—as they apply in nursing practice. These strategies can be considered as a resource pool from which a nurse can draw but not be limited.

Conley (1973) distinguished modes from media by designating *modes* as types of conversations between teacher and learner and *media* as devices or props used in instruction to extend what is discussed. Conley provided the types of modes and media; this author amplifies each in nursing practice, when appropriate.

---

[1]From *Curriculum and Instruction in Nursing*, by V. Conley. Copyright ©1973 by Little, Brown and Co., Inc. Reprinted with permission.

Modes

1. *Lecture.* This is the most widely used mode in education systems and consists mainly of one-way communication—teacher to learner. In one-to-one teaching situations, this framework has little application. It is useful, however, in reaching large groups of clients who share a particular learning need and works best when followed by group discussion, thus reinforcing the intended learning.

2. *Individual or group discussion.* This is a learning format that facilitates integration of new material by enabling two-way conversation between teacher and learner(s) and between learner(s). It is one of the best means for development and discussion of ideas, feelings, beliefs, and experiences around a particular content area. In this mode, the teacher is often seen as a facilitator of learning with expertise in the topic. Group discussion has been found to be most beneficial when learners share a particular problem or disability and support can be given and shared. It tends to destroy the myth of being alone and can build bonds of assistance between clients, staff, and colleagues.

3. *Panel discussion.* This is a somewhat formal method that can be used in teaching client groups. An interplay or mini-group discussion can occur among panel members, with the audience being listeners and occasionally raisers of questions addressed to members of the presenting panel.

4. *Seminar.* In nursing practice, the seminar is most useful for self-learning situations with groups of peers. The typical format involves one or two members presenting an idea, problem, or issue, with everyone then discussing it. The team conference, as discussed in Chapter 11, can be equated with this mode.

5. *Demonstration.* The demonstration involves use of media by the teacher in showing what is to be learned by the audience. This can occur with any number of participants from large groups. An example would be a nurse demonstrating the administration of insulin, using the necessary equipment, and an orange, doll, or other client substitute. Steps and procedures of the task are the foci, and the learners may be given the opportunity to practice the skill after the demonstration. This latter aspect is reflective of the next mode.

6. *Laboratory instruction.* Instruction in a laboratory is usually used in formal student learning where self-discovery is the primary basis for the learning. Simulations may be involved, and didactic presentation may precede or follow the event. In nursing practice, laboratory instruction may follow teacher demonstration, thereby providing the opportunity for "trying on" the new behaviors in a safe environment with assistance, if this is required.

7. *Team teaching.* Team teaching occurs when two or more professionals carry the responsibility for fulfilling specific teaching objectives with a client or group. In reality, this is most often the case in nursing-practice situations, especially with a team-nursing model of delivery. Communication among teachers on the team is essential, and the learner has the opportunity to experience several perspectives in a given area. Learning can be enhanced if the team concept is truly put into operation, but two separate people doing the same thing can be oppressive. Thus, team teaching mandates coordination and integration of all efforts.

Media

Media are devices chosen and used to amplify the aforementioned modes of teaching.

1. *Programmed instruction and computer-assisted instruction.* Both of these media comprise teaching machines or books that carry a learner step by step through the content. They offer immediate feedback to the learner in terms of correct responses to questions that usually follow the presentation of theory. Two-way communication occurs indirectly between the author of the material and the learner. This method has benefit as an augmentor of learning in nursing-practice environments, but it works best when preceded and followed by group discussion or one-to-one talks with the teacher.

2. *Television.* Closed-circuit and public television are becoming increasingly popular in education. Closed-circuit television can employ videotapes prepared by teachers in a given content area for teaching a specified audience. This medium is commonly found in medical and dental offices to help clients in learning. Public television involves many areas; some are specific in content, and others provide vicarious experience of direct health education. Hospital-situation dramas are a prime example of the latter; television specials addressing such topics as rape, or life after death, for instance, are examples of the former.

3. *Motion pictures.* These can be useful in learning when they are specific to the content requiring teaching. Conley (1973) described motion pictures as similar to demonstration when the films amplify content.

4. *Simulations.* These are primarily involved with laboratory learning and demonstration. Everything that must be achieved is presented in a hypothetical situation, with low risk and a safe environment provided by the teacher. Cognitive, affective, and psychomotor aspects of learning are all amplified, and group or one-to-one discussion usually precedes and follows the simulation. Furthermore, these simulations can be videotaped and used as media in future endeavors. The humanistic exercises in this book are examples of simulations.

5. *Pictorial presentations and printed language.* These forms of media are the ones most often employed by nurses. Pictures and figures with adjacent explanations are helpful in reinforcing learning that has occurred via another mode. They should be used to augment learning. Filmstrips and slides are other examples of this teaching mode.

6. *Tape and disc recordings.* These can be helpful in self-learning, group discussions, and seminars when what is recorded focuses on a situation or presentation that addresses the topic in focus. Often, tape or disc recordings provide narration or an explanation of slides.

7. *Models.* These are usually representations of objects needed in a demonstration. For example, a model may be a plastic female pelvis that can be taken apart in order to explain childbirth. Again, as with other media, models illustrate what one wishes to teach.

It should be recognized that whatever mode or method is chosen for teaching objectives, personality aspects of both the learner and the teacher should be considered. If the client is shy and uncomfortable with groups, that mode is contraindicated. Moreover, if the nurse is inexperienced or nervous in demonstrating with groups, another mode is indicated. The decisions about modes and media must create the best possible learning environment for all the interactors in the situation. There is no substitute, however, for a teacher who enjoys what is being done and how it is being done; the excitement is catching.

SUMMARY

The discussion of teaching/learning began with its pertinence in nursing practice. Principles gleaned from learning theory were presented, followed by specific teaching strategies. Within these teaching strategies, a variety of modes and media were presented.

REFERENCES

Bruner, J. (1960). *The process of education.* Cambridge, MA: Harvard University Press.

Conley, V. (1973). *Curriculum and instruction in nursing.* Boston: Little, Brown.

Dewey, J. (1963). *Experience and education.* New York: Macmillan.

Dewey, J. (1966). *Democracy and education.* New York: Free Press.

Ginsburg, H., & Opper, S. (1979). *Piaget's theory of intellectual development* (2nd ed.). Englewood Cliffs, NJ: Prentice-Hall.

Guthrie, E. (1952). *The psychology of learning*. New York: Harper and Row.

Hilgard, E. (1956). *Theories of learning*. New York: Appleton-Century-Crofts.

Hull, C. (1942). Conditioning: Outline of a systematic theory of learning. In *The psychology of learning*. Forty-first Yearbook of the National Society for the Study of Education, Part II. Chicago: University of Chicago Press.

Maslow, A. (1970). *Motivation and personality* (2nd ed.). New York: Harper and Row.

O'Connor, A. (1978). Diagnosing your needs for continuing education. *American Journal of Nursing, 78*, 405–406.

Rogers, C. (1969). *Freedom to learn*. Columbus: Merrill.

von Bertalanffy, L. (1969). *General system theory*. New York: George Braziller.

Wadsworth, B. (1979). *Piaget's theory of cognitive development* (2nd ed.). New York: Longman.

Watson, J. (1916). The place of the conditioned reflex in psychology. *Psychological Review, 23*, 89.

Watson, J. (1972). *Psychological care of infant and child*. New York: Arno.

Wertheimer, M. (1945). *Productive thinking*. New York: Harper and Brothers.

SELECTED READING

The following article by O'Conner describes the process of assessing one's own learning needs. O'Connor provides a means for studying one's own needs for continued education; this process can stand alone in its purpose. It can also be applied, however, in situations involving the assessment of learning needs of others.

Diagnosing Your Needs for Continuing Education

Andrea B. O'Connor

The increased interest in continuing education has resulted in a proliferation of formal continuing education programs, self-study devices, as well as inservice education offerings to provide learning resources for nurses. The learning needs of nurses as a whole have been surveyed, but little is available to help the individual practitioner design a continuing education program to meet personally determined needs.

Too often, nurses who recognize continuing education as necessary enroll in programs simply because they "seem interesting" or "are available" or "offer CEUs." Most of us would agree that selection from the learning resources available should be based on an assessment of learning needs that will provide a basis for improving skills and adding knowledge for use in present or future practice. To do this one must know how to diagnose one's own learning needs.

There are three areas nurses can examine in their self-diagnostic process: the present level of their practice competence; their future professional goals; and their professional awareness, which includes issues and trends in the health care field in general and in nursing in particular. By assessing individual learning needs in each area, the nurse should be able to determine those needs and develop an education program that can be revised and expanded as old needs are satisfied and new ones emerge.

In his book *On Self-Directed Learning*, Malcolm Knowles[1] provides an approach to self-assessment of learning needs that is applicable in these three areas. This involves

1. Developing a model of required competencies;

2. Assessing one's practice in relation to the model;

3. Identifying the gaps between one's own knowledge and skills and those required by the model.

There are numerous models that can be used to assess one's present level of practice.

Such formal criteria of competence as the American Nurses' Association's Standards of Nursing Practice give a broad picture of the knowledge, skills, and behaviors which constitute competent professional practice. These standards include those for nurse practitioners and standards formulated by the divisions of Community Health Nursing, Gerontological Nursing, Maternal and Child Health Nursing, Medical/Surgical Nursing, and Psychiatric and Mental Health Nursing. Specialty nursing organizations have also developed other statements or standards either for nurses now practicing or those entering a specialty.

Nursing journals frequently publish articles on "ideal" nursing practice in particular care situations, and these constitute an additional model source.

Self-administered tests, such as "Test Yourself," which appears monthly in the *American Journal of Nursing*, the nursing examination review books published by the Medical Examination Publishing Co.,[2] and "Nursing Decisions," published by Docent Corp.,[3] provide a model of competence in terms of a knowledge base required in specific practice settings.

Peers or coworkers offer an at-hand source of model identification that can be used in two ways to identify an "ideal" practitioner whom one might wish to emulate, or, in group meetings with peers, to identify a model of practice that might serve as an "ideal" in a particular setting.

The model against which a nurse can assess her present practice may be one or a combination of these models, depending on the practice situation. For example, a nurse working in an acute neurosurgical setting may select aspects of models identified in the American Nurses' Association standards, in literature, and in and by peers and coworkers to construct a picture of competent nursing practice in a neurosurgical setting.

Diagnosing one's own level of practice is a difficult aspect of self-directed learning. Traditional educational experiences provided a built-in assessment in the form of grading: one knew where one was and took little formal responsibility for determining competence. Objective examination of one's weaknesses and strengths in practice is a skill that takes time to develop.

A beginning approach to self-assessment most obviously occurs in the course of practice. During one week, a nurse might focus on her professional competencies by jotting down questions that come to mind while giving nursing care. Perhaps it is a new drug whose actions are unknown to her, or the realization that she is uncertain about the normal values of test results to be interpreted. I'm sure we have all thought to ourselves, "I'll have to look that up later," but never do. By making notes of such questions as they come up, a nurse can begin to formulate a list of knowledges valuable to her in the clinical setting.

Also important in assessing one's practice is an awareness of those nursing activities one tends to avoid or that make one uncomfortable.

Later examination of these situations can provide clues regarding areas of deficiency.

Another obvious basis for assessment is identification of skills one wishes to improve or knowledges that seem superficial.

In the course of self-diagnosis one must be careful to take note of those aspects of practice which represent competence and skill; that is, both positive and negative practices should be recognized, assessed and recorded.

The opinions of others also can be helpful. These may be presented in formal performance ratings by superiors or be elicited from peers or superiors.

Once a model of practice has been identified and one has completed a self-assessment of present practice competence, the two should be compared. Knowles suggests listing those "performance elements" (knowledges, skills, and behaviors) identified in the model and then rating oneself on a scale of 1 to 10 (low to high) for each of the identified elements. Such a rating would reveal areas that need work and form the basis for planning continuing learning projects.

A similar approach to that outlined above can be used in assessing learning needs for future practice. A first step would be the nurse's identification of what expanded or extended roles might be pursued for the future. For example, a nurse in an acute medical setting may decide she would like to become a respiratory care nurse specialist in the future; a nurse working in a delivery room may be attracted to midwifery; or a nurse in a clinic setting or a doctor's office may identify a family nurse practitioner role as a possible future career.

Having decided on one or more goals or possible areas for extended or expanded practice, the nurse should locate models to determine the competencies and educational criteria for these roles. Such models may exist, again, in formal standards or nursing literature and certainly can be found in nurse specialists who are practicing in these areas.

The nurse's self-assessment in relation to such models should extend to the practical aspects of pursuing an educational program to attain such goals. For example, a clinical specialty role may require a master's degree. The nurse must determine whether pursuit of such a degree is feasible. Or, an intensive continuing education program may be requisite for entry into an extended role. Will time and finances or personal considerations permit attendance at such a program?

The area of "professional awareness," encompassing issues and trends in the health care field and in nursing, and including legislative and legal problems, is a more nebulous area for needs assessment in terms of continued learning. The nurse who is satisfied with her present level of practice competence or is pursuing a continuing program of learning to maintain or update practice skills may still feel some deficiencies in terms of involvement with or understanding of issues and trends affecting professional nursing practice.

Here, one can turn to journals and publications of nursing associations for news of the profession or health care in general. Attendance at meetings of professional groups, such as district or state nurses' associations, the local chapter of the National League for Nursing, or a local group of specialty practitioners can provide information on emerging issues and trends important to the profession.

With "professional awareness" thus enhanced, the nurse can now go on to develop a list of knowledges required to actively pursue a solution to a problem or to broaden understanding and awareness of a trend. Pursuit of a learning program to achieve such knowledges coupled with active engagement in programs to solve problems in the profession will serve to further broaden the nurse's "professional awareness" and provide yet another program for continued learning.

REFERENCES

1. Knowles, Malcolm. *On self-directed learning.* New York: Association Press, 1975.

2. Medical Examination Publishing Co. 65–36 Fresh Meadow Lane, Flushing, N.Y. 11365.

3. Docent Corp. 430 Manville Rd., Pleasantville, N.Y. 10570.

Humanistic Exercises

Exercise 11

Teaching—A Beginning

Purposes	1. To begin the experience of teaching.
	2. To gain experience in using different instructional modes and media to teach a content area.
	3. To experience a variety of teaching strategies.
Facility	Large room to accommodate class.
Materials	Specified by the students in their teaching module.
Time Required	Ten minutes per member.
Group Size	Under 25.
Design	1. As a homework assignment, ask students to think of anything (skill, philosophy, belief) that they know or do well.
	2. Have them prepare a five-to-seven minute teaching module on the area chosen. The module should include objectives as well as teaching modes and media.
	3. Request that preparation be made for a class presentation.
	4. At a subsequent class, have students teach the module to small groups of peers.
	5. Encourage group discussion of the experience, focusing on both the teacher's experience and on the learner's.
Variations	Nursing skills or competencies as well as nursing theory can be substituted for the content in the original design.

Exercise 12

Teaching—Applying the Process

Purposes	1. To apply the teaching process.
	2. To broaden experience in diagnosing the teaching needs of clients and colleagues in a health environment.
	3. To increase awareness of the teaching diagnoses that others perceive in the same situation.
	4. To identify appropriate objectives and the most effective teaching strategies to accomplish them.
	5. To evaluate a teaching intervention.
Facility	Large room to accommodate participants seated in groups of six.
Materials	Worksheet A: Scenarios
	Worksheet B: Instructional Analysis
	Paper and pencils.
Time Required	One to two hours.
Group Size	Unlimited groups of six.
Design	1. Participants should consider themselves as head nurses. Using all or any combination of the scenarios, ask participants to individually respond to the following in each situation:
	a. Is there a teaching need? If the answer is yes, use Worksheet B to complete step 1. (Worksheet B may have to be duplicated.)
	b. If there is a teaching need, what needs to be taught and to whom? Give rationale for response.
	c. Identify objective(s) for teaching.
	d. Specify strategy: mode(s) and medium (media).
	e. Delineate how the accomplishment of objectives would be evaluated.
	2. In groups of six, participants should share and discuss their responses. Different perceptions among the learners should receive particular attention.
Variations	1. Step 1 may be done as a homework assignment.
	2. Individuals or small groups can develop and actually carry out the teaching strategy with their peers, as in Exercise 11.
	3. The students' actual clinical placement can be the scene for identifying a learning need and carrying out the process, even to the point of teaching the staff and having them evaluate the program.

Exercise 12   Worksheet A
Scenarios

1. Three times in the past two days you've found that elderly patients who have been gotten out of bed rather early in the morning have stayed up sitting in chairs for the rest of the morning. In each case when you noted this, the patient's respiration was either labored or rapid. The pulse also was rapid, and the patient appeared tired and admitted to feeling tired.

2. A patient on your unit has been on a Stryker frame for two weeks. You have been told that tomorrow a newly employed graduate nurse and two senior nursing students will be with you for the first time.

3. A patient on your unit has been on a Stryker frame for two weeks. Today when you go in to help turn her, two beginning sophomore students ask if they may come with you to see what you are doing.

4. During afternoon conference, a patient was mentioned who had just returned from the operating room following "repair of a fractured hip." A nurse said, "We'll have to be careful of his back since he'll have to stay on it for some time."

5. When making rounds on your unit after lunch, you notice that, although many patients are in their beds, most of the beds are elevated, and in many cases the linen is rumpled. A television set is audible through most of the area, and three of your staff members are talking rather loudly in the corridor.

6. On Monday, Mr. Smith tells you that his doctor has told him he might be going home in a couple of days. Mr. Smith has congestive heart failure, has been on digitalis and a diuretic, still has some peripheral edema, and is on a low-sodium diet. He lives alone.

7. Ms. Jones has asked for and received a prescribed narcotic for pain for several days prior to and following her surgery. The nurse assigned to give medications and the one assigned to care for her yesterday both questioned "whether she really needed it." The doctor was told of this and gave permission for a PRN placebo. Today it is discussed by others on the team. Ms. Jones responded well the first time the placebo was given but then seemed to "want the other medicine" (she recognized that a different injection had been given). The medicine nurse today said she believed Ms. Jones had no real need for the narcotic, but another nurse said he thought Ms. Jones acted as if she really had pain.

8. When an aide attempting to change a patient's position was experiencing evident difficulty, a graduate nurse came over to the aide, assisted, and then explained the procedure to the aide and the patient.

9. You observe a patient walking down the corridor in a coat and hat, carrying a suitcase; an aide is walking beside the patient. A graduate nurse leaves the nurse's station, greets the patient, takes the suitcase, and hands it to the aide. The nurse discusses the patient's plans for discharge as they walk down the hall. The situation was discussed with the aide after the aide returned from taking the patient to the hospital lobby.

Scenarios were received by this author at the College of
Nursing, University of Florida, 1966. Author is unknown.

10. A team leader asked an aide to do a sugar and acetone test for a patient and reminded the aide not to obtain the urine for testing from the patient's tube (indwelling Foley catheter). The aide took a sample from the drainage bottle and reported the test to the team leader, who then recorded the results.

11. A patient is shaking the side rails and is stating in a loud voice that he wants to go to the bathroom. The aide and practical nurse remove the side rails, explaining to the patient why side rails are necessary. (He had slipped out of bed yesterday.) The practical nurse escorts the patient to the bathroom and waits to escort him back to bed.

12. A graduate nurse wheels a patient into the solarium, places the wheelchair close to another patient, and introduces them to each other. The nurse then asks each patient to demonstrate active and passive exercises of their arms. As the nurse leaves the room, the patients continue the exercises and discuss each other's progress.

Exercise 12   Worksheet B
Instructional Analysis

Scenario No. _____

What needs to be taught and to whom?

Program objectives:

Teaching strategy—mode(s) and medium (media):

Evaluation procedure:

Part V

Evaluating: Determining Extent of Goal Attainment

Chapter 11

Evaluation

Chapter 11 will discuss the evaluation process, followed by its application to the case examples developed for this section. Tools used in the evaluative process will then be discussed. It should be noted here, however, that this discussion will be limited to evaluation of direct patient care and the effectiveness of nursing care plans. The broader aspect of nursing-service quality assurance will be covered in Chapter 12.

Evaluation is theoretically the concluding step of the nursing process, nursing's scientific method. It is the act of discovering whether plans were fulfilled and goals were met. Conley (1973) elaborated on the meaning of evaluation from an educational perspective. She stated that the purpose of a nursing curriculum is to bring about changes in certain directions within students; this should be a planned, rational activity. The analogy in nursing care is explicit, for the practitioner desires changes in the client and self; these changes are conscious, planned, and directed. It logically follows that evaluation is the process of going back to the nursing diagnoses and goals and determining whether the needs they signified are now met and determining what other assistance is necessary, based on the outcomes of the care plan for each client's system. Kozier and Erb (1983) identified four possible outcomes of evaluation: (1) the patient responded as expected; (2) short-term goals were achieved but intermediate and/or long-term goals need further intervention; (3) goals were not met; and (4) new diagnoses have been delineated.

THE PROCESS OF EVALUATION

The simplicity of the evaluative process has a positive relationship with the clarity and comprehensiveness of the nursing-care plan—nursing diagnoses, goals, and objectives. If the nursing-care plan is clear, it becomes the base for evaluation. Moreover, when care plans are not explicit, the evaluation process cannot take place since there are no established controls of goals and/or objectives. It is impossible to measure success without being aware of intent.

Broadly speaking, the goal of nursing is to assist the client to fullest health potential, thus eliminating the need for professional assistance. Again, this is based on the definition of a nursing diagnosis as an actual or potential health problem with which the client requires nursing assistance. Hersey and Blanchard (1982) referred to maturity (in other words, a client's fullest potential) as that stage where neither task nor relationship behavior is required from the leader; in nursing words, the client can and will carry out functions and act independently, dependently, and interdependently, according to his own direction.

All parts of the designated system involved in client care require evaluation as each fits into the nursing diagnoses and orders. Yura and Walsh (1983) underscored this point when they stated that the nurse and client are the agents of the process, with involvement of nursing personnel, health-team members, and family. It follows that several facets of care must be evaluated:

1. Restoration of health of the client, with alleviation of problems delineated in the nursing diagnoses;

2. Level of maturity of caregivers and care-receivers in relation to the skills and competencies necessary to implement care (Are they willing and able to carry out the skills required in care?); and

3. Effectiveness of the leadership style used in implementing care (Hersey & Blanchard, 1982)

Based on outcomes of this evaluative process, the nurse becomes aware of additional data on which to plan or adapt subsequent nursing care.

The most frequently used method of evaluation in nursing is a behavioral method involving direct observation by the nurse who is planning the care. However, since evaluation by one person lends less validity to the results because of the normally limited perceptual field of the individual, evaluation of nursing care is best when several health personnel are involved in the process. The larger the number of competent people observing the same effect, the more valid are the results.

The evaluative process can be formal or informal. An example of a formal evaluation is one in which specific outcome criteria in nursing care are delineated and written down prior to implementation. These then become the bases for evaluation. Griffith and Christensen (1982) referred to this type as a formative evaluation. Another example of formal evaluative processes is the retrospective, or summative evaluation (Griffith & Christensen, 1982) in which the nurse makes a point-by-point review of the client's response to care after the nursing plan has been initiated; in retrospective evaluations, outcome criteria are not formally delineated before implementation. Informal processes lack specific written outcome criteria. Professional judgment, explicit observed phenomena such as "no arrhythmias" and "stable vital signs," and intuition derived from knowledge and experience are bases for evaluation. Informal processes are used more often than formal ones.

The evaluative process also can be objective, subjective, or both. *Objective* in this instance refers to evaluation that is based on specific facts, such as a record of a client's vital signs, rather than on an evaluation based on intuitive concerns, feelings, or emotional responses to the client. Those evaluations that involve the nurse's thoughts, rather than hard facts, are *subjective* evaluations. Both are valuable for different reasons. Objective methods of evaluation are most prevalent in nursing-audit literature (Lindeman, 1976a, 1976b; McGuire, 1968; Phaneuf, 1966; Rubin, Rinaldi, & Dietz, 1972); however, subjective methods are most often used in daily practice. This is unfortunate because, even though subjective evaluations are valuable in individualizing and personalizing care as well as in responding to clients, objective evaluations are more reliable and valid and less subject to bias on the part of the evaluator. A combination of an objective evaluation and a subjective evaluation is the best method because it integrates facts with intuition; it eliminates the tendency of an objective evaluation to be automatic and the tendency of a subjective evaluation to be vague or one-sided. In addition, it is a good way to check for error. For example, a client whose temperature registers normal but who says to the nurse that she feels chilled may need to have her temperature measured again; the first reading may have been in error. Objective and subjective evaluations also provide other dimensions to the process. Subjective data may include input from secondary sources, which may prove valuable in determining client outcome; both objective and subjective data can lead to development of research questions and nursing theory.

For an excellent discussion on conceptual issues in the appraisal of the quality of nursing care, refer to Hagan (1975). The author, Elizabeth P. Hagan, is a specialist in measurement and evaluation and has been a consultant and leader in nursing and nursing evaluation for the past several decades. She raises many questions on evaluation of nursing services that reflect expertise in an underdeveloped nursing area.

The paper can also be found in the first edition of this book (La Monica, 1979).

CASE EXAMPLES

Table 11-1 illustrates how to write objective outcome criteria based on two examples. (Note that *objective* used in this way is a descriptive word meaning "factual," whereas an *objective* used in the phrase "to develop an objective for the nursing plan" is a noun meaning "aim or goal.") The objective (factual) outcome criteria in the examples are based on the nursing diagnoses derived from the case study used previously in this book. At the top of each section of the table are the nursing diagnoses, goals, and objectives that need to be dealt with. In the first column are the "Objective Outcome Criteria"—that is, the specific signs expected to be observed before the patient can be considered at fullest health potential; in the second column, labeled "Nursing Observations," are the actual signs noted by the nurse. By comparing objective outcome criteria with the nursing observations, the nurse can evaluate the client's progress toward maximum health potential.

Subjective outcome criteria may be developed and used in the same way. The nurse may write down explicit patterns of attitude and behavior to look for when evaluating the client. Thus, even though this is an intuitive, emotional judgment, it is based on specific observations to be made. For example, the nurse may use subjective criteria to evaluate the client's visiting needs. If the client appears anxious or depressed when the nurse asks visitors to leave because of unit requirements, the nurse may deduce that the client needs more company or needs someone to talk to. The nurse can then make arrangements accordingly: personally talk to the client; move the client into a visiting area for awhile if possible; or introduce the client to another client in the same unit. The nurse also uses subjective outcome criteria to determine whether the client's attitude is congruent with the client's behavior.

Table **11-1**   Evaluation of Nursing Care Using Objective Outcome Criteria:
Case Example

Nursing Diagnosis: Cardiac output, alterations in: decreased

Nursing Goal: To be free of signs and symptoms of cardiac complications

Nursing Objectives: To be free of complications relating to the disease states of MI and diabetes
To be free of pain

Objective Outcome Criteria	Nursing Observations
1. Physical signs should be monitored, with normal ranges noted for five days for the following: a. B/P, P, R, T b. ECG pattern (no arrhythmias) c. heart and lung sounds (no congestion) d. laboratory reports e. respiratory patterns f. urine sugar and acetone g. no dyspnea h. no pain in chest	1. Physical signs monitored for five days show: a. normal B/P, P, R, T b. ECG pattern—no arrhythmias c. heart and lung sounds—no congestion d. laboratory reports—normal e. respiratory patterns—normal f. urine sugar and acetone—normal g. no dyspnea h. no chest pain
2. Client should state that he feels well	2. Client states that he feels well
3. Client's appearance should be normal: a. good color b. skin warm, dry c. alert	3. Client appears normal: a. good color b. skin warm, dry c. alert

---

Nursing Diagnosis: Nutrition, alterations in: Less than body requirements

Nursing Goal: To ingest balanced nutrients within a 2000 calorie diabetic diet

Nursing Objectives: To be free of anorexia
To adapt to a special diet
To adapt to hospital's food patterns, when necessary

Objective Outcome Criteria	Nursing Observations
1. Client should be able to interpret diabetic diet to nurse and family	1. Client interprets diabetic diet to nurse and family accurately
2. Client should plan balanced meals from diet sheet and eat the chosen food on time	2. Client plans balanced meals from diet sheet with dietician and eats chosen food when served—9-2-7

Table **11-1**   (continued)

3. Client should be able to care for his own dietary needs with respect to his diabetic condition	3. Client cares for himself with respect to diabetic condition; requests more information on disease; seeks more knowledge; reads material given to him; discusses information learned with nurse and/or dietician; asks informed questions

With regard to evaluating the level of maturity of caregivers and care-receivers in relation to the skills and competencies necessary to implement care, the intent is to be both willing and able to do whatever is required. Simply ask a "yes/no" question of each state: Are you *able*, for example, to interview a client? Do you have the knowledge and experience that is required, together with a full understanding of possible outcomes? Further, are you *willing* and confident to take responsibility, having a need to achieve effectively, feeling committed, and being fully accountable?[1] These same types of questions can be asked of the care-receiver.

TOOLS IN EVALUATION

There are formal tools that can be used by the nurse to assist in and amplify the evaluative process. These include progress notes, team conferences, and discharge summaries.

Progress Notes

Progress notes take many forms, such as nurse's notes, notes written on the "Progress Notes" sheet by all health personnel involved in the client's care, and the SOAP method discussed in Chapter 8. Many health-care systems require that personnel record routine care in addition to deviations from the normal health states of the client. Whatever the form, however, progress notes should contain statements concerning the nursing diagnosis of the client and the client's progress to date. The movement should be in relation to the goals of care explicated previously and should be changed whenever indicated.

Progress notes provide for continuity of care between health workers, as the entire team works to assist the client in reaching fullest health potential.

Team Conferences

At its best, the team conference involves all persons involved in the care of a client and family. It is a time to discuss the entire care plan, problem-solve, explain, gain competence in skills, and evaluate. With many people sharing expertise and perceptions in a given area, the results can be more reliable and creative and have a broader foundation than a single person's efforts. Team conferences also tend to solidify the system's approach by including everyone in the client's health-plan system. This group approach also can become the bond builder between health workers so that each can become a teacher and learner for and with one another. It strengthens *team* work and creates a support system for all people who are part of it.

Discharge Summaries

Discharge summaries can be used as referrals or summaries of the client's progress to date. They should include a synthesis of client data,

---

[1]Descriptions of the states "willing" and "able" are from Hersey and Blanchard's (1982) leadership model. This author has added the nursing applications.

nursing diagnoses and orders, evaluation of nursing care to date, and recommendations for future nursing care, if appropriate. This is important in continuing care so that the ladder effect in nursing—that is, moving from simple to complex, from low to high maturity—can be facilitated and subsequent caregivers will not have to regress to a zero base.

The summary generally and simply states the patient's progress in relation to the priority diagnoses and may give reference to those areas that are expected to emerge for priority in another time and place. Should clients be readmitted to a health facility, the discharge summary serves as a secondary source of data.

CONTINUOUS EVALUATION, FEEDBACK, AND DATA COLLECTION

The last step of the nursing process, evaluation, is bridged by feedback to the first step; the process begins again, and it is important that it continue dynamically. Actually, the nursing process should not be thought of as linear but as circular, as denoted in Figure 11–1.

Each facet of the nursing-process "pie" is intersected with feedback, which relates to all parts of the system. For example, the results of evaluation become new sources of data that must be processed. This data processing may change a nursing diagnosis, which must then be reflected in the nursing orders. Different orders may require changes in implementation, and all must then be reevaluated, producing additional data. This cyclic process occurs continuously.

SUMMARY

Chapter 11 discussed evaluation and concluded the section on the methods involved in the nursing process. Evaluation was discussed theoretically as it applies in nursing practice, followed by examples of formal and informal

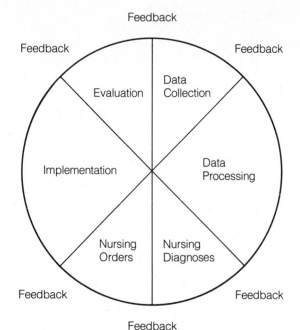

Figure 11–1

The Dynamic Nursing Process

evaluation processes. Team conferences, progress notes, and discharge summaries were discussed as tools in evaluation. The nursing process was then portrayed as a dynamic method of delivering quality, comprehensive, individualized nursing care. Chapter 12 is a discussion of nursing-service quality assurance—a broader aspect of evaluation.

REFERENCES

Conley, V. (1973). *Curriculum and instruction in nursing.* Boston: Little, Brown.

Griffith, J., & Christensen, P. (1982). *Nursing process: Application of theories, frameworks, and models.* St. Louis: Mosby.

Hagan, E. (1975). Conceptual issues in the appraisal of the quality of care. In *Assessment of Nursing Services*, report of the conference sponsored by the Division of Nursing, Department of Health, Education, and Welfare. Bethesda, MD: U.S.D.H.E.W., Publication No. (HRA) 75-40, May.

Hersey, P., & Blanchard, K. (1982). *Management of organizational behavior: Utilizing human resources* (4th ed.). Englewood Cliffs, NJ: Prentice-Hall.

Inzer, F., & Aspinall, M.J. (1981). Evaluating patient outcomes. *Nursing Outlook, 29,* 178–181.

Kozier, B., & Erb, G. (1983). *Fundamentals of nursing: Concepts and procedures* (2nd ed.). Menlo Park, CA: Addison-Wesley.

La Monica, E. (1979). *The nursing process: A humanistic approach.* Menlo Park, CA: Addison-Wesley.

Lindeman, C. (1976a). Measuring quality of nursing care—Part One. *The Journal of Nursing Administration, 6* (5), 7–9.

Lindeman, C. (1976b). Measuring quality of nursing care—Part Two. *The Journal of Nursing Administration, 6* (7), 16–19.

McGuire, R. (1968). Bedside nursing audit. *American Journal of Nursing, 68,* 2146–2148.

Phaneuf, M. (1966). The nursing audit for evaluation of patient care. *Nursing Outlook, 14,* 51–54.

Rubin, C., Rinaldi, L., & Dietz, R. (1972). Nursing audit—Nurses evaluating nursing. *American Journal of Nursing, 72,* 916–921.

Yura, H., & Walsh, M. (1983). *The nursing process: Assessing, planning, implementing, evaluating* (4th ed.). Norwalk CT: Appleton-Century-Crofts.

SELECTED READING

The selected reading for this chapter is a description of a small study designed to assist nurses to develop evaluative outcome criteria. It contains some specific examples of how to break down outcome criteria so that achievement can be measured on a five-point scale.

Evaluating Patient Outcomes

Frances Inzer
Mary Jo Aspinall

Every nurse who has ever developed a care plan knows the importance of formulating patient goals. In the past, nursing activities were often included in these goals; however, in recent years nurses have developed goal statements in terms of patient outcome behavior. The word "outcome" is generally accepted to mean the end result of an activity, rather than the activity itself. Examples of goal statements for patient outcome behavior are: "will be free of chest pain," "will ambulate the length of the hall," and "will demonstrate colostomy care." These goals indicate a focus on the patient's end behavior, not the nurse's action.

Currently, considerable attention is being given to the development of outcome criteria as a measurement tool in the evaluation process. Such criteria are being utilized in quality assurance programs, nursing audits, standards for accreditation of hospitals, and standards for nursing practice. For instance, Standard IV of the American Nurses' Association's *Standards for Medical-Surgical Nursing Practice* stipulates that in evaluation of the nursing care plan, "patient response is compared with observable outcomes which are specified in the goals."[1]

OBJECTIVE MEASUREMENTS

As with all new concepts, however, the ideas are intellectually adopted before they are actually put into practice. In reviewing a number of

patient (medical) records, we found that most nurses record patient responses in judgmental, interpretive terms—such as "seems to be more comfortable," "wound appears to be healing"—instead of in specific behavioral terminology. Upon closer examination, the identification of specific criteria that could be used as an index for evaluation by all nurses who recorded the patient's response was strikingly absent. For example, one nurse may have recorded that the patient was increasing in ambulation when he could walk from the bed to the chair, whereas another nurse may have stated he achieved this goal when he could walk the length of the corridor. Without specificity, recordings are unreliable as indicators of patient progress.

In searching the literature, a number of articles identified the need to refine objective methods of measuring patient progress as basic to building the science of nursing. For the most part, however, there are relatively few articles describing tools that operationalize evaluation of goal attainment. In one article, Zimmer and others describe prototype sets of health outcome criteria that they developed for specific patient populations.[2] They defined increment measurements for each criterion and demonstrated how each could be scaled for measurement purposes.

Since there has been limited scientific testing of scales to measure patient progress, we raised the question: Is it feasible to utilize observable patient behavioral data to develop a practical incremental scale for measuring patient outcome behavior in relation to goal attainment? The answer to this question came, in part, from a study in which a group of RNs on three surgical wards at the Veterans Administration Medical Center, Long Beach, California, participated. The study, reported by Hefferin, evaluated the effectiveness of experimental treatment by the degree and rate of the patient's goal attainment.[3]

FORMULATING GOALS

Prior to the study period, patient goals which were recorded on nursing care plans in the study wards were surveyed in order to determine the type of goals that would require scaling. Since many goals were stated in general, nonspecific terms such as "will be able to care for self after discharge," "will return to board and care home," it was apparent that nurses would first need help in learning to state goals in specific, measurable terms.

Once they had mastered formulating goal statements, the next task was developing scales to measure the attainment of the goals. A modified version of the standard Goal Attainment Scaling (GAS) method, described by Kiresuk, was utilized.[4] This method calls for a goal-continuum of five relatively equal increments for each goal. For the study, the patient's initial status was made Step 1. Four other steps or levels, depicting progressive goal achievement, were then developed with Step 5 indicating goal attainment. Through this five-point scale, measurement of the patient's progress toward the goal could be made at specified time intervals.

EXAMPLE 1.   GOAL: TO LOSE 10 POUNDS OF WEIGHT

Step 1	Step 2	Step 3	Step 4	Step 5
weighs 190 pounds (present weight)	weighs 187–189 pounds	weighs 184–186 pounds	weighs 181–183 pounds	weighs 180 pounds or less (desired weight)

EXAMPLE 2.   GOAL: TO CARE FOR COLOSTOMY WITHOUT ASSISTANCE
Subgoal: To remove soiled bag

Step 1	Step 2	Step 3	Step 4	Step 5
Cannot do task without assistance	Can do 25% of task without assistance	Can do 50% of task without assistance	Can do 75% of task without assistance	Can do 100% of task without assistance

EXAMPLE 3.   GOAL: TO CARE FOR COLOSTOMY WITHOUT ASSISTANCE

Step 1	Step 2	Step 3	Step 4	Step 5
Unable to do any care without assistance	Able to remove soiled bag without assistance	Able to remove soiled bag and irrigate without assistance	Able to remove soiled bag, irrigate, and cleanse stoma without assistance	Able to remove soiled bag, irrigate, cleanse stoma, and apply new bag without assistance

EXAMPLE 4.   GOAL: TO CARE FOR COLOSTOMY WITHOUT ASSISTANCE
Four components —remove soiled bag—irrigate—cleanse stoma—apply new bag

Step 1	Step 2	Step 3	Step 4	Step 5
Does none of above without assistance	Does one of above without assistance	Does two of above without assistance	Does three of above without assistance	Does four of above without assistance

EXAMPLE 5.   GOAL: TO WALK WITH CRUTCHES (RIGHT LEG TOE TOUCHING ONLY)
                          ON LEVEL SURFACES AND STAIRS

Four components —do 10 consecutive quad sets and 10 consecutive straight leg raises
                        —transfer from bed to chair (or guerney)—walk with crutches on stairs
                          parallel bars with right leg toe touching

Step 1	Step 2	Step 3	Step 4	Step 5
Does none of the above	Does one of above	Does two of above	Does three of above	Does four of above

EXAMPLE 6.   GOAL: TO WALK WITH CRUTCHES (PATIENT WITH 2ND STAGE SYMES, LEFT FOOT)

Seven components —transfer from bed to chair by self—rise from chair and stand—balance on right foot
                         without support—stand on toes of right foot while holding to chair—hop on one
                         foot while holding to a stationary chair—hop on one foot while moving along
                         parallel bars—walk with crutches

Step 1	Step 2	Step 3	Step 4	Step 5
Does none of above	Does one or two of above	Does three or four of above	Does five or six of above	Does all of above

EXAMPLE 7.   GOAL: TO INCREASE THE RANGE OF MOTION OF THE LEFT SHOULDER
                          (PATIENT WITH LEFT TRANSCERVICAL FRACTURE)

Four components —can extend left upper extremity forward—can extend left upper extremity sideways
                        —can do circular motion of left upper extremity—can raise and lower shoulders

Step 1	Step 2	Step 3	Step 4	Step 5
Does none of above	Does one of above	Does two of above	Does three of above	Does four of above

EXAMPLE 8.   GOAL: TO INCREASE RANGE OF MOTION OF RIGHT ARM
                          (PATIENT WITH THORACOTOMY AND RIGHT LOWER LOBE LOBECTOMY)

Four components —can raise arm straight in front—can raise arm straight to side
                        —can raise arm straight overhead—can raise arm and reach to back

Step 1	Step 2	Step 3	Step 4	Step 5
Does none of above	Does one of above	Does two of above	Does three of above	Does four of above

EXAMPLE 9.   GOAL: TO HAVE A HEALED STUMP

Four components —no swelling—no drainage—no pain or exceptionally tender spots
                        —presence of granulation tissue

Step 1	Step 2	Step 3	Step 4	Step 5
Has none of above	Has one of above	Has two of above	Has three of above	Has four of above

EXAMPLE 10.   GOAL: TO GET OUT OF BED WITHOUT ASSISTANCE

Four components —move to side of bed without assistance—swing both legs over side of bed without
assistance—get to a sitting position on the side of bed without assistance
—push self up to a standing position without assistance

Step 1	Step 2	Step 3	Step 4	Step 5
Does none of above	Does one of above	Does two of above	Does three of above	Does four of above

DEVELOPING SCALES

Goals involving a numerical component were fairly easy to scale, while other goals were more difficult because of their abstract nature. Examples of goals with a numerical component are: "to lose 10 pounds," "to reduce the blood pressure by 10 mm Hg." Scaling a numerical goal is illustrated in Example 1.

After this relatively easy task, we directed our attention to finding a system to evaluate non-numerical goals such as "to care for colostomy without assistance." However, in reaching this goal, several activities are involved—that is, removing the bag, irrigating the colon, cleansing the stoma, and applying a new bag. Mindful of the old adage about mixing apples and oranges, it was decided to experiment with a separate subgoal for each component and use a scale to measure attainment for each. Example 2 illustrates one subgoal attainment scale.

This method of scaling subgoals did not seem to be a feasible solution, however, because it was difficult to gauge what 25 percent, 50 percent, etc., would be. Another problem was how to measure the patient's total ability to accomplish all the subgoals without assistance, since a patient could be at Step 2 of one subgoal and Step 5 of another at the same point in time.

We then tried another approach to scale the main goal by incorporating attainment of each subgoal in a progressive manner as shown in Example 3. But, we quickly recognized the problems with this method: some patients did not progress in the order in which elements of the steps were written. For instance, some patients could apply a new bag without assis-

tance, but they could not remove the soiled bag without assistance.

The format that was finally adopted listed all components of the goal. Each step indicated the number of components the patient could perform, regardless of the sequence in which the patient accomplished the task (see Example 4). This method seemed to differentiate effectively between levels of goal achievement and was easily understandable to the nurses.

USING PATIENT OUTCOMES SCALES

A few of the nurses, after seeing one example of this method, could independently identify components of a goal and develop a scale to measure its achievement. Others had difficulty in analyzing activities that a patient had to complete to achieve a goal. The problems ranged from those nurses who could not identify any integral activities to those who identified too many activities, most of which did not pertain to the goal.

Obviously, many of the nurses needed to develop skills in both analyzing patient goals and synthesizing essential elements or activities into the goal. We used a directed thought process during the training period to help them achieve these skills, that is, we asked the following questions:

"Tell me what a patient will have to do in order to walk on crutches." "Will he be able to get out of bed alone?" "Does he need to learn how to move himself to the side of the bed?" "Are quad set exercises essential to his walking?" "What is the outcome you expect of the patient as a result of your using the Nelson bed?" "If he needs to climb stairs as well as walk on level surfaces, then shouldn't the goal be stated 'to walk with crutches on level surfaces and stairs'?"

With guided practice, all of the nurses developed the ability to analyze a goal and divide it into component parts, which were stated as patient outcomes rather than nursing actions. They also learned to synthesize essential elements into a comprehensive goal when certain activities were not included in the original goal statement. The complexity of this task is shown in Example 5, which was written for a patient with right total hip prosthesis.

We were concerned that the nurses would tend to use the same scale, perhaps inappropriately, for another patient with the same goal. Although some duplication occurred, the nurses individualized the scale if different component activities were involved. For example, a patient with a Symes procedure needs to learn to walk with crutches as does a patient with a total hip prosthesis. However, since most patients with a Symes procedure have no problem with quad sets and straight leg raising, this is not an appropriate activity for them. Instead, they need to learn balancing, since they cannot toe touch. The goal for a patient with this condition is scaled in Example 6.

Another demonstration of individualizing a scale is shown in Examples 7 and 8. These two scales evaluate range of motion of the upper extremity for patients with different surgical conditions. Although only one goal was needed to assess progress in a few patients in the study, most patients were evaluated in attaining two or three goals. For instance, a patient with an amputation might have a goal for stump healing for prosthesis fit in addition to the goal of walking with crutches. In this situation, both Example 5 and Example 9 goals would be evaluated for this patient.

In using the scales, it became obvious that a five-point scale was easier with four components or multiples of four. Many nurses had a tendency to list four components, omitting a fifth if it did not seem too vital. This practice did not seem to be a disadvantage, since components usually were carefully weighed to select the most essential. We consistently used a five-point scale because the data were being statistically evaluated in a research project. However, any combination of intervals of four, six, or other numbered scales could be used in most practice settings.

Most of the examples cited are discharge goals, which are usually appropriate for most surgical patients because of the short length of their hospitalization. For a few patients who had complications, a longer stay in the hospital was required. In these instances, the nurses had to learn to write more basic goals because these patients progressed more slowly. For example, ambulating without assistance would require a considerable period of time for a 78-year-old male, weighing 200 pounds, who had a resection of an abdominal aortic aneurysm. One goal for this patient is stated in Example 10.

SUMMARY

In this study, nurses effectively demonstrated that in addition to stating goals in observable outcomes, they could develop rating scales to measure a patient's progress toward goal attainment. An unexpected finding was that improvement in evaluation was accompanied by corresponding improvement in other components of the nursing process. For example, prior to the study period, nurses rarely listened to chest sounds or measured ventilatory volume to assess lung congestion, even though many had received training in physical assessment and a respirometer was available on the unit. During the study period, however, there was a flurry of auscultation and spirometric measurement activities for patients whose goals were to decrease lung congestion. When one such patient failed to progress as rapidly as the nurse anticipated, greater assistance was given to pulmonary physiotherapy and assistance with coughing.

Although nursing has not given sufficient attention to the development of patient evaluation tools, recent legislation as well as consumers' demand for quality care are providing the impetus for developing such mechanisms in a scientific way. This fact may significantly contribute to refining clinical data for the objective evaluation of patient progress. Since most nurses receive some theoretical education in the evaluation process, the challenge may well be to provide nurses, in both educational and service settings, with practical experiences in developing and implementing evaluation techniques.

REFERENCES

1. AMERICAN NURSES' ASSOCIATION. *Standards of Medical-Surgical Nursing Practice.* Kansas City, Mo., The Association, 1974.

2. ZIMMER, M. J., AND OTHERS. *Development of Sets of Patient Health Outcome Criteria by Panels of Nurse Experts.* (Final Report Project No. 7) Madison, Wisconsin Regional Medical Program, University of Wisconsin Hospitals Nursing Service, and University of Wisconsin-Milwaukee School of Nursing, 1974.

3. HEFFERIN, ELIZABETH. Health goal setting: patient-nurse collaboration at Veterans Administration Facilities. *Military Med.* 144: 814–822, Dec. 1979.

4. KIRESUK, T. J., AND SHERMAN, R. E. Goal attainment scaling: a general method for evaluating comprehensive mental health programs. *Community Ment. Health J.* 4:443–453, Dec. 1968.

Chapter 12

Nursing Audit

The purpose of Chapter 12 is to discuss the nursing audit, a program having the primary goal of assuring quality of nursing practice. In this chapter, the historical development of the audit is briefly traced, followed by a definition of the audit. Characteristics of an effective audit (quality-assurance) system are discussed. The chapter closes with methods for executing an audit, followed by a discussion of the benefits for the consumer and nurse.

HISTORICAL DEVELOPMENT

Pioneering work in medical assessment dates back to 1918 (Deeken, 1960), when the American College of Surgeons concluded that reliable and valid methods of evaluation did not exist. Prior to this time, however, the audit concept had been introduced by managers of industrial corporations who believed that objective criticism of their fiscal status was important (McGuire, 1968).

The seeds of the health-care audit first took root in the field of medicine, and application to the field of nursing was not addressed until the middle fifties (Deeken, 1960). This occurred in nursing despite a book by Finer (1952) that cautioned against it. Finer devoted an entire book to rather convincingly portraying nursing care as quality that could not be quantified. Nevertheless, writings on the nursing quality-assurance program flourished (Doughty & Mash, 1977; Lesnik & Anderson, 1962; McGuire, 1968; Phaneuf, 1964, 1966, 1968, 1976; Rubin, Rinaldi, & Dietz, 1972). Today, a multidisciplinary audit is a requirement mandated by the Joint Commission on Accreditation and Hospitals, and nurses have been highly creative in applying the concept of quality assurance to the specific settings and groups in which nurses function.

NURSING AUDIT DEFINED

Schmadl (1979) provided a conceptual definition of quality assurance:

> Quality assurance involves assuring the consumer of a specified degree of excellence through continuous measurement and evaluation of structural components, goal-directed nursing process, and/or consumer outcome, using preestablished criteria and standards and available norms, and followed by appropriate alteration with the purpose of improvement (p. 465).

Quality assurance is a concept; the nursing audit is a process for studying quality assurance. The term *audit* usually connotes an objective check on the balancing of accounts, as well as a check on financial appropriations and expenditures. The nursing audit is similarly objective but differs because of the nonfinancial operations to which it is applied.

The nursing audit is a program used to assist nurses and nursing in assessing the quality of services provided. It is designed to relate to the functions of nursing as well as to established standards that define quality care. By definition, the term *audit* means a formal, methodical examination of a record by objective,

outside observers. This is followed by a written report of the findings. In a nursing audit, the procedure takes many forms—which are discussed in the methods portion of this chapter—and compares the care given to clients with established nursing standards. This is done by an objective observer. Its purposes are simple (Tinubu, 1976):

1. To constitute a tool for evaluating, verifying, and improving the quality of nursing practice;

2. To provide a basis for client and staff educational programs;

3. To provide a self-evaluative means for developing and improving nursing records;

4. To reveal specific areas of strengths and weaknesses in nursing care, as measured against standards;

5. To reduce the incidence of medical/nursing/legal complications arising from inaccurate or incomplete records and practices.

CHARACTERISTICS OF AN EFFECTIVE EVALUATION SYSTEM

The Joint Commission on Accreditation of Hospitals—JCAH—(1983) explicated the following as the essential requirements for an acceptable client-care evaluation:

1. *Objectivity.* In measuring whether caregivers are functioning at an appropriate level, standards and criteria must be established prior to the evaluation.

2. *Clinically sound.* Given the expertise and resources available, the standards and criteria must reflect optimum care for the client, achievable by the system of caregivers.

3. *Efficient.* Professional nursing time must be used when necessary; nonprofessional time should be allocated to those parts of a program that require no professional judgment.

4. *Flexible*. In the evaluation, variations from standards and criteria are permitted—with reported, good cause.

5. *Documented*. All decisions and evaluations must be written, signed, and reported to the responsible person(s) of quality care.

6. *Action-oriented*. Confirmed deficiencies that may result from an audit must be analyzed and appropriate corrective interventions built.

The JCAH further delineated seven components, or steps, of a quality-assurance program; this author adds an eighth (Step 2—Standards), based on the eloquent words of Hagen (1975). These eight components are as follows:

1. *Criteria*. The kind of variables that are to be appraised.

2. *Standards*. Established expected-performance levels of nursing care (Hagen, 1975).

3. *Measurement*. The retrieval of and methods for collecting patient and nursing data to show conformance with the pre-established criteria and standards.

4. *Evaluation*. The analysis of variations between collected data and standards; deduction of deficiencies and the probable rationale for them.

5. *Action*. Specified corrective measures or programs to eradicate deficiencies.

6. *Follow-up*. Evaluation of the effectiveness of actions (Step 5).

7. *Report*. Written, signed rendition of the entire audit, sent to appropriate, responsible, accountable leaders of the client-care system.

8. *Repeat of the audit process*.

It becomes obvious, then, that the nursing audit is progressive, that all steps interact, and that it establishes a scientific, methodical approach to the problem of securing quality in care.

GENERAL CRITERIA FOR THE NURSING AUDIT

The nursing audit must reflect the goals of the organization and the expertise within the organization relevant to the care rendered. In other words, the audit must be personalized by the system in which it is to be used. For the purpose of learning, however, general variables that are common subjects of the audit can be delineated. Phaneuf (1966) specified seven functions with 50 descriptive statements as a basis for an audit. Her list is not meant to be inclusive of every system, but it provides a foundation upon which agencies can elaborate. Tucker, Breeding, Canobbio, Jacquet, Paquette, Wells, and Willman (1980) provided a complete itemization of variables that may be used when developing audit criteria for specific conditions. Phaneuf's (1966) audit criteria follow:

1. Application and execution of physician's legal orders
   a. Medical diagnosis complete
   b. Orders complete
   c. Orders current
   d. Orders promptly executed
   e. Evidence that nurse understood cause and effect
   f. Evidence that nurse took medical history into account

2. Observations of symptoms and reactions
   a. Related to course of above disease(s) in general
   b. Related to the course of above disease(s) in this patient
   c. Related complications due to therapy (each medication and each treatment)
   d. Vital signs
   e. Patient to his condition (attitude)
   f. Patient to his course of disease(s)

3. Supervision of the patient
   a. Evidence that initial nursing diagnosis was made
   b. Safety of patient
   c. Security of patient
   d. Adaptation (support of patient in reactions to condition and care)
   e. Continuing assessment of patient's condition and capacity
   f. Nursing plans changed in accordance with assessment
   g. Interaction with family and with others considered

4. Supervision of those participating in care (except the physician)
   a. Care taught to patient, family, or other nursing personnel
   b. Physical, emotional, mental capacity to learn considered
   c. Continuity of supervision to those taught
   d. Support of those giving care

5. Reporting and recording
   a. Facts on which further care depended were recorded
   b. Essential facts reported to physician
   c. Reporting of facts included evaluation thereof
   d. Patient or family alerted as to what to report to physician
   e. Record permitted continuity of intramural and extramural care

6. Application and execution of nursing procedures and techniques
   a. Administration and/or supervision of medications
   b. Personal care (bathing, oral hygiene, skin, nail care, shampoo)
   c. Nutrition (including special diets)
   d. Fluid balance
   e. Elimination
   f. Rest or sleep
   g. Physical activity
   h. Irrigations (including enemas)
   i. Dressings and bandages
   j. Formal exercise program
   k. Rehabilitation (other than formal exercises)
   l. Prevention of complications and infections
   m. Recreation, diversion
   n. Clinical procedure—urinalysis, B/P
   o. Special treatments (such as care of tracheostomy, use of oxygen, colostomy or catheter care, and so forth)

7. Promotion of physical and emotional health by direction and teaching
   a. Plans for medical emergency evident
   b. Emotional support to patient
   c. Emotional support to family
   d. Teaching preventive health care
   e. Evaluation of need for additional resources (such as spiritual, social service, homemaker service, physical or occupational therapy)
   f. Action taken in regard to needs identified*

It is noted that all of Phaneuf's components relate to the areas of responsibility of nurses discussed in Chapter 5 of this book. *Nurses are accountable for each and every one.*

JCAH (1983), in association with the Associated Hospital Service of New York (Blue Cross), specified three recommended parts of the nursing-audit report and inclusive items of each:

---

*Copyright 1966 American Journal of Nursing Company. From *Nursing Outlook*, June, Vol. 14, No. 6.

Part 1: Patient identification data and key administrative-policy questions intended to safeguard the rights of patients and institutions. This part can be completed by a trained clerk.

Part 2: Judgment entry made by the nursing-audit committee member who reviewed the chart.

Part 3: Specific comments on the functions of professional nurses according to criteria and standards, in the care of patient(s) in focus.

NURSING-AUDIT METHODS

The most widely used method of collecting data for a nursing audit is the retrospective method. In this, the charts of clients are studied and measured against established criteria and standards. Client-care outcome is the primary focus, even though specific processes such as catheterization may be pointedly studied. In a process audit (Sundeen, Stuart, Rankin, & Cohen, 1981) a direct observational method may be used to observe the nurse providing direct client care.

A variety of methods may be used in the audit, however, and it is important to be aware of them in each specific organization. Even though the term *audit* connotes retrospective study, reality says that this is neither always the case nor always indicated. Methods chosen for evaluation must reflect the purpose for which used, the time given for the project, and the availability of data. Given all three, the best method for achieving goals should be chosen. For more information on methods, the reader is referred to Thorndike and Hagen (1977) for a complete discussion of testing methods and evaluation procedures.

BENEFITS OF A NURSING QUALITY-ASSURANCE PROGRAM

Aside from the fact that a multidisciplinary quality-assurance program is required by JCAH,

it is and should be recognized as valuable for nurses and clients.

With public officials' and consumer demands for health-care quality reaching an all-time high, standards and criteria must be shared and accepted by all. A quality-assurance program in nursing suggests clarity and agreement on nursing care among all parties. It determines the extent to which standards are met and points out needed improvements. Elimination of poor practices is also facilitated through the documentation that occurs during the audit. Furthermore, with the recent law establishing a national prospective-payment system for Medicare inpatient hospital care that is based on "diagnosis-related groupings" (DRGs), it becomes imperative that nursing-care plans be fully documented and audited (Joel, 1983; News, 1983, 1984; Shaffer, 1984). Only in this way can nursing be assured of the staff required to carry out the nursing interventions that are essential for safe, early discharge of the client.

Toward the goal of quality in nursing practices, the audit lends reliability and validity to the changes in procedures, policies, educational priorities, staffing needs, and other aspects that may result, as suggestions or needs, from the auditing process. In other words, documentation through the nursing audit, using a sound research method, is a firm basis for pointing out needed changes in the system.

SUMMARY

Chapter 12 discussed the nursing audit as the quality-assurance program in professional nursing practice. The protocol for an effective evaluation system was delineated, followed by explicit criteria applicable in nursing. The usual method for executing the audit was described, and a discussion of the benefits of the program concluded the chapter. The next chapter is on the rights of patients, a necessary consideration in evaluating nursing care.

REFERENCES

Deeken, Sr. M. (1960). *Guide for nursing service audit.* St. Louis: Catholic Hospital Association of the United States and Canada.

Doughty, D., & Mash, N. (1977). *Nursing audit.* Philadelphia: F. A. Davis.

Finer, H. (1952). *Administration and the nursing services.* New York: Macmillan.

Hagen, E. (1975). Conceptual issues in the appraisal of the quality of care. In *Assessment of nursing services,* report of the conference sponsored by the Division of Nursing, Department of Health, Education, and Welfare. Bethesda, MD: U.S.D.H.E.W., Publication No. (HRA) 75-40, May.

Joel, L. (1983). DRGs: The state of the art of reimbursement for nursing services. *Nursing & Health Care, 4,* 560–563.

Joint Commission on Accreditation of Hospitals. (1983). *Accreditation manual for hospitals.* Chicago: Author.

Lesnik, M., & Anderson, B. (1962). *Nursing practice and the law* (2nd ed.). Philadelphia: Lippincott.

McGuire, R. (1968). Bedside nursing audit. *American Journal of Nursing, 68,* 2146–2148.

News. (1983). The DRG revolution gets rolling; Hospitals already cutting back. *American Journal of Nursing, 83,* 1607–1610+.

News. (1984). New nursing role will be vital to DRG success, says NCFA's Davis. *American Journal of Nursing, 84,* 112–113.

Phaneuf, M. (1964). A nursing audit method. *Nursing Outlook, 12,* 42–45.

Phaneuf, M. (1966). The nursing audit for evaluation of patient care. *Nursing Outlook, 14,* 51–54.

Phaneuf, M. (1968). Analysis of a nursing audit. *Nursing Outlook, 16,* 57–60.

Phaneuf, M. (1976). *The nursing audit: Profile for excellence* (2nd ed.). New York: Appleton-Century-Crofts.

Rubin, C., Rinaldi, L., & Dietz, R. (1972). Nursing audit—nurses evaluating nursing. *American Journal of Nursing, 72,* 916–921.

Schmadl, C. (1979). Quality assurance: Examination of the concept. *Nursing Outlook, 27,* 462–465.

Shaffer, F. (1984). A nursing perspective of the DRG world, Part 1. *Nursing & Health Care, 5,* 48–51.

Sundeen, S., Stuart, G., Rankin, E., & Cohen, S. (1981). *Nurse-client interaction: Implementing the nursing process* (2nd ed.). St. Louis: Mosby.

Thorndike, R., & Hagen, E. (1977). *Measurement and evaluation in psychology and education* (4th ed.). New York: Wiley.

Tinubu, A. (1976). *Nursing audit.* Unpublished paper, Teachers College, Columbia University, New York.

Tucker, S., Breeding, M., Canobbio, M., Jacquet, G., Paquette, E., Wells, M., & Willman, M. (1980). *Patient care standards* (2nd ed.). St. Louis: Mosby.

Chapter 13

Patient Rights

From 1965 to the present, increasing attention has been paid to the rights of health-care consumers. This trend was amplified as public awareness grew regarding health-care activities and the health caregiver's response in desiring more effective, humanistic care with greater client satisfaction. Besides client benefits, all members of the health system also reaped benefits: physician, client, nurse, allied health workers, and organizations that provide services.

The most important work accomplished in securing patients' rights was delivered by the American Hospital Association's (AHA) Board of Trustees' Committee on Health Care for the Disadvantaged. This group has long been recognized as an advocate on behalf of the health-care-consumer population. On February 6, 1973, the AHA House of Delegates approved the original Patient's Bill of Rights, a revised statement of which is presented in this chapter (American Hospital Association, 1975). In addition, Chapter 13 discusses the advocacy role of the nurse in putting this document into operation in all health-care settings. Both concepts—patient rights and advocacy—point out the goal of increased humanism in health practices.

DEFINITION OF ADVOCACY

Advocacy is defined by Webster as an active act of pleading for, supporting, or recommending. The advocate is the person who fills this role; the advocate is one who pleads for or on behalf of another—an intercessor.

It should be noted, however, that the pure concept of advocacy does not imply merely a hierarchical structure, such as a mother defending her child or a nurse interceding for a client in a hospital system. Peers can be advocates of one another, and children can be advocates for parents. Advocacy can work in any necessary direction between people and in any area of life.

A PATIENT'S BILL OF RIGHTS

The American Hospital Association Board of Trustees' Committee on Health Care for the Disadvantaged, which has been a consistent advocate on behalf of consumers of health care services, developed the *Statement on a Patient's Bill of Rights*, which was approved by the AHA House of Delegates February 6, 1973. The statement was published in several forms, one of which was the S74 leaflet in the Association's S series. The S74 leaflet is now superseded by this reprinting of the statement (AHA, 1975).

The American Hospital Association presents a Patient's Bill of Rights with the expectation that observance of these rights will contribute to more effective patient care and greater satisfaction for the patient, his physician, and the hospital organization. Further, the Association presents these rights in the expectation that they will be supported by the hospital on behalf of its patients, as an integral part of the healing process. It is recognized that a personal relationship between the physician and the patient is essential for the provision of proper medical care. The traditional physician-patient relationship takes on a new dimension when care is rendered within an organizational structure. Legal precedent has established that the institution itself also has a responsibility to the patient. It is in recognition of these factors that these rights are affirmed.

1. The patient has the right to considerate and respectful care.

2. The patient has the right to obtain from his physician complete current information concerning his diagnosis, treatment, and prognosis in terms the patient can be reasonably expected to understand. When it is not medically advisable to give such information to the patient, the information should be made available to an appropriate person in his behalf. He has the right to know, by name, the physician responsible for coordinating his care.

3. The patient has the right to receive from his physician information necessary to give informed consent prior to the start of any procedure and/or treatment. Except in emergencies, such information for informed consent should include but not necessarily be limited to the specific procedure and/or treatment, the medically significant risks involved, and the probable duration of incapacitation. Where medically significant alternatives for care or treatment exist, or when the patient requests information concerning medical alternatives, the patient has the right to such information. The patient also has the right to know the name of the person responsible for the procedures and/or treatment.

4. The patient has the right to refuse treatment to the extent permitted by law and to be informed of the medical consequences of his action.

5. The patient has the right to every consideration of his privacy concerning his own medical care program. Case discussion, consultation, examination, and treatment are confidential and should be conducted discreetly. Those not directly involved in his care must have the permission of the patient to be present.

6. The patient has the right to expect that all communications and records pertaining to his care should be treated as confidential.

7. The patient has the right to expect that within its capacity a hospital must make reasonable response to the request of a patient for services. The hospital must provide evaluation, service, and/or referral as indicated by the urgency of the case. When medically permissible, a patient may be transferred to another facility only after he has received complete information and explanation concerning the needs for and alternatives to such a transfer. The institution to which the patient is to be transferred must first have accepted the patient for transfer.

8. The patient has the right to obtain information as to any relationship of his hospital to other health care and educational institutions insofar as his care is concerned. The patient has the right to obtain information as to the existence of any professional relationships among individuals, by name, who are treating him.

9. The patient has the right to be advised if the hospital proposes to engage in or perform human experimentation affecting his care or treatment. The patient has the right to refuse to participate in such research projects.

10. The patient has the right to expect reasonable continuity of care. He has the right to know in advance what appointment times and physicians are available and where. The patient has the right to expect that the hospital will provide a mechanism whereby he is informed by his physician or a delegate of the physician of the patient's continuing health care requirements following discharge.

11. The patient has the right to examine and receive an explanation of his bill regardless of source of payment.

12. The patient has the right to know what hospital rules and regulations apply to his conduct as a patient.*

No catalog of rights can guarantee for the patient the kind of treatment he has a right to

---

*Reprinted with permission of the American Hospital Association, copyright 1975.

expect. A hospital has many functions to perform, including the prevention and treatment of disease, the education of both health professionals and patients, and the conduct of clinical research. All these activities must be conducted with an overriding concern for the patient, and, above all, the recognition of his dignity as a human being. Success in achieving this recognition assures success in the defense of the rights of the patient.

ROLE OF THE NURSE AS A PATIENT ADVOCATE

Since the American Hospital Association passed the Patient's Bill of Rights, hospitals and other community agencies have paid closer attention to the matter of patients' rights. Many hand out brief versions of the rights of clients in pamphlet form upon admission; others post the rights in frequented client areas of the facility. The intent is to make the public aware and to elaborate on the client's control of care by letting the client know these rights and then have avenues through which to ensure them.

Large hospitals are beginning to employ someone in the position of "Patient Advocate" or "Ombudsman." The latter term is often more familiar in academic settings; the philosophic framework of both, however, is congruent. This person is employed primarily for the consumer and acts as liaison between the consumer with problems and the organizational structure, clarifying and, it is hoped, satisfying all involved people regarding their rights.

Even with someone specifically designated as the advocate, however, a responsibility of advocacy always rests with nursing personnel because they are most closely in contact with clients. This contact and relationship can be the source of frequent questions, expression of fears, and teaching activity with the client. It is, therefore, necessary for the nurse to assume the coordinator role in carrying out the advocacy function in response to a system (Marriner, 1983; Yura & Walsh, 1983). If a designated Patient Advocate is available, questions of clients may be referred to the official Advocate. Should diagnostic medical information be requested, the physician should be notified and a written notation made by the nurse. In any area that a professional nurse feels comfortable with knowledge and experience in answering questions and informing the clients—within the confines of the nurse's legal responsibility—the nurse should and must do so. Informed consent and the protection of human subjects are *ethical* rights of all consumers.

Since the Patient's Bill of Rights very often involves interpretation in application to the unique consumer, any questions that the professional nurse has must be answered. Peer teaching and discussion is often necesary, and advice from colleagues with more experience and knowledge should be sought whenever a question exists in interpretation of application. Ethical standards of the nursing profession must *always* be followed.

Annas (1975) elaborated on the Patient's Bill of Rights in his recent publication entitled *The Rights of Hospitalized Patients*. He specified that, in addition to the AHA items, clients should

1. Have round-the-clock telephone access to an advocate who can answer their questions;

2. Participate in all decisions regarding their health-care program;

3. Be knowledgeable of research and experimental protocols involved in their care;

4. Have access to an interpreter if they do not speak English;

5. Have the right to consult a specialist at their request and expense;

6. Have the legal right to refuse treatments performed on them with primary emphasis on educational purposes, rather than direct personal benefits; and

7. Have a right to be accessible to visitors and have access to a telephone—parents and family of terminally ill clients being able to come and go totally at their will.

Annas (1975) did not deviate from the AHA (1975) statements, but he did become more specific.

SUMMARY

Client rights have been discussed, with emphasis on the role of the professional nurse in carrying out the statements on rights passed by the American Hospital Association in 1973. The responsibility of the nurse varies within the institution in which the nurse is employed and depends on the complement of personnel attending the advocacy function. Coordination of all aspects of this facet of client care, however, rests with the nurse; the nurse must ensure that all client needs in this area are met.

A closely allied area of patient rights is ethics. Chapter 14, written by Dr. Maxine Greene, contains a poignant discussion of this concept. Dr. Greene is an internationally recognized scholar of philosophy.

REFERENCES

American Hospital Association. (1975). *A patient's bill of rights*. Chicago: Author.

Annas, G. (1975). *The rights of hospital patients*. New York: Avon Books.

Marriner, A. (1983). *The nursing process: A scientific approach to nursing care* (3rd. ed.). St. Louis: Mosby.

Yura, H., & Walsh, M. (1983). *The nursing process: Assessing, planning, implementing, evaluating* (4th ed.). Norwalk, CT: Appleton-Century-Crofts.

Chapter 14

Ethical Choosing

by Maxine Greene

In Leo Tolstoy's (1875–1877/1946) *Anna Karenina*, as in other great novels, there are many descriptions of people falling ill and of the challenges their illnesses pose to other people. They are the kinds of challenges that put those around the sufferer to the test, that reveal people to themselves. On one occasion, Levin's embittered, unappealing brother Nikolay falls desperately ill in a roadside hotel. When Levin goes to visit him, he finds he cannot be natural and calm in the sick man's presence. "He smelt the awful odor, saw the dirt, disorder and miserable condition, and heard the groans, and felt that nothing could be done to help" (p. 560). It never occurs to him to consider how Nikolay's "emaciated legs and thighs and spine were lying huddled up, and whether they could not be made more comfortable, whether anything could be done to make things, if not better, at least less bad" (p. 560). He is sure that nothing can be done for Nikolay to prolong his life, and the thought of the details of his brother's situation makes his blood run cold. Fearful and

Maxine Greene, A.B., Ph.D., L.H.D., is Professor of Philosophy and Education and the William F. Russell Professor in the Foundations of Education, Teachers College, Columbia University, New York, New York.

270

powerless, he keeps thinking of excuses to go out of the room. Levin's wife Kitty, in contrast, feels an instant desire to act when she sees Nikolay, even though she has no particular training or skill. "And since she had not the slightest doubt that it was her duty to help him, she had no doubt either that it was possible, and immediately set to work. The very details, the mere thought of which reduced her husband to terror, immediately engaged her attention" (pp. 560–561). She sends for the doctor, sends out for medication, has the room cleaned, changes the sheets, makes Nikolay comfortable, restores a kind of hope. She chooses herself— although she is not compelled to do so—as a kind of nurse, a healer, and something is disclosed to her about her own identity.

In Albert Camus's (1948) *The Plague*, which is full of dreadful scenes of suffering and separation, Dr. Rieux has repeatedly to deal with the relatives of the plague-stricken in "fever-hot, nerve-ridden sickrooms," where he treats the ill as well as he can even as he arranges for their removal. For a while he defends against the horror of it with indifference and abstraction. At most, he is determined to reject the "scheme of things" and simply go on struggling against death. "The essential thing," he and his co-workers in the sanitary squads decide, "was to save the greatest possible number of persons from dying and being doomed to unending separation. And to do this there was only one resource: to fight the plague" (p. 122). When the plague has receded, the doctor is no longer so abstract, and he decides that he has to bear witness in favor of those afflicted: ". . . to state quite simply what we learn in time of pestilence: that there are more things to admire in men than to despise" (p. 278). He knows there is no final victory, that joy will always be imperiled, and that everything they had done would have to be done again and again "in the never ending fight against terror and its relentless onslaughts, despite their personal afflictions, by all who, while unable to be saints but refusing to bow down to pestilences, strive their utmost to be healers" (p. 278.)

DUTY AND PERSONAL AGENCY

These are two quite different renderings of what it signifies to strive to be a healer, but they are linked by a sense of "duty" or "oughtness" or "obligation." They are linked, too, by the suggestion that significant choices of the kind described are free choices. People cannot be coerced to be healers, if to be a healer entails paying attention, feeling concern, taking action for the good of another, striving "to be." People surely can be ordered to—or compelled to, or required to—make beds, use syringes, administer medications, fill out charts, maintain life-support machines. They can do what they "have" to do routinely, indifferently, correctly. In the one case, they are choosing themselves freely in the light of some conception of good or right, some idea of what they ought to do and be. In the other cases, they are probably behaving properly, conforming to command or to external rule. They are not, we shall be insisting, acting as moral agents, for all the likelihood that what they do is "right."

The difference lies partly in the degree of personal agency experienced by the individual (whether this person is a physician, nurse, nurse-practitioner, administrator, or layperson) in situations where there are perceived alternatives. Kitty, for instance, had no doubt "that it was her duty to help" even though she knew full well that, like her husband, she could have run out of the room. Dr. Rieux freely decides to save as many people as he can, although he could just as easily have stayed in his office and avoided the "nerve-ridden" rooms. Both were able to take initiatives; they *acted*; they did not simply behave. Both, as it were, chose to choose with a conception of what was right or good in mind.

NURSING DECISIONS

To consider what is involved in health ethics— or nursing ethics, or medical ethics—is to think not only about the kinds of situations that call for the making of moral decisions. It is to think about the ways those situations are attended to, the ways in which they are experienced and interpreted by men and women who, theoretically, are responsible. One peculiarity of the decision making required is that it is almost always specific and concrete. There are factors in each situation that are inevitably unique, since human beings and their predicaments vary almost infinitely. Should the truth be told to a terminally ill patient, begging to know whether she is going to survive? Much depends, of course, on the orders given by the physician, but there is also the question of how the nurse, let us say, chooses to deal with those orders. As important is the nurse's attitude to the whole matter of truth-telling and the alternatives to telling the truth. There is, as well, the nature of the patient asking the question: her age, intelligence, and psychic strength. There is also the *look* of the patient; there is the way the sound of her voice affects the nurse, the way her hands gesture, the way she glances toward window or door. The nurse may have had numerous encounters with patients making the same request under similar conditions, but there are elements in this situation (as there were in every other) that are new, urgencies for which the nurse could not conceivably have prepared.

In deciding what to do, any practitioner is bound to look for guidance somewhere. More than likely, this person will try to consult guidelines that seem relevant, or a set of principles, or some more or less general idea or ideal of the good. Wherever he or she turns, however, the prescription or norm is bound to seem abstract, since it is presumably applicable to a whole category of cases, not invented for this one alone. Because of that, it may not seem to apply precisely. (Think, for instance, of the guidelines that call upon the nurse always to await the physician's instructions. Think of universal principles, like the one that calls on human beings always to tell the truth. Think of prohibitions like the one forbidding actions that might cause unnecessary suffering. Think of the Golden Rule.) To add to the complexity, the guidelines or principles or norms that come to mind may conflict with one another. Surely, we ought to tell the truth, but we ought not to inflict the pain accompanying the anxiety the patient will undoubtedly feel if the terrible truth is told. We ought to show our respect for the dignity of the patient by spelling out precisely what we know, but we are professionally obligated to await the physician's word. Acknowledging the possibility of conflict, we also have to acknowledge that there is no court of last resort.

As has been said above, to set all this aside and react automatically or indifferently to the patient's question is to evade or avoid moral responsibility. Another alternative is simply to act in accord with inclination, or in terms of what "feels right," or on pure intuition. A sensitive, empathic nurse might well decide to let emotion be his or her guide. Situations like this, the nurse might think, cannot be settled cognitively. How, after all, can one measure or analyze despair? How can one weigh pros and cons when a person in trouble is pleading for a response? Are not moral decisions primarily subjective in any case? The difficulty with this approach is that it makes it nearly impossible to account for whatever action is chosen *or* to justify it. Justification depends upon having good reasons, and reasons require reference points. It is never enough, especially in social or institutional situations, to say, "Well, I *felt* that way."

THE UNCERTAINTIES OF CHOICE

It is seldom easy, and we must begin with a recognition of the uncertainties, the tensions, associated with ethical choosing. We must begin with some awareness that the ability to act morally demands what Kierkegaard (1843/1947) described as a particular kind of courage, the courage to be (pp. 106–107). That means a capacity to recognize when one stands at a crossroads in life, a place where—usually without guarantees—one is bound to move one way or another. Robert Frost's (1972) poem, "The Road Not Taken" comes to mind. It begins, the reader may recall:

> Two roads diverged in a yellow wood,
> And sorry I could not travel both
> And be one traveler, long I stood
> And looked down one as far as I could
> To where it bent in the undergrowth
> (p. 171).

Both roads were equally fair, both were covered with leaves "no step had trodden black," and the poet knows that, even if he saved one for another day, it was doubtful he would ever come back. He had, nevertheless, to choose one, never sure that it was the right one or the best one. "I took the one less traveled by, / And that has made all the difference" (Frost, 1972). Looking back later, unable to retrace his steps, he could say nothing else. The alternative, of course, was to turn his back and avoid the problem of diverging roads. If he had done that, he would have been like Levin, thinking of excuses. He would have been like the people in Camus's novel who resigned themselves to the plague and stayed at the bars or the card tables, bowing down (as the doctor would have put it) to pestilence. There are always those who do not choose to choose, but here we are concerned with the ones willing to acknowledge "the road not taken," the risk, the uncertainty, the problem of choice. How *does* one decide what choice to make, what (in particular situations) one ought to do?

Now, it must be clear that questions like this cannot be answered with statements of fact. Values, unlike facts, cannot be empirically verified; statements of value cannot be demonstrated to be true or false. We are in the domain of values once we begin talking about moral choice. Values may be thought of as conceptions of the desirable, of what appears worthy of appreciation or cherishing, of that which is believed to be good or right. Not all values, of course, have to do with morality: we may value certain objects, works of art, modes of recreation, ways of proceeding in solving problems or affirming truths. When value words are applied to human conduct, we make what might be called moral judgments about others or ourselves. To describe a person or a course of action as decent, humane, honest, courageous, fair, or compassionate is ordinarily to make such a judgment. It is to express approval or to recognize that some standard or norm is being complied with, that a person (given what is valued in the culture) can be described as a good person or that the course of action can be described as right.

CULTURAL CONTEXT

Judgments of this sort cannot be made in a vacuum. We are all born into cultures identified by certain moral codes and practices. Our earliest experiences of acculturation are experiences of being inducted into what has been called the "moral institution" that has developed in our society over time (Frankena, 1963, p. 5). This is the case whether the society is an authoritarian society, a slave society, or a free society. In *The Adventures of Huckleberry Finn* (Twain, 1885/1959), the focal event highlights this fact with particular poignancy. Huck and the runaway slave Jim have been on the river together for many weeks; they have become, as it were, brothers, if not surrogate father and son. Then Huck sees a handbill offering a reward for Jim's return. Hard as it is for the contemporary reader to accept, Huck abruptly realizes that he has offended against the moral code of the community. He would, he now sees, be doing "the right thing and the clean thing" if he wrote and reported Jim's whereabouts. Only if he turns him in, will he feel "all washed clean of sin." But he cannot do what he should do, and, at length, he concludes, "All right, then, I'll *go* to hell . . ." (pp.209–210). Not only have the dominant institutions in the slave society defined complicity with a runaway slave as a sin; Huck has internalized official notions of the good and right; his very conscience tells him he is wrong. He acts *against* his own conscience when he refuses to comply; he does not challenge existing codes. He is a boy, after all, and in no position to effect significant change.

There is something analogous to this in the plight of the nurse two decades or so ago. The "moral institution" that prevailed in the world of clinics and hospitals required nurses to follow physicians' orders without questioning or protest. Here, too, there existed a network of customs, codes, and rules, if not laws. If a nurse refused an order or asserted a contrary opinion, she might not have felt sinful, but she surely would have felt guilt or fear, no matter what the degree of her frustration or rage. Like Huck, she might have refused to comply (at the risk of losing her job), but, in refusing, she would have known that she was fundamentally wrong. Most nurses were female in those days; as women, they were in no better position than the adolescent Huck Finn. Very few, it would appear, challenged the institution itself. Most behaved prudentially. They did not view themselves as people free to consider alternative courses of action (apart from the course of leaving the profession); they did not view themselves as moral agents, free to choose.

THE SCOPE OF CHANGE

Even as in the case of Southern society, things have fundamentally changed for health professionals. It is certainly true that they must cope with administrative bureaucracies and status hierarchies in the institutions where they do their work, but the traditional legitimation systems are no longer taken for granted as givens. For one thing, they no longer accord with technological and attitudinal changes occurring throughout the society. The claims of expertise have been repeatedly questioned, along with paternalism and all that that implies. What long showed itself as "benevolence" has been shown to have its "limits" (Gaylin, Glasser, Marcus, & Rothman, 1978). As respect for and trust in authorities have eroded, more and more

excluded populations have affirmed their human rights. The origin of recent "rights revolutions" can be found in the civil rights movements of the 1960s, soon followed by struggles for woman's rights, children's rights, the rights of the handicapped, and patients' rights (Dorsen, 1971; Rothman, 1971). At times, it may appear that the hard-won victories in these areas are being eroded, but it is extremely unlikely that society will slip back into conditions of taken-for-granted submission, discrimination, and bigotry. The rejection, for example, of even well-meaning control and management is likely to increase, rather than decrease. More and more people will feel entitled to be consulted in matters concerning their welfare. Before treatment (or counseling, or guidance, or rehabilitation) of any sort is given, they will say they are entitled to be asked for their consent.

Technological developments and the growth of technical expertise have had profound effects as well. Perhaps even more influential, however, has been the proliferation of what Jacques Ellul (1967) once called "self-generating" or "self-augmenting" technique. He wrote that "technique has arrived at such a point in its evolution that it is being transformed and is progressing almost without decisive intervention by man" (p. 85). Dialysis machines, cat scans and brain scans, life-support mechanisms, lasers: all have increased the range and efficacy of the health professions, but they daily alter the roles and functions of practitioners. Lewis Thomas (1983) reminds us that "the mechanization of scientific medicine is here to stay," that the doctor/patient relationship is no longer "a long conversation" with the patient at the "epicenter of concern" (pp. 59–60). Computerized diagnoses and projections have replaced such conversation; arrays of complex machines have taken the place of "hands-on" medical care. Thomas does not lament this or wish it otherwise, because it has obviously made medical treatments more scientific, precise, and effective. But it has clearly changed the physician/patient relationship and imposed upon the nurse a range of new responsibilities, some of them responsibilities for "conversation," many for ethical choice.

Few nurses are unfamiliar with the case of Karen Quinlan and the difficult moral challenges it presented. It is true that no individual nurse was burdened with the responsibility of deciding whether or not to release Karen Quinlan from the life-support apparatus, but enough nurses have been witness to similar situations to perceive the dilemmas involved. Some have been obligated to care for brain-dead infants or hopelessly burned patients; they know how narrow the line may be between choosing to sustain life and choosing to let people die. They know, in other words, that both alternatives may be in some sense "right," and there are those who have been either directed to take the responsibility to decide or who have seized the opportunity themselves. Increasing numbers of nurses, too, have had to face the personal and moral difficulties involved in maintaining the vital functions of those who are potential organ donors. Others have had to confront the painful alternatives facing professional staffs in cases of child abuse, especially sexual abuse. All these situations dramatize, on some level, the need to pay attention to ethical questions and concerns. On another level, however, they dramatize the temptations of what has been called "technicism" in dealing with such problems. "Technicism" means, as Manfred Stanley (1978) puts it, the tendency to ignore the need "to pay attention to the *discontinuities* between the human world and other worlds that are also the objects of scientific attention" (p. 13). It is one thing to see a Karen Quinlan in terms of statistical probabilities or scientific variables and simply to act in accord with them. It is quite another to recognize the discontinuity, or the difference, between a Karen Quinlan, say, and a faulty machine. Even so, there are those who tend to believe that it is best to turn to science when faced with problems of that sort. It is not at all uncommon, in these times, for people to accept scientific

assumptions and scientific truths as in some way ultimate, to view scientific method as universally applicable. To function scientifically or empirically, after all, is to be in a position to test certain hypotheses, to consult available evidence, and to demonstrate the truth of one's conclusions.

The nursing profession is in no way immune to this tendency. The alternative to a kind of low-level vocational or practical approach, we are told, can only be one that is rigorously scientific. That means, for many, trying to be unbiased and value-free in all the domains of practice. Reliability and fairness (not to speak of efficiency) appear to be more likely if individuals remain neutral, "rational"—in some manner removed. There are new professionals who are convinced (perhaps through having been taught) that valuing ought to be separated from knowing and inquiry, especially professional inquiry. It is as if the introduction of value judgments or feelings (compassion, sympathy, kindness) would inevitably interfere with clear thinking and the application of techniques. For some, to be cool and efficient and impersonal is to challenge the old sexist stereotypes so long pervasive in nursing. They aspire to the kind of autonomy Lawrence Kohlberg (1973, pp. 29–30) tells us defines the fifth and sixth stages of moral development. Interestingly enough, when Kohlberg describes the individual (almost always a male) who attains one of those stages, he says he moves "to a perspective outside that of his society" and, in doing so, identifies morality with justice. The very notion of an "outside" perspective suggests a release from the kinds of relationships some people think make it so difficult to function according to a scientific paradigm.

SCIENCE AND BEYOND

Leaving aside the question of whether Kohlberg's (1973) description adequately accounts for women's experiences (Gilligan, 1982, pp. 18–19), we need to recall John Dewey's (1958) comment that "the realm of meanings is wider than that of true-and-false meanings; it is more urgent and more fertile. When the claim of meanings to truth enters in, then truth is indeed preeminent. But this fact is often confused with the idea that truth has a claim to every everywhere, that it has a monopolistic jurisdiction. Poetic meanings, moral meanings, a large part of the goods of life are matters of richness and freedom of meanings, rather than of truth; a large part of our life is carried on in a realm of meanings to which truth and falsity as such are irrelevant" (pp. 410–411). Dewey would never deny that matters of fact or questions having to do with the existing state of things were to be dealt with empirically. Take the issue of whether the disease AIDS is contagious and whether a nurse taking care of an AIDS victim is thus in danger of infection. Or the question of whether garbled speech is, in a specific instance, a sign of drunkenness, or whether the common cold can be cured by a high dosage of Vitamin C, or whether a potential blood donor has a blood type that matches that of a dying child. All, quite clearly, call for the application of what Dewey understood to be the scientific method.

Yet, as is generally recognized, many of the nurse's crucial decisions have to be made in realms of meaning where "truth and falsity are as such irrelevant." We have already suggested that value judgments cannot be proven true or false; they belong to the realm "of richness and freedom of meanings, rather than of truth." There are occasions when realms seem to overlap, and these may pose considerable challenges to the practitioner. In the case of AIDS victims, a nurse may find himself or herself so overcome with either fear or prejudice that the nurse must make what actually constitutes an ethical decision in *choosing* to acknowledge the problem as one that can only be empirically settled. He or she may have to decide between a long-held "conviction"—say, that homosexuals should be punished for what they do (or be denied the attention of respectable society)—and a commitment to professionalism or to compliance with hospital regulations. And, indeed, this is not unusual. The case of a dishevelled, unpleasant derelict whose speech is garbled may also demand a choice to take an empirical approach, perhaps even a choice to be ethical. People who are technicist in their attitudes forget this; they assume that science has indeed "monopolistic jurisdiction." If arguments or conclusions cannot be demonstrated to be true or false, they either ignore them or term them "meaningless." Too often, this tendency to overlook the "discontinuity" between the AIDS victim or the derelict and a material object or machine, even though expressed in acceptable behavior, erodes personal concern and becomes a rationale for indifference. When a moral issue *does* arise—as, for example, when there is a shortage of staff on a Sunday and a decision has to be made between answering the call of the appealing, soon-to-be-discharged young woman and that of the hopelessly ill, pain-ridden AIDS victim—the road simply may not be taken. It will not occur to the technicist thinker that there *is* a moral issue involved when he or she hears the bells and (most probably) takes the easy way. A situation demanding choice will not arise for this person, partly because of what Hannah Arendt (1976) once called a distinctive kind of "thoughtlessness" (pp. 4–5), partly because there is no dependable evidence to indicate that one way is "better" than another.

PERSONAL HISTORIES

Nonetheless, the individual who has to make decisions regarding the jurisdiction of "truth" is never a disembodied mind; nor is he or she uninvolved in social relationships, acknowledged or not. Each person has a life history that inevitably affects how he or she perceives situations, identifies relevant themes, responds to what is felt to be a demand. Early experiences, examined and unexamined beliefs cannot but affect the ways in which a practitioner addresses events as they occur. They may even affect the kind of cognitive action he or she endeavors to take, as they may influence the very course of moral reasoning. Consider the familiar case of the Catholic nurse working in a city hospital and finding himself or herself continually confronting cases of abortion. Opposed though this nurse may be on religious grounds, he or she may still (because the hospital requires it) present abortion as an option to, for example, teen-age adolescents, prepare them for the necessary procedures, take care of them afterward. In some instances, Catholic nurses do this because they "have to" do so; in others, they deliberately choose what they view as professional obligation over personal religious faith. This does not mean, however, that their faith or any other fundamental belief may be set aside; nor does it mean that early memories are totally repressed. Biographical considerations (images, voices, dogmas of the past) inevitably color reasoning processes in the present, determine the shape of decisions made, affect the degree of compassion the nurse allows himself or herself. If this were not the case, if persons had no memories, they could scarcely manage a personal presentness to situations. After all, the sense of identity depends upon the binding work of memory. Lacking a sense of identity, an individual is unlikely to experience personal responsibility, and, without a consciousness of responsibility, no one is likely to make ethical choices.

Now this leaves open the question of whether human beings are capable of the purely rational, universalizable decisions that, for some, define morality. Whether they are or not, whether morality is to be conceived in such a fashion or not, there is certainly psychological warrant for saying that it makes a difference in later life if a nurse has known trust and connectedness in childhood and adolescence, if he or she has been valued as a person (Erikson, 1950). It makes a difference, too, if the individual has grown up wearing "masks," warding off feeling, risking only formal and distant contacts with those who come near. Literature and drama, which are significant sources for the understanding of human histories (Putnam,

1979, pp. 83–94), repeatedly dramatize the rootedness of "character" in early experience. George Eliot's Dorothea Brooke (Eliot, 1871–1872/1965), Edith Wharton's Lily Bart (Wharton, 1905/1964), James Joyce's Stephen Dedalus (Joyce, 1922/1946, 1916/1947), F. Scott Fitzgerald's Jay Gatsby (Fitzgerald, 1925/1974), Thomas Wolfe's Eugene Gant (Wolfe, 1929), Arthur Miller's Willy Loman (Miller, 1949/1968), Eugene O'Neill's Tyrones (O'Neill, 1955), and countless other imagined personalities disclose in great and delicate detail the influences of early life and environment on what individuals turn out to be, to cherish, and to choose. That is why an amount of insight or self-reflectiveness is necessary if the practitioner is to be free to function—and, perhaps, to be rational. There must be some capacity to reflect upon and understand one's "self-formation" (Habermas, 1971, p. 310) if moral situations are to be fully grasped as moral situations, requiring some ethical commitment, some kind of choice. Surely, the cry of the cancer patient for more medication than the doctor ordered is heard differently by a nurse whose own relative has died of cancer. The need to attend to a life-support machine to which a "crib-dead" infant is attached is grasped differently by someone who has had a child than by one who has not. The pleas and complaints of a senile patient are listened to in one way by the one who has tended to an aged parent or grandparent, another way by the one who has not. The hearing, the grasping, the listening do not themselves dictate whether a choice has to be made or what kind of choice it is likely to be. The point is that personal experiences cannot but mediate what is heard, grasped, and listened to and, in turn, have much to do with how people constitute situations as offering alternative possibilities of action—each one referring to a value, a principle, a notion of right or wrong. Observed behaviors may be very similar in an emergency room, an intensive care unit, a ward; all the practitioners may appear to be functioning "professionally." But our concern is as much with the *quality* of the attention paid, the ethical sensitivity, the degree of altruism or "regard for the good of another person for his own sake" (Blum, 1980, p. 9). And none of this can be grasped by a mere accounting of the observed.

NURSES AND PHYSICIANS

Does it really matter? There are numerous physicians who would prefer that nurses not be acquainted with theories of ethics or moral conduct. They are prone to assert that nurses do not have (and should not have) opportunities to make consequential decisions. Underlying this, more often than not, is the belief that—because of entirely different expectations and degrees of expertise—nurses should function as informed and skillful subordinates. Within the bureaucratic structure of many hospitals as well, the nursing practitioners are assigned generally inferior places in the hierarchy, and the institutional roles defined for them exclude self-chosen autonomy. On the other hand, as nurses realize increasingly today, there are all sorts of unpredictable situations that do indeed call for consequential decisions. It is not simply that nurses perceive themselves differently, not simply that old legitimations are no longer taken for granted. For one thing, there is the vacuum Lewis Thomas (1983) suggested, the vacuum left when physicians no longer treat their patients as "the epicenter of concern." For another, there are the unprecedented responsibilities inherent in the presence of life-support and other machines. For still another, there are the challenges posed by "patient consent," by the newly recognized rights of patients and their families who will no longer view physicians as high priests, unbiased "patient advocates," repositories of benevolence and truth. And there is the simple pragmatic fact that nurses in their various specialties do indeed come up against situations involving moral conflict—where there is insufficient time to ask for "orders," where there is a crucial need to choose. Finally (and surely as important), there

is the gulf between our time and the time in the past when "right" action was thought of as compliance with a set of pieties. These included, of course, kindness, mercy, humility, gentleness, generosity, even gratitude, and they were communicated by means of a type of preaching. As in most preaching, there was a coerciveness beneath the words of reminder, exhortation, and inspiration: if the nurse did not conform, that nurse would be expelled, excluded, shamed, punished, conceivably damned. Today we know that people are not rendered capable of ethical conduct through such handling; we have to face the need to create situations in which individuals may learn what it is to make decisions of principle (Hare, 1964, pp. 56–78), to give good reasons for their decisions, or to *choose* to be virtuous within a world that may not care.

FAITH AND OBLIGATION

There are, then, diverse existential actualities that create the problematic contexts in which individual practitioners attend to matters of good and bad, right and wrong. (Attend, or may attend, depending on whether or not they feel free enough and responsible enough to risk "the road not taken.") It seems fairly evident that most people's conscious moral careers began in reliance on some mode of revelation: the Scriptures, the Ten Commandments, the Sermon on the Mount, the Talmud. First, of course, there was purely instinctual behavior; then, in early childhood, desire and inclination were controlled by various rewards and punishments, including the withholding of approval and love. In many cases, the true source of love, and abandonment as well, was identified as the deity (who watched at all times, who could see through closed doors). This became, then, the first acquaintance with what could be called justification: the good and the right were not merely what one *wanted* to do; they were what one *ought* to do, and the sense of "oughtness" derived from a belief in something higher, more encompassing than oneself. The Ten Commandments, for instance, begin with the assertion, "I am the Lord thy God who has brought you out of the land of Egypt," and that implies that we ought to abide by the Commandments in gratitude. Gratitude, surely, is stressed as one of the primary motivations for obedience to the Word. Oftentimes, the point is also made that the love of God is the ground of all loving, that the capacity to love others is a kind of testimony to an experience with God. Almost everyone is familiar, also, with the idea that God's Word (or command, or prescription, or law) finds expression through the individual conscience; one "knows" intuitively what is right; one suffers guilt or shame when one offends against what conscience is said to require.

As we realize, however, what has been interpreted as the Word of God has meant a great variety of things. We need only recall the case of Huckleberry Finn, whose Sunday School training and (consequently) whose conscience dictated that slavery accorded with God's will. The problem, of course, is that there is no public way of demonstrating what God's will "truly" demands, just as there is no universally acceptable "reading" of the Scriptures. (How, indeed, does one prove to a Fundamentalist that he or she is wrong when it comes to censorship, sexual preference, abortion, and school prayers? How does one convince a devoted member of "Right to Life" that the Scriptures allow for the right to choose?) In a pluralist society like American society, one is constantly faced with dilemmas of this sort, and there is no way of resolving them except through resort to some inner, private certainty. This is not to suggest that one is required to give up one's faith in order to engage in ethical decision making. It is to argue that life in a diverse community demands something more than reference to conscience, private certainty, or an arbitrary invocation of the Word of God.

There is no denying that some of our greatest prophets and moral exemplars justified their actions in that fashion. We need only recall the work of the Reverend Martin Luther King, Jr., whose "dream" was founded in a conception

of what the moral law demanded. His appeal to intuitive knowledge was in a long and noble tradition, carried on by Henry David Thoreau, Leo Tolstoy, and Mahatma Gandhi, and there is no question but that some of the highest human achievements were made possible by that kind of glowing certainty. But Thoreau, Tolstoy, Gandhi, and King were highly principled persons, committed to a belief in the dignity of all human beings and in universal human rights, and there are those who are convinced that, for all their appeal to intuition and to an immediate grasping of the "good," their moral superiority ought to be attributed to their highly developed rational capacities and to their attainment of full autonomy as they matured. Whatever the explanation, their ethical orientations have to be distinguished from those of Governor George Wallace (when he barred the door of the University of Alabama), from those of the Ku Klux Klan, and from the claims of certain members of the Moral Majority. They, too, have often pleaded private certainty or intuitive knowledge, and they are reminders of the complexities involved in any morality justified by a presumed ability to "see" or to "grasp" some quality or relation or truth invisible or incomprehensible to others sharing similar experiences in the same place and time. Any nurse who has had to try to convince a member of Jehovah's Witnesses to allow a transfusion for a deathly ill child well knows the blind alleys to which this approach can lead.

JUSTIFICATIONS

Much more widespread among those concerned with morality and ethics is the belief that only rational persons can act in accord with a moral law that is expressed as a sense of "ought." Most influential on modern thinking, of all the philosophers of the past, has been Immanuel Kant (1785/1964) and his view of principled action. To be rational, he said, actually means being responsive to a moral law that acts as an imperative in the mind. It follows that moral principles must be understood to be universal, to be valid for all. Kant would have found it inconceivable for a rational person *not* to feel compelled by, say, the principle that promises ought always to be kept and by the necessity to universalize that principle, assuming it to be applicable to all rational agents. (After all, if promise-keeping were dependent on individual taste or judgment, the very notion of a promise would be meaningless.) For Kant, morality has to do with obligation, with a sense of duty: one does the right thing because one is obligated to do it and to do it for its own sake, not because of any consequences that might be beneficial and not because of any desires or emotions or attachments one may have. In the case of a cardiac arrest in the emergency room, a nurse would be expected to do his or her duty no matter what. Compassion would have nothing to do with it; nor would altruism; nor would loyalty; nor the simple desire to be of help. The act would be morally right if and only if inclination and self-interest and sympathy were put aside. A rational person knows that every human being must be treated as an end, never as a means. A human being is suffering a cardiac arrest; the categorical imperative demands that, without exception, action must be taken to save that life.

Nurses have had the experience of seeing hopeless burn cases revived after cardiac arrests, and some, because of pure human sympathy, have felt outraged. Indeed, this suggests one of the difficulties of a strict Kantian (Kant, 1785/1964) approach. Not only does it exclude feelings from moral action; it does not allow for variations in situations. Kant himself would have said that action that is emotionally motivated is likely to be unreliable, if not irrational, and that it is ordinarily occasioned by a particular situation or emergency. It cannot, therefore, be generalized or universalized and, for that reason, cannot be described as moral. We have already expressed our dissatisfaction with entirely formal, depersonalized approaches and our belief that moral or ethical action involves a personal presentness, for all the

fallibility that may introduce. We have also expressed doubt with respect to action based entirely in impulse or feeling, the kind of action that escapes justification. Even though an unqualified Kantianism is difficult to accept, the questions still remain open. There are additional problems with Kant's view, however, when looked at from a modern vantage point. One is that it presumes a type of rationality and a sense of duty universally characteristic of human beings, something long since denied by anthropological studies, for all the "universals" anthropology has found. Another is that Freudianism and other psychoanalytic inquiries have made it impossible to believe in a capacity of "pure" reason unaffected by repression, sublimation, or the distortions attributable to the unconscious mind. Psychoanalysts also lay stress on the value of rational insight and on the need to replace the demands of the "id" with the rational reality-orientation of the "ego," but they would consider rationality of this sort to be a hard-won attainment, not an original endowment, and certainly not the same in quality for everyone.

THE PLACE OF PRINCIPLE

For all this, the Kantian (Kant, 1785/1964) notion of principle remains significant for anyone pondering the ethical domain. A principle, as we have seen, may be understood to resemble an imperative statement with a directive or prescriptive force. It may, for many people, function as a suggestion or a proposal referring to kinds of action considered right and obligatory. It indicates that what ought to be done in any particular situation or by any individual person ought to be done in any other situation, and in that sense it is universalizable. Now, it is important to realize that principles of this sort are not to be identified with orders issued from without, with external edicts, or with written rules. Moral principles are incarnated, somehow internalized. This need not mean that they necessarily constitute imperatives inherent in rationality itself. They may be grasped as far-ranging, universal in scope, and thereby "understood" to be the only appropriate criteria for moral judgments. They may be chosen by individuals in their efforts to define themselves as moral beings. They may be, as it were, invented by a group of people to govern the way they live together and work together, and they may be freely accepted as binding by the members of whatever community results. Or, like "life, liberty, and the pursuit of happiness," they may represent the fundamental norms of a society, some shared conception of the way things ought to be. However they are construed, they are not to be seen as the causes of behavior; nor does their acknowledgment guarantee that they will be acted on by all affected or concerned. Moral principles become meaningful, however, only as individual agents accept them as directives for their own conduct, and in this sense they are internalized.

There are many who believe that, without principles, we would have nothing to refer to in moments of moral uncertainty or disagreement. We might recall the AIDS victim once again and consider what might be said to persuade a prejudiced and recalcitrant colleague that he or she should, indeed, provide the necessary care. We might refer to the principle of fairness, meaning that distinctions among patients ought not to be made on the ground of irrelevant differences (in this case, a difference in sexual orientation). We might refer to the principle having to do with regard for each person's dignity, no matter who or what that person is, or respect for his human rights. The reasons we would offer would be given point and relevance through reference to such principles. To tell a colleague that he or she should attend to a patient because we want him or her to do so, or because it is "only right," is quite different from an appeal on the ground of some shared commitment to principle. "We think you should," we might say, "because this patient is a human being, and we know that, like the rest of us, you believe that each human being is worthy of regard." This would not force or cause the colleague to act, but it would constitute an address to him or her as moral agent capable of voluntary decision. It might also imply that the colleague belonged to a certain kind of moral community and that, by deciding not to care for the AIDS victim, he or she would be breaking with community norms.

With the principle of justice or fairness in mind, we might consider a somewhat more complex situation, one not unfamiliar in the American South during the days of widespread segregation there. Black children were frequently excluded, not only from public schools but from pediatric wards, solely because of the color of their skin. To exclude a child because that child had a particular type of infectious disease might have been justifiable because of a documented danger to those around, but to exclude the same child because of skin color was manifestly unjust, since skin color is hardly a relevant ground for making distinctions among children in need of care—at least in a situation where any sort of justice rules. If, in those days, a nurse were to arrange for the admission of a sick Black child to an all-White hospital, among the ostensibly good reasons the nurse might give for such an action would be the principle of justice or fairness. The nurse might have so internalized that principle that it would have seemed unthinkable for others to reject it and, to make things worse, to deny the human rights of the sick Black child.

Two things, at least, might have happened in that time. The nurse might have been informed that the hospital administration or the community read the principle of fairness differently than he or she did (meaning that they happened to think it fair for people to be with "their own kind"), or the point might have been made that the principle of fairness, in that circumstance, was in conflict with an equally important principle having to do with self-determination, or freedom of choice for the adults concerned. It is also conceivable that the practitioner might have been told that his or her duty as an employee required that the sick Black child be dispatched to another clinic or hospital, no matter what the nature of the illness. The nurse, therefore, might be confronted with a range of perplexities, and, in some fashion, the nurse would have to choose.

On the matter of what was called "duty": much would depend on the fabric of codes, customs, and values in which duty was defined. It is conceivable that the practitioner, disturbed in any case about racism and discrimination, might simply deny that his or her "duty" was as defined. What would follow, of course, would be partly up to the hospital administration, and, if threatened, the nurse would have to decide whether her principles were more powerful than expediency (or the need, under any circumstances, to keep a job). The matter of the conflict among principles is in some way more interesting and more common. Few would deny that the freedom to choose is as important to human beings as fairness (which John Rawls has described as the primary value "of the polity," 1971, p. 4). People have suffered and died, in fact, for freedom—as they have for the idea of human rights—and it is difficult to make it secondary to justice.

SUSTAINING MEMBERSHIPS

When two principles of that sort conflict (no matter what the motivations of those who hold them), resolution in logical terms is extremely difficult, and we have already pointed to the fact that there exists no court of last resort. In the situation under discussion, the nurse might be fortunate enough to be a member of a moral community within the hospital itself, a community strong enough to sustain his or her point of view and make its influence felt. Beyond that, there is only the possibility of conversation or discussion with those who stand for the alternative principle. There is only the possibility of appealing to their own general sense of what is right and what is wrong, of suggesting ways in which the two principles might be reconciled (at least in the pediatric

ward), and of trying to widen the discourse so that self-interest (at least) could be set aside.

Conflict between principles is not unusual in the nurse's world today, as we have already noted. Ordinarily, the handling of such conflict depends on agreements shared, on mutual trust, on the quality of the existing community, and oftentimes on friendship. But it must be recalled that it is finally up to the individual practitioners to choose or not to choose, either alone or in association. If they have developed a strong sense of obligatoriness, of "oughtness," it will be extraordinarily difficult not to take some kind of position, some kind of risk. If they find themselves to be so administered, so manipulated as to be deprived of freedom of action, they may be outraged, even rebellious, but they may not make any kind of significant move. They will not make an ethical choice. This sort of predicament is not unusual either, and it cannot be resolved from outside. Individual decision, grounded in a commitment to principle in some consciousness of what may follow after, is required. If people do not live under totalitarian control, if they are not imprisoned, they themselves have to choose what is possible. Often, the conviction of being thwarted or manipulated is itself a kind of choice or an excuse. There is a need to be honest, a need to be clear.

ANTICIPATIONS AND CONSEQUENCES

Choices governed solely by preexistent principles, however, are not the only kinds of choices made in the ethical domain (Frankena, 1963, p. 13). It is not uncommon for people, perhaps particularly in the medical profession, to make their decisions mainly in the light of the consequences they anticipate. In the case of the Black child in the South, these people would be more inclined to speak about the damage (or lack of damage) that might be done to the child by refusing him admission than they would be to refer to a principle of fairness or of freedom. This end-oriented (or results-oriented) attitude is geared more nearly to the specific and concrete case than it is to the general or the universalizable. What is general in the approach harks back to the utilitarian approach devised by John Stuart Mill (1861/1949) in the 19th century. Moral decisions, according to this view, are validated by the degree they contribute to human happiness or pleasure or satisfaction. This does not mean any kind of happiness or satisfaction; the human beings the utilitarian had in mind were primarily rational—capable of controlling their desires, seeking out what might be called the "higher" pleasures. It is at least conceivable, for example, that someone normally prejudiced might choose to offer equal treatment to a Black child because of the pleasure involved in feeling self-esteem. But the basic criterion for the utilitarian was the balance of good over evil; he or she sought, in each instance, "the greatest good for the greatest number." An act was considered right if it or the rule that led to it produced as great a balance of good over evil as any available alternative.

In the case of the cancer patient who is asking to be told the truth, the utilitarian approach (customary among physicians) would involve a determination of the relative harm done by provoking anxiety and the relative benefit achieved by treating the patient as a rational, dignified being capable of informed consent. An obvious difficulty here has to do with the often unacknowledged fallibility of the physician. How is he or she to calculate the degree of anxiety? How is the physician to ascertain the physical harm it will cause? How is the relative value of respect for the patient as a rational agent to be measured? Very often, of course, the physician selects the alternative that will mean the least discomfort for physician and staff, and that ordinarily means a relieving of anxiety, even if the truth is obscured. As has been suggested, the nurse is frequently left with the persisting questions of the patient, with his or her own felt need to choose between the demands of the truth-telling principle and concern for the patient's ease of mind, if not happiness. The problem is often exacerbated when the nurse realizes that the patient has unfinished business of importance not merely to that patient but to the lives of relatives and associates. If the truth were told to her, the patient might be able to make arrangements she would not make under the solace of false promises.

According to John Dewey (1957), ethical issues of this kind ought to be handled through a careful anticipation of future consequences (pp. 44–45). He would have people go over, in their imaginations, various alternative courses of action and pay as much attention as possible to impinging circumstances and existing "interests." He would have recommended that the nurse faced with the uncertainties of dealing with the cancer patient inform himself or herself as fully as possible about the patient's actual situation. Attending to whatever explanations the patient chose to give, the nurse might be able to come to some intelligent understanding of the several interests affected by the patient's ignorance of what was to occur and some intelligent evaluation of the good to be achieved if the patient were fully informed. As for principles, Dewey (1957) did not believe that *only* principles (or duty, or the categorical imperative) should be taken into account. Principled people, though often admirable, are too often rigid, overly righteous, unable to bend with the wind. He spoke of a principle as a "cautionary standard" (pp. 21–22), enabling a person to select those facets of a given situation that were relevant and that might contribute to the securing of values considered good and right. There is no finality in such a view, nor is there a dependence upon the universal. There is, rather, an open-endedness, a quasi-experimentalism, a tentativeness, even as there is an orientation to situations in their wholeness and their incompleteness. Objections to this view have focused, first of all, on the likelihood that the Deweyan moves too easily from the "is" to the "should," and there is a general agreement among ethical theorists that ethical recommendations cannot be based on empirical generalizations. In other words, a factual description (no matter how detailed) of the patient's life situation and responsibilities cannot lead logically to conclusions about what *ought* to be. Conclusions about what ought to be can be drawn only from statements that include value judgments. One cannot say, for instance, that a person has a variety of business responsibilities and that, therefore, she ought to be told the truth about her condition. One *can* say that a person has a variety of responsibilities, that responsibilities ought to be met if at all possible, and that (since they can only be met if the patient is told the truth) the patient ought to be given the facts about her condition.

Other objections have focused on the matter of appraisal. How is one to know that the consequence one chooses as the best is, in fact, the most desirable? Does one not need a principle (or a criterion, or a norm) to help one determine the alternative to be preferred? Is there not a danger of total relativism in situations of this sort? Dewey (1957) would have responded that what is really good is the good reflected upon, viewed in its interconnectedness not solely with the wishes of the agents concerned nor with the interests of those affected, but also with the principles by which the agents have chosen to live. In no sense, therefore, was he proposing an approach that placed the person "outside" relationships and contingencies, nor was he making desire or inclination the wellspring of moral action.

REFLECTION AND CONNECTION

In that respect, Dewey's (1957) work relates to that of Carol Gilligan (1982) and others who have taken issue with purely rational, rule-governed orientations. Moving from an account of how women, in contrast to many men, structure their realities in terms of responsibility and social concern, Gilligan (1982) works

toward an ethic reconciling what she calls "justice and care" (p. 149). This would appear to be of special relevance to the nursing profession, interested as many practitioners are in rights as well as responsibilities, in equality as well as mercy—or concern. It is difficult to imagine how moral clarity and commitment can be achieved without conditions of reciprocity that allow nurses to enter into ongoing dialogue with one another on how they wish to live their professional lives, on claims they wish to make, on obligations they choose freely to incarnate and to act upon as they do their work in the world.

Hannah Arendt (1958), describing what she called a "web of relations" that might bind individuals into a plurality, spoke of "interests" as what lay between people, relating and binding them together. Most action and speech, she wrote, are concerned with this "in-between," which is overlaid with "deeds and words" and originates in distinctive individuals' "acting and speaking directly to one another" (p. 182). It may be within such a web, where situated and self-aware persons communicate with one another, that significant ethical thinking begins. This possibility in no way diminishes the importance of the sense of human agency, nor does it make irrelevant the ways in which certain moral situations connect with themes in individuals' biographies. To speak in what Hannah Arendt described as "agent-revealing" voices and to speak directly "*to* one another" demands a subjective involvement Kantians, later rationalists, utilitarians, and even Deweyans ignored.

To be subjectively engaged is not to be closed off from the common, nor is it to be left to a noncognitive orientation to practice and choice. Human beings grasp the appearances of things through acts of consciousness. The acts are multiple (including intuiting, imagining, perceiving, believing, judging, feeling), and the objects of these modes of grasping form "networks of relationship" brought into existence by individuals themselves. Indeed, as has been said, "we are ourselves these networks of relationship" (Merleau-Ponty, 1962, p. 456). When

Levin walks in terror out of his brother's room, when the positivist excludes valuing from the process of inquiry, when the rationalist separates feeling from principled behavior, when the person is subsumed under the universal, those networks are unraveled. Functioning one-dimensionally very often, the individual may find it very difficult to achieve the sort of agency he or she needs for moral action and at once be in the world impinging on him or her. Such a person may find it particularly difficult to incarnate significant principles and make them his or hers to act upon—and difficult to exist in reciprocity.

Network, dialogue, presentness, reflectiveness, and concern: these may be the watchwords when it comes to the ethics of nursing. To confront nurses with logical dilemmas, to presume that they are disembodied minds, to expect them to act in disinterest and autonomy: all this may result in a kind of virtuosity, an ability to reason and to explain, but it will not address them as living beings participant in the human condition. Nor will it allow for the ambiguities, the persistent uncertainties that haunt the ethical domain. We would want to suggest, as others have, that nurses engage themselves as much as possible in the several arts in order better to tolerate ambiguities and, at once, to come in contact with the idea of alternative realities. Coming to know the work, say, of Virginia Woolf or Toni Morrison or Ralph Ellison or Wallace Stevens, learning to be present to Rothko's paintings or Hopper's or Cezanne's, nurses may find themselves discovering what it can mean to look through the windows of the actual, to look at the ordinary and the taken-for-granted as if it could be otherwise. They may find themselves rediscovering what it means to be *interested*, how it feels to imagine untapped possibilities. They may find themselves, at once, attending more intensely to the world around them—becoming more sensitive to the look of faces, of bodies in motion, of trees moving in the wind, of shadows lengthening, of the sound of breathing, of the silences in empty rooms. Surely, attentiveness

and a heightened consciousness of alternative possibilities have something to do with moral wide-awakeness. They may be as significant as the understanding of guidelines, the incarnation of principles, the anticipation of consequences, the feeling of resolve.

SITUATIONAL DEMANDS

Everything turns, finally, on the capacity to respond to the demand implicit in moral situations. Such situations, however, do not come labeled or predefined. Attention has to be paid if the predicament of the pregnant adolescent is to be perceived as a predicament and if the situation in which the young woman is involved is to be viewed as one in which there are alternative courses of treatment or of action, one better or more just or more humane than the others. The nurse has to *be* there as a concerned and compassionate person if he or she is to resonate to the despair of the battered wife, the plea of the dying old man, the guilt and pain of the old man's son. But the nurse has to do more than sympathize. Somehow, he or she has to know how to constitute (where at all appropriate) situations as situations demanding choice; heed actualities, nuances, contesting forces—recognize what is at stake. If the practitioner feels that he or she ought to take some kind of action, the practitioner is bound, as it were, to look both ways. There is the concrete complexity of the situation; there are the relevant guidelines; there are other people—colleagues and superiors; there are the overarching principles (justice, regard for persons, respect for human rights) by which he or she may have chosen to live; there are the relationships within whatever moral community has been formed. And, at once, there are virtues—decency, honesty, compassion, generosity—that have marked the tradition of nursing and that must be personally chosen each time a new life story begins (MacIntyre, 1981). The nurse may look to the future, trying to anticipate what will result from what is done; he or she can reflect on what still works within because of the forgotten past; he or she can turn to fellow participants in dialogue.

But then there is the leap, the risk. There is the recognition of the road not taken. There is the choice—and all we can ask is that it be a decent one, reflected-on, authentic, concerned. It is finally a choice of the self, not as victim but as agent, a choice of the self in its freedom, a way of being in the world.

REFERENCES

Arendt, H. (1958). *The human condition.* Chicago: University of Chicago Press.

Arendt, H. (1976). *The life of the mind: Volume 1. Thinking.* New York: Harcourt Brace Jovanovich.

Blum, L. (1980). *Friendship, altruism and morality.* London: Routledge and Kegan Paul.

Camus, A. (1948). *The plague.* New York: Knopf. (Originally published 1947).

Dewey, J. (1957). *Human nature and conduct.* New York: Modern Library.

Dewey, J. (1958). *Experience and nature.* New York: Dover.

Dorsen, N. (Ed.). (1971). *The rights of Americans.* New York: Pantheon.

Eliot, G. (1965). *Middlemarch.* Baltimore: Penguin. (Originally published 1871–1872).

Ellul, J. (1967). *The technological society.* New York: Vintage Books.

Erikson, E. (1950). *Childhood and society.* New York: Norton.

Fitzgerald, F. (1974). *The great Gatsby.* Franklin Center, PA: Franklin Library. (Originally published 1925.)

Frankena, W. (1963). *Ethics.* Englewood Cliffs, NJ: Prentice-Hall.

Frost, R. (1972). The road not taken. In O. Williams (Ed.), *American verse.* New York: Washington Square Press.

Gaylin, W., Glasser, I., Marcus, S., & Rothman, D. (1978). *Doing good: The limits of benevolence.* New York: Pantheon.

Gilligan, C. (1982). *In a different voice.* Cambridge: Harvard University Press.

Habermas, J. (1971). *Knowledge and human interests.* Boston: Beacon Press.

Hare, R. (1964). *The language of morals.* New York: Oxford University Press.

Joyce, J. (1946). *Ulysses.* New York: Random House. (Originally published 1922.)

Joyce, J. (1947). *A portrait of the artist as a young man.* New York: Viking. (Originally published 1916.)

Kant, I. (1964). *Groundwork of the metaphysics of morals* (H. Paton, Trans.). New York: Harper and Row. (Originally published 1785.)

Kierkegaard, S. (1947). Either/Or. In R. Bretall (Ed.), *Kierkegaard.* Princeton, NJ: Princeton University Press. (Originally published 1843.)

Kohlberg, L. (1973). Continuities and discontinuities in childhood and adult moral development revisited. In *Collected papers on moral development and moral education.* Cambridge: Moral Education Research Foundation, Harvard University.

MacIntyre, A. (1981). *After virtue.* Notre Dame: Notre Dame University Press.

Merleau-Ponty, M. (1962). *Phenomenology of perception.* New York: Humanities Press.

Mill, J. (1949). *Utilitarianism.* New York: Liberal Arts Press. (Originally published 1861.)

Miller, A. (1968). *Death of a salesman.* New York: Viking. (Originally published 1949.)

O'Neill, E. (1955). *Long day's journey into night.* New Haven: Yale University Press.

Putnam, H. (1979). *Meaning and the moral sciences.* Boston: Routledge and Kegan Paul.

Rawls, J. (1971). *A theory of justice.* Cambridge: Harvard University Press.

Rothman, D. (1971). *The discovery of the asylum.* Boston: Little, Brown.

Stanley, M. (1978). *The technological conscience.* New York: Free Press.

Thomas, L. (1983). *The youngest science: Notes of a medicine-watcher.* New York: Viking.

Tolstoy, L. (1946). *Anna Karenina.* Cleveland: World Publishing. (Originally published 1875–1877.)

Twain, M. (1959). *The adventures of Huckleberry Finn.* New York: New American Library. (Originally published 1885.)

Wharton, E. (1964). *The house of mirth.* New York: New American Library. (Originally published 1905.)

Wolfe, T. (1929). *Look homeward, angel.* New York: Modern Library.

Humanistic Exercises

Evaluating: Determining Extent of Goal Attainment

Exercise 13

Self-Evaluation and Diagnosis

Purposes	1. To diagnose one's own strengths and weaknesses in nursing practice.
	2. To diagnose one's own learning needs in relation to nursing practice.
	3. To develop strategies for meeting one's own learning needs.
Facility	None.
Materials	Worksheet A: Self-Evaluation and Diagnosis Form Pen or pencil
Time Required	One and one-half hours.
Group Size	Homework assignment.
Design	1. Request that learners respond to the instrument out of class.
	2. Set up individual appointments between instructor and learner to discuss the responses.
Variations	Both teacher and learner can respond to the instrument. The teacher will be evaluating the learner and offering suggestions on ways to meet the indicated learning needs that the teacher perceives. Differences in perceptions by self and others could form a basis for discussion.

Exercise 13　　　Worksheet A

Self-Evaluation and Diagnosis Form*

Part I

Directions:　Select the *three* areas in which you think you perform the best.
Then select the *three* areas in which you (comparatively) perform the poorest.
This is an evaluation of *your* comparative strengths and weaknesses, *not*
one comparing you with others. Indicate in the column on the right your
comments regarding your choices. (You may comment on as many other
areas as are important to you.)

Area of Competency	Best	Poorest	Comment
A.　Nursing Process			
1.　Data collection			
a.　Nursing histories			
b.　Interviewing			
c.　Interpretation of clinical data			
d.　Consultation with other professionals			
e.　Talking with families			
f.　Physical assessment			
2.　Processing data			
3.　Nursing diagnosis			
a.　Determining diagnosis			
b.　Setting priorities			
4.　Writing nursing orders			
5.　Evaluating outcomes			

*This form is a modification of the original used by
Professor Virginia Earles at the University of Massachusetts, Division of Nursing, 1975.

Worksheet **A** (continued)

Area of Competency	Best	Poorest	Comment
B. Providing Care			
1. Direct physical care			
2. Effective use of interpersonal processes			
3. Technical skills			
4. Teaching			
5. Being an advocate of the client/family			
6. Making referrals			
7. Coordinating care			
8. Supervising nursing personnel			

Part II

Discuss ways in which your thinking about the nursing process and its role in nursing practice has developed since you began this course/program.

Part III

What do you plan to do about your poorest areas?

Part IV

What are you planning to do about further development of your strengths?

Part V

List your personal course objectives and how you originally intended to meet them. Describe how you actually met them, with an evaluation of each objective.

Objectives	How you intended to meet them	How you met them	Evaluation

Exercise 14

The Advocacy Role of the Nurse

Purposes	1. To raise consciousness of the various implications for nurses regarding patients' rights.
	2. To become aware of various perceptions of the advocacy role.
	3. To identify major nursing implications of the Patients' Bill of Rights.
	4. To identify and discuss problem areas relative to patients' rights.
Facility	Classroom to accommodate groups of ten.
Materials	Patients' Bill of Rights (Chapter 13) Paper and pencils. Worksheet A: Individual Diagnosis Worksheet B: Group Diagnosis
Time Required	Two hours.
Group Size	Unlimited groups of ten.
Design	1. Ask group members to individually read the Patients' Bill of Rights and write down five areas or instances in which there are direct implications for nursing practice.
	2. Have individuals write down three problems relative to being a patients' advocate. For Steps 1 and 2, use Worksheet A (allow 20 minutes).
	3. In the group of ten, have members share their individual implications and problem areas (20 minutes).
	4. Request that the group compile a list of ten major implications and five most significant problem areas from individual presentations (Worksheet B). Discussion should then focus on possible solutions to the problem areas—that is: What would alleviate the problem? Is the problem relative to my personality/position, or can it be generalized? What do I/we do? (45 minutes).
	5. The balance of the time can be used by having each group share with the total class its list of major implications, problems, and solutions. Someone could write responses on the blackboard.
	6. Discuss findings.
Variations	Each group could write its list of major implications, problems, and solutions on large newsprint paper with magic markers. These could be displayed during Step 4.

Exercise 14   Worksheet A
Individual Diagnosis

Implications in Nursing Practice

1.

2.

3.

4.

5.

Problem Areas

1.

2.

3.

Exercise 14　　　　Worksheet　B
Group Diagnosis

Major Implications in Nursing Practice

1.

2.

3.

4.

5.

6.

7.

8.

9.

10.

Problem Areas	Solutions
1.	
2.	
3.	
4.	
5.	

Exercise 15
Evaluation of the Course

Purpose

To provide feedback to the course planner/instructor.

Facility

Regular classroom setting.

Materials

Evalutions A, B, and/or C.
Pen or pencil

Time Required

Approximately ten minutes.

Group Size

Unlimited

Design

The course evaluations may be used when the instructor desires feedback from the learners. Each can be administered in class or taken home for completion.

1. Evaluation A: Usable at any point during the semester in which the class is given. It provides a means for evaluating the needs of students midway through the semester in order for adjustments to be made as indicated by the responses. Instructors must list in the left-hand column the broad content areas covered to date.

2. Evaluation B: This is a short end-of-course evaluation.

3. Evaluation C: Evaluation C provides a more descriptive end-of-course report. All evaluations can be either anonymous or identifiable with the students and/or openly discussed or not with relevant participants or the entire group.

Exercise   15   Evaluation   A
Course Content Evaluation

Circle the number that best describes each content area.

Course Content Areas	Too Little 1	Just Right 2	Too Much 3
	1	2	3
	1	2	3
	1	2	3
	1	2	3
	1	2	3
	1	2	3
	1	2	3
	1	2	3
	1	2	3
	1	2	3
	1	2	3
	1	2	3
	1	2	3
	1	2	3
	1	2	3
	1	2	3
	1	2	3

Exercise 15　　　　Evaluation B
End-of-Course Evaluation

For each item, circle the number that best represents your evaluation.

	Poor			Average			Excellent		
A. Subject content									
Interesting in terms of new knowledge	1	2	3	4	5	6	7	8	9
Valuable in terms of daily activities	1	2	3	4	5	6	7	8	9
Up-to-date in terms of current trends, issues, and problems	1	2	3	4	5	6	7	8	9
B. Instructor/Program leader									
Attitude toward participants	1	2	3	4	5	6	7	8	9
Command of subject matter	1	2	3	4	5	6	7	8	9
Ability to hold participants' interest	1	2	3	4	5	6	7	8	9
Organized presentation of material	1	2	3	4	5	6	7	8	9
Coverage of material	1	2	3	4	5	6	7	8	9
Use of handouts	1	2	3	4	5	6	7	8	9
C. Overall evaluation of program	1	2	3	4	5	6	7	8	9

D. Course/Program comments

1. What was of most value to you in the course/program? _____

_____

_____

_____

_____

_____

2. What was of least value? _____

_____

_____

3. Do you have any specific suggestions about how to improve this course/program? _____

_____

_____

4. Reflecting on the best instructor you have had, how did your present instructor compare?

_____

_____

_____

Why? _____

_____

_____

Exercise 15   Evaluation   C*
End-of-Course Evaluation

Course Number & Title:

Professor:

Date:

Using the scale provided, rate each item on its overall idea, rather than on specific parts.

CONTENT	Strongly disagree	Moderately disagree	Slightly disagree	Slightly agree	Moderately agree	Strongly agree
1. Objectives are appropriate for the course content.	1	2	3	4	5	6
2. Objectives were met through class seminars, clinical practicum, and course design.	1	2	3	4	5	6
3. The course has provided me with extensive knowledge in the content area and is applicable in my professional practice.	1	2	3	4	5	6
4. Course requirements cover essential aspects of the course and have learning value.	1	2	3	4	5	6
5. This course has increased my learning, given me new viewpoints and appreciation, and increased my capacity to think and to formulate questions.	1	2	3	4	5	6
6. Contrasting viewpoints, current developments, and related theory were integrated into class topics.	1	2	3	4	5	6

---

*Adapted from a Faculty Evaluation Form used at the University of Massachusetts, 1975.

PROCESS	Strongly disagree	Moderately disagree	Slightly disagree	Slightly agree	Moderately agree	Strongly agree
1. The instructor is clear, states objectives, summarizes major points, presents material in an organized manner, and has extensive knowledge of subject.	1	2	3	4	5	6
2. The instructor is sensitive to the response of the class, encourages student participation, and facilitates questions and discussion.	1	2	3	4	5	6
3. The instructor is available to students, conveys a genuine interest in students, and recognizes their individuality in learning.	1	2	3	4	5	6
4. The instructor enjoys teaching, is enthusiastic, and makes the course content stimulating and alive.	1	2	3	4	5	6
5. The instructor has provided a class environment that increases my motivation to do my best and acquire knowledge independently.	1	2	3	4	5	6
6. This course, as taught by this instructor, is one that I would recommend. On the whole, the course was excellent.	1	2	3	4	5	6

Evaluation C (continued)

What was of most value in the course?

What was of least value in the course?

Other suggestions/comments.

Part VI

Nursing: A Helping Profession

Chapter 15

Helping

The nursing process, as the scientific foundation upon which all nursing practice is built, is applicable to any client population in any setting. It provides the framework within which the art and science of nursing can be carried out so as to assure individualized, quality nursing care. To facilitate fuller understanding of what the nursing process means today, Part VI views the present and future development of nursing, as well as the theoretic concepts that provide the foundation for humanistic nursing practice.

PROFESSIONS

This past decade has brought continuous and seemingly unending conflict over what a "profession" is. Since everyone from pest controllers to building contractors currently advertises services as "professional," it is not surprising that nurses, as well as other dedicated humanists, are in the process of defining their services explicitly in an attempt to discern the meaning of this commonly used term. Nursing literature abounds with authors who have defined professionalism in nursing, and one has only to look in the nursing indices to discover an array of existing beliefs—all similar, yet different. The strongest common bond is the conclusion that being a professional means different things to different people. It is based on the individual backgrounds, experiences, expectations, and practices of varied nurses. Yet, in respect to scholarship, it becomes necessary to be able to state beliefs in concrete terms usable by growing professionals as each builds his or her own theory of nursing.

A general review of writings on the subject yields three essential components to a profession:

Area of responsibility   +   Authority   +   Autonomy

The content of the area of responsibility depends solely upon the field and carries with it the legal authority to set standards and administer services. All professions are based on an extensive body of knowledge, both pure and applied. Perhaps the key difference between the nursing profession and the rest of the "professional" world is that nursing is based on directly assisting and supporting the total individual.

According to Flexner (cited in Metzger, 1975), there are six distinct attributes that qualify an occupation as a profession:

1. Possession of a body of knowledge relevant to problems in its area;

2. Conjoining knowledge and skills in an intellectual enterprise;

3. Applying knowledge in response to an area of human need;

4. Striving to acquire and improve the knowledge bank through research efforts;

5. Acquiring knowledge and experience primarily through formal university educational systems, culminating with an earned academic degree; and

6. Formulating a code of ethics and character of the profession.

Other theorists would argue that a full commitment of time and energy is essential (Moore, cited in Metzger, 1975), as well as a licensing mechanism and independent practice design (Wilson, cited in Metzger, 1975).

Items one through five of Flexner's criteria feature knowledge, which can be derived in three ways: (1) applied theory from other disciplines; (2) pure theory from research discoveries in the specific area; and (3) experimental knowledge developed through individual practice. Adding to Flexner's fifth attribute, a mode for knowledge acquisition implies a definitive, transferable method that can be taught and learned. *The nursing process provides such a method.*

A profession becomes an integral part of one's existence. The personality of the profession is reflected in the personality of the professional, and this person is a scholar who is continuously learning. Mandated by the profession, nursing must be based on all the scientific and human knowledge available. Because knowledge is the necessary base, the roots of the profession are in formalized educational systems.

In viewing the nursing profession today, it is apparent that the study and elaboration of nursing attributes and components must continue. Three essential learning and practice dimensions become evident: cognitive, psychomotor, and affective. Cognitive learning involves the theory and knowledge base, psychomotor learning involves the skills, and affective learning involves the process and feelings associated with each of the first two. The humanistic approach in learning encompasses all three dimensions and will be addressed more fully in a subsequent chapter. It is necessary, however, to study the theory of helping in order to understand fully the concepts of a *helping profession.*

HELPING MODEL

A generally accepted viewpoint is that most of human behavior is learned; it evolves as a consequence of persons interacting with all facets of their environment. In essence, one learns to be the kind of being one is through past and present relationships. It is through furthering such relationships that one grows into tomorrow's self (Otto, 1970).

The conceptual model of helping upon which this book is based stems primarily from the writings of Carl Rogers. As will be noted, several authors have extended his original work and also conducted substantiating investigations. Foremost in this amplification are the studies of Robert Carkhuff.

Carkhuff (1973) used the analogy of an infant and an aging person to emphasize that the way in which one's environment and one's relationships with important people evolve largely determines one's self-perception: An infant who is totally dependent would likely not live more than a few hours if left alone. An aging person seizes life's last opportunity to understand, be understood, and develop meaning for self at that time. Each one, then, depends on himself or herself and on others in the environment, at the same time. A crisis in one's life may lead to greater growth or to greater deterioration, depending on what is done by the individuals involved and on the skills available to them in helping one another. Weigand (1971, p. 247) wrote: "How we interact, relate and transact with others, and the reciprocal impact of this phenomenon, form the single most important aspect of our existence."

Carl Rogers (1961) developed a general hypothesis regarding the facilitation of personal growth based on what he had learned during his experiences and encounters in all human relationships. The essence of this hypothesis involved his ability as a helper to create a relationship characterized by genuineness, warmth, and sensitivity. Within this environment, the other individual would then be able to grow effectively. Moreover, the degree to which he could create relationships that facilitated the growth of others as individuals would be a measure of the growth he himself had achieved. This was based on his hypothesis that the optimal helping relationship is that created by a psychologically mature person.

Based on this general hypothesis, Rogers (1961, p. 41) further posed the questions: "What are the characteristics of those relationships which do help, which do facilitate growth?" and "Is it possible to discern those characteristics which make a relationship unhelpful, even though it was the sincere intent to promote growth and development?" There was not a large amount of empirical research that would give objective answers at the time Rogers asked these questions. Studies had focused, instead, on the attitudes of the helper that either promoted or inhibited growth.

Baldwin, Kalhorn, and Breese (1945) made a careful study of parent/child relationships. They concluded that, of the various attitudes exhibited by parents toward children, the "acceptant-democratic" one seemed most growth facilitating. These children showed accelerated intellectual development, more originality, and emotional security. In direct contrast to this, children whose parental attitudes were classified as "actively rejectant" showed opposite effects.[1]

Rogers suggested that those findings of Baldwin, Kalhorn, and Breese most likely apply in other relationships as well. Stated Rogers (1961, p. 42): "The counselor or physician or administrator who is warmly emotional and expressive, respectful of the individuality of himself and of the other, and who exhibits a nonpossessive caring, probably facilitates self-realization much as does a parent with these attitudes." He drew the analogy from parental attitudes to helper attitudes and added that the helper must express "acceptant-democratic" attitudes in his behavior. He did not clearly distinguish attitudes from behavior. It is important to point out that Hersey and Blanchard

---

[1]"Acceptant-democratic" and "actively rejectant" were phrases used by the authors to describe the dichotomy between open, loving parents who listened to the individual aspects of their children versus rigid, controlling parents who saw their children only as extensions of themselves.

(1982) addressed the attitudes or predispositions of the helper/manager as different from behavior, which tends to be the actions perceived by others. Attitudes of empathy, respect, warmth, and concern can then be viable only if the behavior of the helper is perceived as such by the helpee.

Whitehorn and Betz (1954) investigated the degree of success physicians found while working with schizophrenic patients on a psychiatric ward. They found that helpful physicians primarily made use of active personal participation. They tended to see the schizophrenic client in terms of the personal meaning that various behaviors had to the client and worked toward goals rooted in the personality of the client. They developed a rapport in which the client felt trust and confidence in the physician. These approaches were in contrast to those of the physician who used procedures such as interpretation, instruction, advice, or emphasis on practical care.

Another study investigated the way in which a person being helped perceived the relationship. Heine (1950) studied the individuals who had undergone psychotherapeutic treatment. The clients reported similar changes in themselves regardless of the orientation of the therapist. The major elements they found helpful in their environment centered on the trust they had felt for the therapist, the feelings of being understood, and the independence they had in making decisions. The therapist's procedures found to be most helpful were clarification and open communication of the feelings that the client had approached hesitantly. The identified unhelpful elements included lack of interest, remoteness, superfluous sympathy, and emphasis on past history, rather than on present problems.

Fiedler (1953) found that expert therapists, regardless of their orientation, formed client relationships characterized by similar elements: empathy, a sensitivity to the client's attitudes, and a warm interest without emotional over-involvement. Seeman (1954) noted that psychotherapeutic success is closely tied to a mutual

liking and respectful interaction between the client and therapist. Rogers (1961, p. 44) discovered that "the attitudes and feelings of the therapist, rather than his theoretical orientation" are what is important. It is also "the way in which his attitudes and procedures are perceived which makes a difference" (Rogers, 1961, p. 44). Halkides (1958) also affirmed that a high degree of empathic understanding was significantly associated with successful therapy, as were a high degree of unconditional positive regard and the counselor's genuineness.

It was with this background that Carkhuff (1969) went on to state and empirically document the core conditions necessary to promote facilitative human relationships—namely, empathy, respect, warmth, genuineness, self-disclosure, concreteness, confrontation, and immediacy of relationship.

Carkhuff's (1969) work stemmed from the basic assumption that counseling and psychotherapy are aspects of interpersonal and relearning processes or, generally, human relations. From this assumption, research has documented that human encounters may have constructive or destructive effects and that all effective processes share a common bond of conditions that are conducive to facilitative human experiences (Berenson & Carkhuff, 1967; Berenson & Mitchell, 1968; Carkhuff & Berenson, 1977; Rogers, Gendlin, Kiesler, & Truax, 1967).

Effective and Ineffective Cycles

From the previously cited research findings, Carkhuff (1969) proposed a model for effective and ineffective functioning. At each point in one's life during which one has contact with another person, the encounter either enables one to grow further or causes one to deteriorate; there is no neutrality. Thus, the severely deteriorated person who seems to be functioning ineffectively in all relationships can be viewed as a product of prolonged, nonhelpful relationships that hinder growth. By comparison, the person who has experienced a series of facilitative relationships will function at high or effective levels in most areas of the person's existence. Those persons who are neither totally effective nor totally ineffective in coping with life's processes are those who have had a series of mixed relationships—some effective, some harmful. According to Carkhuff (1969, p. 22), "Each significant encounter, then, between more knowing and less knowing persons[2] may be considered a crisis in the lives of both groups. Whether an individual grows or deteriorates is dependent in large part upon the interaction of the activities of both the more knowing and the less knowing persons."[3] A person's basic direction—toward growth or toward deterioration—depends a great deal upon what happens at each critical stage in the person's development, even though different resources and predispositions of individuals are involved (Carkhuff, 1969). This can be equated to Hersey and Blanchard's (1982) "effective and ineffective cycles."

The *effective cycle* in organizational theory is one of which high expectations by leaders produce high performance by followers. This process spirals upward and builds upon itself. The *ineffective cycle* is one during which low expectations imposed on followers produce low performance; it spirals downward (Hersey & Blanchard, 1982). Human relationships can be analyzed in the same way if one would add to the effective/ineffective cycles the variable of the leader's ability to communicate effectively. Constructive and facilitative experiences with other persons during crisis points in one's life produce a spiral upward and provide a new level from which to continue growth. Ineffective or deteriorating experiences produce the opposite effects, spiraling downward, thus placing a person on a lower level of functioning from which

the person must then regrow. It is possible to project, then, that a series of helpful relationships reinforces one at an elevated level, whereas a series of ineffective relationships can be extremely harmful.

Going back to Hersey and Blanchard's (1982) theory, it appears logical to conclude, therefore, that, if a leader's high expectations of followers are coupled with facilitative communication skills, this may initiate an effective cycle. Similarly, if one joined low expectations with poor communicative skills, a deleterious downward cycle might result. High expectations paired with ineffective communications or low expectations paired with facilitative skills might act much like an acid/base buffer system, one factor neutralizing the other and thereby retarding outcome. It follows, however, that effective process must be synchronized with realistic goals. In line with Beck's (1963) existential view that the total human organism reacts to any situation, one cannot react either intellectually or emotionally to the exclusion of the other. Also, humans behave in terms of their subjective view of reality, not according to some externally defined objective. Each person has heredity and experiences unique to that person, and from these it is to be expected that each person will behave differently from others whose experiences are different.

FACETS OF THE HELPING RELATIONSHIP

Carkhuff (1969) provided a description of facets in a helping relationship: helper, helpee, and environmental variables.

The Helper

The helper's contribution can be divided broadly into two phases—understanding and action. The first phase, understanding, enables the helpee to probe inwardly by exploring and experiencing the core of his or her existence. The facilitative conditions of empathy, respect, warmth, and self-disclosure employed during

---

[2]"More knowing and less knowing persons" refers to the relationship between helper/helpee, parent/child, teacher/student, and so forth.

[3]From *Helping and Human Relations: A Primer for Lay and Professional Helpers,* Volume I, by R. R. Carkhuff. Copyright © 1969 by Human Resource Development, Inc. This and all other quotations from the same source are reprinted with permission.

this phase offer the helpee both a stimulus and a reinforcement. In turn, this serves to lower the helpee's defenses, thereby enabling the helper to elicit more meaningful material (Carkhuff, 1969). "High levels of facilitative conditions enable the helper to understand the helpee and the helpee to experience the feeling of being understood" (Carkhuff, 1969, p. 42).

The second phase of the helper's contribution is the action-oriented dimension. Carkhuff and Berenson (1977) called this the upward phase, or period of "emergent directionality." After having explored self, the distressed person experiences a need to act on the world in a more effective manner than in previous encounters. Since trust and understanding have already been established in the first phase, the helper can now be a guide in this action-oriented dimension (Carkhuff, 1969).

The two phases of helping have been shown to be essential components of a comprehensive helping model. They may not be sequential and distinctive; they must operate together within the helper/helpee relationship. The helper must be functioning at a level at which the helper has been established by the helpee as a model for effective living (Carkhuff, 1969).

It is important to note that studies of helper-trainee characteristics have suggested that traditional feminine response patterns have been demonstrated in helper trainees.[4] Farson (1954), McClain (1968), and Patterson (1967) have discovered that helpers tend to get high scores on social-service interests and nurturant inclinations, as well as on indexes of more traditionally feminine personality dispositions such as restraint, friendliness, deference, and affiliation. Low scores were observed on more aggressive, assertive, and achievement-oriented traits. However, a comprehensive model for the helping process should be viewed as containing both types. Carkhuff (1969, p. 34) expressed this succinctly: "The effective helper is both

mother and father. The whole person has incorporated both the responsive and assertive components. He (or she) can understand his internal and external physical, emotional, and intellectual world with sensitivity and can act upon these worlds with responsibility."

The Helpee

Since an interaction requires more than one person, it is necessary to look also at the *helpee*. According to Carkhuff (1969), contributions made by the helpee can be delineated as follows: (1) what the helpee brings to the experience, (2) how the helpee reacts within the process, and (3) what changes are elicited in the helpee as a result of the process.

The first set of factors—what a helpee brings to the situation—is divided into (1) the demographic characteristics of the helpee's system and (2) the helpee's level of functioning. There is little or no research relating helpee demographic characteristics to treatment outcome, but social class and racial variables have been studied. Banks, Berenson, and Carkhuff (1967) found that the counselors who either were similar or could generate perceived similarity were seen by Black college students as more effective change agents. Anderson and Anderson (1962), Banks (1972), Carkhuff and Pierce (1967), and Correll (1955) found that racial similarity was a source of increased client self-exploration while social class had no statistical significance. Winder and Hersko (1955) and Hollingshead and Redlich (1958) reported that both counselors and psychologists, themselves middle class, facilitated self-exploration in clients of similar social status and discouraged it in clients of lower social status. Gardner (1972) investigated the variables of race, education, and experience as significant factors in the degree to which counselors are perceived as effective by Black college students. He found all three to be significant sources of effect for student ratings. The implications of the research are that counselors with backgrounds similar to that of the client are most effective.

---

[4]The use of a "feminine" description of any trait refers only to usage of the term by the authors cited.

However, the works of Rogers et al. (1967) and Truax and Carkhuff (1967) gave evidence that helpees who were seen by motivated helpers, regardless of social class or demographic characteristics, had an opportunity for constructive change.

The helpee's level of functioning is the second division of what the helpee brings to the relationship. There is little evidence to indicate that assessments of levels of functioning are in any way correlated with differential treatment (Carkhuff, 1968; Carkhuff & Berenson, 1977; Pagell, Carkhuff, & Berenson, 1967; Spiegel & Spiegel, 1967; Thorne, 1967; Truax and Carkhuff, 1967). "Traditional diagnosis does not make a difference" (Carkhuff, 1969, p. 50). In other words, the theoretic framework on which a helper bases practice and diagnosis is far less important to counseling outcome than is the helper's level of functioning in communication skills.

The second set of factors of the helpee's contribution to the counseling relationship is how the helpee reacts within the relationship. This includes the helpee's process variables, sets, expectancies, and motivations. These variables are internal in the helpee. What a helpee perceives (sets) and the expectations of therapy together produce motivation, and the energy resulting from motivation affects the process of counseling itself. Carkhuff (1969, p. 52) stated that "basically what the helpee expects and, indeed, needs are a high level of understanding in his life." Helping-process variables—which include helpee self-exploration, problem expression, and the immediacy of experiencing—are essential to constructive helpee change or gain (Carkhuff, 1969; Carkhuff & Berenson, 1977). Stated Carkhuff (1969, p. 54), "The degree to which the helpee can explore himself within the helping process is related to the degree to which he changes constructively." Writings of Carkhuff and Berenson (1977) and Truax and Carkhuff (1967) confirmed this point.

The last contribution of the helpee involves the changes the relationship elicits in the helpee. The outcome of the helping relationship is a reflection of the goals of counseling. Carkhuff stated (1969, p. 62), "The helper's task is thus to serve as a guide on the helpee's journey toward finding himself and acting upon who he is. Through the helper's eyes and ears the helpee can come to see and hear the sights and sounds of life; with the helper's hands he can learn to touch and to act; through the helper's life he can come to find his own life."

The Environment

The last set of variables that must be considered in the helping process includes environmental and contextual influences (Carkhuff, 1966; Carkhuff & Berenson, 1977). The helper and helpee do not interact in a vacuum. The setting in which helping takes place, as well as the environment and people to which the helpee must return, incorporate critical variables (Goffman, 1959, 1961; Jones, 1953; Rapaport, 1960; Scheff, 1966, 1967; Shibutani, 1961; Smelser & Smelser, 1963; Wesseu, 1964). Within the rationale for helping, Carkhuff (1969, p. 69) maintained, "what the helpee learns to do within the context of the helping relationship can be generalized to other significant areas of his life."

IMPORTANCE OF EMPATHY

Writings of other authors have clarified the concept of empathy and its primary importance in a helping relationship. Combs, Avila, and Purkey (1978), for example, described empathy as the ability to put oneself in another's shoes so as to perceive the world as he or she does. They further stated that helpers must be able to understand the private world of the helpee in terms of feelings, attitudes, wants, and goals. This requires reaching "inside the skin" of another person.

Blocher (1974) divided empathy into two components. The cognitive component involves psychologic understanding, while the affect component is feeling *with* a person. Buchheimer

(1963) addressed empathy within the context of several dimensions of the helping process:

1. The *tone* of the counseling relationship is an expressive and possibly nonverbal dimension based upon expressions of warmth and spontaneity.

2. The *pace* involves the appropriateness and the flow of the relationship.

3. The counselor's *perception* is related to the counselor's abilities to abstract the core of the client's concerns and respond to these in an acceptable, constructive manner.

4. *Strategy* relates to the predictive or role-playing aspect of the relationship.

5. *Leading* involves the resourcefulness of the counselor in moving the relationship in the direction of the client's concerns.

Jourard (1971) correlated the helper's ability to effect constructive growth in helpees with what Foote and Cottrell (1955) called interpersonal competence. This is described as the ability of the helper to produce valued, desirable outcomes in transactions with people. Professionals who have achieved interpersonal competence are those who are able to achieve desirable outcomes in their encounters with their clients; outcomes are measured in terms of the signs exemplifying the quality of care given the helpees. Professionals must, therefore, possess and use empathy in the helping process as a vehicle to effect overt and measurable changes.

The literature has shown that empathy involves more than a simple understanding and reflection of a client's verbal behavior. La Monica (1981) defined *empathy* as follows: "Empathy signifies a central focus and feeling *with* and *in* the client's world. It involves accurate perceptions of the client's world by the helper, communication of this understanding to the client, and the client's perception of the helper's understanding" (p. 398). Based on recent research using a multitrait-multimethod approach in studying the construct validity of her empathy instrument, La Monica (1981) concluded

that empathy is a hierarchical process beginning with the helper's perception, moving next to the helper's communication, and finally moving to the client's perception of the helper's understanding. Empathy operates throughout the helping relationship.

Having looked at two related, yet distinct, concepts—professions and helping models, we must now integrate these two areas in order to define a helping profession. A helping profession, then, is one that has the following attributes:

1. A unique area of service that fills an area of human need

2. Data-based knowledge derived from research processes

3. Skills that build on knowledge

4. Formal educational avenues for acquisition of knowledge and experience

5. Authority to implement services according to standards set by the unique helping profession

6. Responsibility and accountability for all services provided by the profession

NURSING AS A HELPING PROFESSION

In order to establish that nursing is a helping profession, it is first necessary to define nursing. The literature is replete with descriptive and succinct nursing definitions involving nursing concepts, roles, and actions. These definitions are necessary in setting professional standards and also in providing a frame of reference for learners as each begins the individual journey of practice. They are also helpful in increasing role awareness among the public.

For current purposes, it is necessary to look at established definitions and decide whether nursing qualifies as a helping profession. Perhaps the most widely used and current definition of nursing was written by Henderson (1966, p. 3):

The practice of professional nursing means the performance for compensation of any act in the observation, care, and counsel of the ill, injured, or infirm, or in the maintenance of health or prevention of illness of others, or in the supervision and teaching of other personnel, or the administration of medications and treatments as prescribed by a licensed physician or dentist; requiring substantial specialized judgment and skill and based on knowledge and application of the principles of biological, physical, and social science.

The simplest definition of a nurse, as provided by Webster, is that of a person educated to provide care and curative help or treatment to any in need. Florence Nightingale (1860/1969) considered nursing as the prevention and cure of injury or disease and as the care that put a patient in the best condition for nature to restore health. Stressed throughout her definition was that nursing meant treating the *person*, not the disease.

Reiter (1966) focused professional nursing practice and clinical competence on three "Cs": care, cure, and coordination. These included promotion of health; counseling; responsibility for individuals, families, and the community; supervision; teaching; directing care providers; and collaborating and synchronizing health services. All of these require knowledge of a high order and skill based on a broad framework of theory.

For the purposes of this book, the author defines a nurse as;

A formally educated person who is a provider of knowledge, support, assistance, and/or care to any person who is in need, in any setting, on a twenty-four-hour basis, in collaboration with other health professionals as appropriate and in conjunction with the current American Nurses' Association Standards of Practice.

It has been shown that nursing, by all of its own definitions, is indeed a helping profession. The attributes of a helping profession can be seen throughout nursing education and practice. Basically speaking, there are four parts of nursing education and practice:

1. *Knowledge.* Our primary knowledge begins and ends with our client(s) and what is known about human behavior, health, sickness, and treatment. In formal and informal educational systems, applied theory from the pure sciences, the humanities, and the behavioral sciences is integrated into client care. Nursing research, our pure science, is carried on continuously as nursing theory is expanded.

2. *Skills.* The skills and competencies necessary for the delivery of nursing care are basic in education and perpetual throughout practice. They include skills relative to nursing's responsibility, including those reflective of helping processes. Service institutions are constantly providing programs for practitioners in which skills and concepts can be learned and/or updated.

Skills and competencies are divided into two broad areas: attitudinal and behavioral learning; they include content and process.

3. *Code of Ethics.* The Code of Ethics in nursing practice is set by our professional organization, the American Nurses' Association (1978, 1980a, 1980b, 1982) and is followed by all nursing administrations and individual practitioners.

4. *Method.* The definitive transferable method in nursing is the nursing process. It is our own scientific method and forms the basis for all nursing care.

The helping model presents the concept of helping as the promotion of growth and constructive change, whereas the nursing model features the meeting of a client's needs. The two models together provide a more comprehensive and humanistic basis for the nursing process than either one by itself. It is crucial to visualize these two areas as harmoniously operating together and at the same time; a nurse meets a client's needs in identified areas by promoting growth and constructive change in the client toward specified goals.

SUMMARY

This chapter has studied the attributes of a helping profession as well as the facets of the action of helping. Nursing was portrayed in terms of its components relative to the entire process. It became evident that the professional and helping aspects of practice are threads in the Gestalt of nursing. The nursing process is the method that enables a practitioner to use a broad base of knowledge and experience in the client/nurse interaction.

"And there are those who give and know
not pain in giving, nor do they seek joy,
nor give with mindfulness of virtue;

They give as in yonder valley the myrtle
breathes its fragrance into space.

Through the hands of such as these God
speaks, and from behind their eyes He
smiles upon the earth."

Kahlil Gibran

REFERENCES

American Nurses' Association. (1978). *Perspectives on the code for nurses*. Kansas City, MO: Author.

American Nurses' Association. (1980a). *Ethics in nursing practice and education*. Kansas City, MO: Author.

American Nurses' Association. (1980b). *Code for nurses*. Kansas City MO: Author.

The Prophet, 1951, p. 20. Reproduced by permission of Alfred A. Knopf, Inc.

American Nurses' Association. (1982). *Ethics references for nurses*. Kansas City, MO: Author.

Anderson, R., & Anderson, G. (1962). The development of an instrument for measuring rapport. *Personnel and Guidance Journal, 41*, 18–24.

Baldwin, A., Kalhorn, J., & Breese, F. (1945). Patterns of parent behavior. *Psychological Monographs, 58*, 1–75.

Banks, W. (1972). The differential effects of race and social class in helping. *Journal of Clinical Psychology, 28*, 90–92.

Banks, G., Berenson, B., & Carkhuff, R. (1967). The effects of counselor race and training upon counseling process with Negro clients in initial interviews. *Journal of Clinical Psychology, 23*, 70–72.

Beck, C. (1963). *Philosophical foundations of guidance*. Englewood Cliffs, NJ: Prentice-Hall.

Berenson, B., & Carkhuff, R. (1967). *Sources of gain in counseling and psychotherapy*. New York: Holt, Rinehart and Winston.

Berenson, B., & Mitchell, K. (1968). *Confrontation in counseling and life*. Unpublished manuscript, American International College, Springfield, MA.

Blocher, D. (1974). *Developmental counseling* (2nd ed.). New York: Ronald Press.

Buchheimer, A. (1963). The development of ideas abut empathy. *Journal of Counseling Psychology, 10*, 61–71.

Carkhuff, R. (1966). Counseling research, theory and practice. *Journal of Counseling Psychology, 13*, 467–480.

Carkhuff, R. (1968). The differential functioning of lay and professional helpers. *Journal of Counseling Psychology, 15*, 117–126.

Carkhuff, R. (1969). *Helping and human relations: A primer for lay and professional helpers* (Vol. 1). New York: Human Resource Development Press.

Carkhuff, R. (1973). *The art of helping*. Amherst, MA: Human Resource Development Press.

Carkhuff, R., & Berenson, B. (1977). *Beyond counseling and therapy* (2nd ed.). New York: Holt, Rinehart and Winston.

Carkhuff, R., & Pierce, R. (1967). The differential effects of therapist race and social class upon patient depth of self-exploration in the initial clinical interview. *Journal of Consulting Psychology, 31,* 631–634.

Combs, A., Avila, D., & Purkey, W. (1978). *Helping relationships: Basic concepts for the helping professions* (2nd ed.). Boston: Allyn and Bacon.

Correll, P. (1955). *Factors influencing communication in counseling.* Unpublished doctoral dissertation, University of Missouri.

Farson, R. (1954). The counselor is a woman. *Journal of Counseling Psychology, 1,* 221–223.

Fiedler, F. (1953). Quantitative studies on the role of the therapists' feelings toward their patients. In O. H. Mowrer (Ed.), *Psychotherapy: Theory and research.* New York: Ronald Press.

Foote, N., & Cottrell, L. (1955). *Identity and interpersonal competence.* Chicago: University of Chicago Press.

Gardner, W. (1972). The differential effects of race, education, and experience in helping. *Journal of Clinical Psychology, 28,* 87–89.

Goffman, E. (1959). *The presentation of self in everyday life.* New York: Doubleday.

Goffman, E. (1961). *Encounters: Two studies in the sociology of interaction.* New York: Bobbs-Merrill.

Halkides, G. (1958). *An experimental study of four conditions necessary for therapeutic change.* Unpublished doctoral dissertation, University of Chicago.

Heine, R. (1950). *A comparison of patients' reports on psychotherapeutic experience with psychoanalytic, non-directive, and Adlerian therapists.* Unpublished doctoral dissertation, University of Chicago.

Henderson, V. (1966). *The nature of nursing.* New York: Macmillan.

Hersey, P., & Blanchard, K. (1982). *Management of organizational behavior: Utilizing human resources* (4th ed.). Englewood Cliffs, NJ: Prentice-Hall.

Hollingshead, A., & Redlich, F. (1958). *Social class and mental illness.* New York: Wiley.

Jones, M. (1953). *The therapeutic community.* New York: Basic Books.

Jourard, S. (1971). *The transparent self* (2nd ed.). New York: Van Nostrand Reinhold.

La Monica, E. (1981). Construct validity of an empathy instrument. *Research in Nursing and Health, 4,* 389–400.

McClain, E. (1968). Is the counselor a woman? *Personnel and Guidance Journal, 46,* 444–448.

Metzger, W. (1975). What is a profession? *Seminar Reports.* New York: Columbia University.

Nightingale, F. (1969). *Notes on nursing: What it is and what it is not.* New York: Dover. (Originally published 1860.)

Otto, H. (1970). *Group methods to actualize human potential: A handbook.* Beverly Hills, CA: Holistic Press.

Pagell, W., Carkhuff, R., & Berenson, B. (1967). The predicted differential effects of the level of counselor functioning upon the level of functioning of outpatients. *Journal of Clinical Psychology, 23,* 510–512.

Patterson, C. (1967). *The selection of counselors.* Paper presented at the Conference on Research Problems in Counseling, Washington University, St. Louis, MO.

Rapaport, R. (1960). *The community as a doctor.* Chicago: Charles C. Thomas.

Reiter, F. (1966). The nurse-clinician. *American Journal of Nursing, 66,* 274–280.

Rogers, C. (1958). The characteristics of a helping relationship. *Personnel and Guidance Journal, 37,* 6–16.

Rogers C. (1961). *On becoming a person.* Boston: Houghton-Mifflin.

Rogers, C., Gendlin, E., Kiesler, D., & Truax, C. (Eds.). (1967). *The therapeutic relationship and its impact: A study of psychotherapy with schizophrenics.* Madison: University of Wisconsin Press.

Scheff, T. (1966). *Being mentally ill: A sociological theory.* Chicago: Aldine.

Scheff, T. (Ed.). (1967). *Mental illness and social processes.* New York: Harper and Row.

Seeman, J. (1954). Counselor judgments of therapeutic processes and outcome. In C. Rogers & R. Dymond (Eds.), *Psychotherapy and personality change.* Chicago: University of Chicago Press.

Shibutani, T. (1961). *Society and personality: An interactionist approach to social psychology.* Englewood Cliffs, NJ: Prentice-Hall.

Smelser, N., & Smelser, W. (Eds.). (1963). *Personality and social systems.* New York: Wiley.

Spiegel, P., & Spiegel, D. (1967). Perceived helpfulness of others as a function of compatible intelligence. *Journal of Counseling Psychology, 14,* 61–62.

Thorne, K. (1967). The etiological equation. In R. Carkhuff & B. Berenson, *Beyond counseling and therapy* (Appendix A). New York: Holt, Rinehart and Winston.

Truax, C., & Carkhuff, R. (1967). *Toward effective counseling and psychotherapy: Training and practice.* Chicago: Aldine.

Weigand, J. (Ed.). (1971). *Developing teacher competencies.* Englewood Cliffs, NJ: Prentice-Hall.

Wesseu, A. (1964). *The psychiatric hospital as a social system.* Chicago: Charles C. Thomas.

Whitehorn, J., & Betz, B. (1954). A study of psychotherapeutic relationships between physicians and schizophrenic patients. *American Journal of Psychiatry, 111,* 321–331.

Winder, A., & Hersko, M. (1955). The effect of social class on the length and type of psychotherapy in a V. A. Mental Hygiene Clinic. *Journal of Clinical Psychology, 11,* 77–79.

SELECTED READING

The selected reading for this chapter is a classic article by Carl Rogers (1958) on the characteristics of a helping profession. Writing as a psychologist, he amplified and extended the theory and rationale for helping that was presented in the chapter.

The Characteristics of a Helping Relationship

Carl R. Rogers

My interest in psychotherapy has brought about in me an interest in every kind of helping relationship. By this term I mean a relationship in which at least one of the parties has the intent of promoting the growth, development, maturity, improved functioning, improved coping with life of the other. The other, in this sense, may be one individual or a group. To put it in another way, a helping relationship might be defined as one in which one of the participants intends that there should come about, in one or both parties, more appreciation of, more expression of, more functional use of the latent inner resources of the individual.

Now it is obvious that such a definition covers a wide range of relationships which usually are intended to facilitate growth. It would certainly include the relationship between mother and child, father and child. It would include the relationship between the physician and his patient. The relationship between teacher and pupil would often come under this definition, though some teachers would not have the promotion of growth as their intent. It includes almost all counselor-client relationships, whether we are speaking of educational counseling, vocational counseling, or personal counseling. In this last-mentioned area it would include the wide range of relationships between the psychotherapist and the hospitalized psychotic, the therapist and the troubled or neurotic individual, and the relationship between the therapist and the increasing number of so-called "normal" individuals who enter therapy to improve their own functioning or accelerate their personal growth.

These are largely one-to-one relationships. But we should also think of the large number of individual-group interactions which are intended as helping relationships. Some administrators intend that their relationship to their staff groups shall be of the sort which promotes growth, though other administrators would not have this purpose. The interaction between the group therapy leader and his group belongs here. So does the relationship of the community consultant to a community group. Increasingly the interaction between the industrial consultant and a management group is intended as a helping relationship. Perhaps this listing will point up the fact that a great many of the relationships in which we and others are involved fall within this category of interactions in which there is the purpose of promoting development and more mature and adequate functioning.

Reprinted with permission from *Personnel and Guidance Journal*, Vol. 37. Copyright 1958 by American Personnel and Guidance Association. This article also appears in Dr. Rogers's book *On Becoming a Person*, Boston: Houghton-Mifflin Company, 1961, pp. 39–58.

THE QUESTION

But what are the characteristics of those relationships which *do* help, which do facilitate growth? And at the other end of the scale is it possible to discern those characteristics which make a relationship unhelpful, even though it was the sincere intent to promote growth and development? It is to these questions, particularly the first, that I would like to take you with me over some of the paths I have explored, and to tell you where I am, as of now, in my thinking on these issues.

THE ANSWERS GIVEN BY RESEARCH

It is natural to ask first of all whether there is any empirical research which would give us an objective answer to these questions. There has not been a large amount of research in this area as yet, but what there is is stimulating and suggestive. I cannot report all of it but I would like to make a somewhat extensive sampling of the studies which have been done and state very briefly some of the findings. In so doing, oversimplification is necessary, and I am quite aware that I am not doing full justice to the researches I am mentioning, but it may give you the feeling that factual advances are being made and pique your curiosity enough to examine the studies themselves, if you have not already done so.

Studies of Attitudes

Most of the studies throw light on the attitudes on the part of the helping person which make a relationship growth-promoting or growth-inhibiting. Let us look at some of these.

A careful study of parent-child relationships made some years ago by Baldwin and others (1) at the Fels Institute contains interesting evidence. Of the various clusters of parental attitudes toward children, the "acceptant-democratic" seemed most growth-facilitating. Children of these parents with their warm and equalitarian attitudes showed an accelerated intellectual development (an increasing IQ), more originality, more emotional security and control, less excitability than children from other types of homes. Though somewhat slow initially in social development, they were by the time they reached school age, popular, friendly, non-aggressive leaders.

Where parents' attitudes are classed as "actively rejectant" the children show a slightly decelerated intellectual development, relatively poor use of the abilities they do possess, and some lack of originality. They are emotionally unstable, rebellious, aggressive, and quarrelsome. The children of parents with other attitude syndromes tend in various respects to fall in between these extremes.

I am sure that these findings do not surprise us as related to child development. I would like to suggest that they probably apply to other relationships as well, and that the counselor or physician or administrator who is warmly emotional and expressive, respectful of the individuality of himself and of the other, and who exhibits a non-possessive caring, probably facilitates self-realization much as does a parent with these attitudes.

Let me turn to another careful study in a very different area. Whitehorn and Betz (2, 18) investigated the degree of success achieved by young resident physicians in working with schizophrenic patients on a psychiatric ward. They chose for special study the seven who had been outstandingly helpful, and seven whose patients had shown the least degree of improvement. Each group had treated about 50 patients. The investigators examined all the available evidence to discover in what ways the A group (the successful group) differed from the B group. Several significant differences were found. The physicians in the A group tended to see the schizophrenic in terms of the personal meaning which various behaviors had to the patient, rather than seeing him as a case history or a descriptive diagnosis. They also tended to work toward goals which were oriented to the personality of the patient, rather than such goals as reducing the symptoms or curing the disease. It was found that the helpful physicians, in their day by day interaction, primarily made use of active personal participation—a person-to-person relationship. They made less use of procedures which could be classed as "passive permissive." They were even less likely to use such procedures as interpretation, instruction or advice, or emphasis upon the practical care of the patient. Finally, they were much more likely than the B group to develop a relationship in which the patient felt trust and confidence in the physician.

Although the authors cautiously emphasize that these findings relate only to the treatment of schizophrenics, I am inclined to disagree. I suspect that similar facts would be found in a research study of almost any class of helping relationship.

Another interesting study focuses upon the way in which the person being helped perceived the relationship. Heine (11) studied individuals who had gone for psychotherapeutic help to psychoanalytic, client-centered, and Adlerian therapists. Regardless of the type of therapy, these clients report similar changes in themselves. But it is their perception of the relationship which is of particular interest to us here. When asked what accounted for the changes which had occurred, they expressed some differing explanations, depending on the orientation of the therapist. But their agreement on the major elements they had found helpful was even more significant. They indicated that these attitudinal elements in the relationship accounted for the changes which had taken place in themselves: the trust they had felt in the therapist; being understood by the therapist; the feeling of independence they had had in making choices and decisions. The therapist procedure which they had found most helpful was that the therapist clarified and openly stated feelings which the client had been approaching hazily and hesitantly.

There was also a high degree of agreement among these clients, regardless of the orientation of their therapists, as to what elements had been unhelpful in the relationship. Such therapist attitudes as lack of interest, remoteness or distance, and an over-degree of sympathy, were perceived as unhelpful. As to procedures, they had found it unhelpful when therapists had given direct, specific advice regarding decisions or had emphasized past history rather than present problems. Guiding suggestions mildly given were perceived in an intermediate range—neither clearly helpful nor unhelpful.

Fiedler, in a much quoted study (7), found that expert therapists of differing orientations formed similar relationships with their clients. Less well known are the elements which characterized these relationships, differentiating them from the relationships formed by less expert therapists. These elements are: an ability to understand the client's meanings and feelings; a sensitivity to the client's attitudes; a warm interest without any emotional over-involvement.

A study by Quinn (15) throws light on what is involved in understanding the client's meanings and feelings. His study is surprising in that it shows that "understanding" of the client's meanings is essentially an attitude of *desiring* to understand. Quinn presented his judges only with recorded therapist statements taken from interviews. The raters had no knowledge of what the therapist was responding to or how the client reacted to his response. Yet it was found that the degree of understanding could be judged about as well from this material as from listening to the response in context. This seems rather conclusive evidence that it is an attitude of wanting to understand which is communicated.

As to the emotional quality of the relationship, Seeman (16) found that success in psychotherapy is closely associated with a strong and growing mutual liking and respect between client and therapist.

An interesting study by Dittes (4) indicates how delicate this relationship is. Using a physiological measure, the psychogalvanic reflex, to measure the anxious or threatened or alerted reactions of the client, Dittes correlated the deviations on this measure with judges' ratings of the degree of warm acceptance and permissiveness on the part of the therapist. It was found that whenever the therapist's attitudes changed even slightly in the direction of a lesser degree of acceptance, the number of abrupt

GSR deviations significantly increased. Evidently when the relationship is experienced as less acceptant the organism organizes against threat, even at the physiological level.

Without trying to integrate the findings from these various studies, it can at least be noted that a few things stand out. One is the fact that it is the attitudes and feelings of the therapist, rather than his theoretical orientation, which is important. His procedures and techniques are less important than his attitudes. It is also worth noting that it is the way in which his attitudes and procedures are *perceived* which makes a difference to the client, and that it is this perception which is crucial.

"Manufactured" Relationships

Let me turn to research of a very different sort, some of which you may find rather abhorrent, but which nevertheless has a bearing upon the nature of a facilitating relationship. These studies have to do with what we might think of as manufactured relationships.

Verplanck (17), Greenspoon (8) and others have shown that operant conditioning of verbal behavior is possible in a relationship. Very briefly, if the experimenter says "Mhm," or "Good," or nods his head after certain types of words or statements, those classes of words tend to increase because of being reinforced. It has been shown that using such procedures one can bring about increases in such diverse verbal categories as plural nouns, hostile words, statements of opinion. The person is completely unaware that he is being influenced in any way by these reinforcers. The implication is that by such selective reinforcement we could bring it about that the other person in the relationship would be using whatever kinds of words and making whatever kinds of statements we had decided to reinforce.

Following still further the principles of operant conditioning as developed by Skinner and his group, Lindsley (12) has shown that a chronic schizophrenic can be placed in a "helping relationship" with a machine. The machine,

somewhat like a vending machine, can be set to reward a variety of types of behaviors. Initially it simply rewards—with candy, a cigarette, or the display of a picture— the lever-pressing behavior of the patient. But it is possible to set it so that many pulls on the lever may supply a hungry kitten—visible in a separate enclosure—with a drop of milk. In this case the satisfaction is an altruistic one. Plans are being developed to reward similar social or altruistic behavior directed toward another patient, placed in the next room. The only limit to the kinds of behavior which might be rewarded lies in the degree of mechanical integrity of the experimenter.

Lindsley reports that in some patients there has been marked clinical improvement. Personally I cannot help but be impressed by the description of one patient who had gone from a deteriorated chronic state to being given free ground privileges, this change being quite clearly associated with his interaction with the machine. Then the experimenter decided to study experimental extinction, which, put in more personal terms, means that no matter how many thousands of times the lever was pressed, no reward of any kind was forthcoming. The patient gradually regressed, grew untidy, uncommunicative, and his ground privileges had to be revoked. This (to me) pathetic incident would seem to indicate that even in a relationship to a machine, trustworthiness is important if the relationship is to be helpful.

Still another interesting study of a manufactured relationship is being carried on by Harlow and his associates (10), this time with monkeys. Infant monkeys, removed from their mothers almost immediately after birth, are, in one phase of the experiment, presented with two objects. One might be termed the "hard mother," a sloping cylinder of wire netting with a nipple from which the baby may feed. The other is a "soft mother," a similar cylinder made of foam rubber and terry cloth. Even when an infant gets all his food from the "hard mother" he clearly and increasingly prefers the "soft mother." Motion pictures show that he definitely "relates" to this object, playing with it, enjoying it, finding security in clinging to it when strange objects are near, and using that security as a home base for venturing into the frightening world. Of the many interesting and challenging implications of this study, one seems reasonably clear. It is that no amount of direct food reward can take the place of certain perceived qualities which the infant appears to need and desire.

Two Recent Studies

Let me close this wide-ranging—and perhaps perplexing—sampling of research studies with an account of two very recent investigations. The first is an experiment conducted by Ends and Page (5). Working with hardened chronic hospitalized alcoholics who had been committed to a state hospital for 60 days, they tried three different methods of group psychotherapy. The method which they believed would be most effective was therapy based on a two-factor theory of learning; a client-centered approach was expected to be second; a psychoanalytically oriented approach was expected to be least efficient. Their results showed that the therapy based upon a learning theory approach was not only not helpful, but was somewhat deleterious. The outcomes were worse than those in the control group which had no therapy. The analytically oriented therapy produced some positive gain, and the client-centered group therapy was associated with the greatest amount of positive change. Follow-up data, extending over one and one-half years, confirmed the in-hospital findings, with the lasting improvement being greatest in the client-centered approach, next in the analytic, next the control group, and least in those handled by a learning theory approach.

As I have puzzled over this study, unusual in that the approach to which the authors were committed proved *least* effective, I find a clue, I believe, in the description of the therapy based on learning theory (13). Essentially, it consisted (1) of pointing out and labeling the behaviors which had proved unsatisfying, (2) of exploring objectively with the client the reasons behind these behaviors, and (3) of establishing through re-education more effective problem-solving habits. But in all of this interaction the aim, as they formulated it, was to be impersonal. The therapist "permits as little of his own personality to intrude as is humanly possible." The "therapist stresses personal anonymity in his activities, i.e., he must studiously avoid impressing the patient with his own (therapist's) individual personality characteristics." To me this seems the most likely clue to the failure of this approach, as I try to interpret the facts in the light of the other research studies. To withhold one's self as a person and to deal with the other person as an object does not have a high probability of being helpful.

The final study I wish to report is one just being completed by Halkides (9). She started from a theoretical formulation of mine regarding the necessary and sufficient conditions for therapeutic change (14). She hypothesized that there would be a significant relationship between the extent of constructive personality change in the client and four counselor variables: (1) the degree of empathic understanding of the client manifested by the counselor; (2) the degree of positive affective attitude (unconditional positive regard) manifested by the counselor toward the client; (3) the extent to which the counselor is genuine, his words matching his own internal feeling; and (4) the extent to which the counselor's response matches the client's expression in the intensity of affective expression.

To investigate these hypotheses she first selected, by multiple objective criteria, a group of 10 cases which could be classed as "most successful" and a group of 10 "least successful" cases. She then took an early and late recorded interview from each of these cases. On a random basis she picked nine client-counselor interaction units—a client statement and a counselor response—from each of these interviews. She thus had nine early interactions and nine late interactions from each case. This gave her several hundred units which were now placed in random order. The units from an early interview of an unsuccessful case might be followed by the units from a late interview of a successful case, etc.

Three judges, who did not know the cases or their degree of success, or the source of any given unit, now listened to this material four different times. They rated each unit on a seven point scale, first as to the degree of empathy, second as to the counselor's positive attitude toward the client, third as to the counselor's congruence or genuineness, and fourth as to the degree to which the counselor's response matched the emotional intensity of the client's expression.

I think all of us who knew of the study regarded it as a very bold venture. Could judges listening to single units of interaction possibly make any reliable rating of such subtle qualities as I have mentioned? And even if suitable reliability could be obtained, could 18 counselor-client interchanges from each case—a minute sampling of the hundreds or thousands of such interchanges which occurred in each case—possibly bear any relationship to the therapeutic outcome? The chance seemed slim.

The findings are surprising. It proved possible to achieve high reliability between the judges, most of the inter-judge correlations being in the 0.80's or 0.90's, except on the last variable. It was found that a high degree of empathic understanding was significantly associated, at a 0.001 level, with the more successful cases. A high degree of unconditional positive regard was likewise associated with the more successful cases, at the 0.001 level. Even the rating of the counselor's genuineness or congruence—the extent to which his words matched his feelings—was associated with the successful outcome of the case, and again at the 0.001 level of significance. Only in the investigation of the matching intensity of affective expression were the results equivocal.

It is of interest too that high ratings of these variables were not associated more significantly with units from later interviews than with units from early interviews. This means that the counselor's attitudes were quite constant throughout the interviews. If he was highly empathic, he tended to be so from first to last. If he was lacking in genuineness, this tended to be true of both early and late interviews.

As with any study, this investigation has its limitations. It is concerned with a certain type of helping relationship, psychotherapy. It investigated only four variables thought to be significant. Perhaps there are many others. Nevertheless it represents a significant advance in the study of helping relationships. Let me try to state the findings in the simplest possible fashion. It seems to indicate that the quality of the counselor's interaction with a client can be satisfactorily judged on the basis of a very small sampling of his behavior. It also means that if the counselor is congruent or transparent, so that his words are in line with his feelings rather than the two being discrepant—if the counselor likes the client, unconditionally, and if the counselor understands the essential feelings of the client as they seem to the client—then there is a strong probabiity that this will be an effective helping relationship.

Some Comments

These then are some of the studies which throw at least a measure of light on the nature of the helping relationship. They have investigated different facets of the problem. They have approached it from very different theoretical contexts. They have used different methods. They are not directly comparable. Yet they seem to me to point to several statements which may be made with some assurance. It seems clear that relationships which are helpful have different characteristics from relationships which are unhelpful. These differential characteristics have to do primarily with the attitudes of the helping person on the one hand and with the perception of the relationship by the "helpee" on the other. It is equally clear that the studies thus far made do not give us any final answers as to what is a helping relationship, nor how it is to be formed.

HOW CAN I CREATE A HELPING RELATIONSHIP?

I believe each of us working in the field of human relationships has a similar problem in knowing how to use such research knowledge. We cannot slavishly follow such findings in a mechanical way or we destroy the personal qualities which these very studies show to be valuable. It seems to me that we have to use these studies, testing them against our own experience and forming new and further personal hypotheses to use and test in our own further personal relationships.

So rather than try to tell you how you should use the findings I have presented I should like to tell you the kind of questions which these studies and my own clinical experience raise for me, and some of the tentative and changing hypotheses which guide my behavior as I enter into what I hope may be helping relationships, whether with students, staff, family, or clients. Let me list a number of these questions and considerations.

1. Can I *be* in some way which will be perceived by the other person as trustworthy, as dependable or consistent in some deep sense? Both research and experience indicate that this is very important, and over the years I have found what I believe are deeper and better ways of anwering this question. I used to feel that I fulfilled all the outer conditions of trustworthiness—keeping appointments, respecting the confidential nature of the interviews, etc.—and if I acted consistently the same during the interviews, then this condition would be fulfilled. But experience drove home the fact that to act consistently acceptant, for example, if in fact I was feeling annoyed or skeptical or some other non-acceptant feeling, was certain in the long run to be perceived as inconsistent or untrustworthy. I have come to recognize that being trustworthy does not demand that I be rigidly consistent but that I be dependably real. The term congruent is one I have used to describe the way I would like to be. By this I mean that whatever feeling or attitude I am experiencing would be matched by my awareness of that attitude. When this is true, then I am a unified or integrated person in that moment, and hence I can *be* whatever I deeply *am*. This is a reality which I find others experience as dependable.

2. A very closely related question is this: Can I be expressive enough as a person that what I am will be communicated unambiguously? I believe that most of my failures to achieve a helping relationship can be traced to unsatisfactory answers to these two questions. When I am experiencing an attitude of annoyance toward another person but am unaware of it, then my communication contains contradictory messages. My words are giving one message, but I am also in subtle ways communicating the annoyance I feel and this confuses the other person and makes him distrustful, though he too may be unaware of what is causing the difficulty. When as a parent or a therapist or a teacher or an administrator I fail to listen to what is going on in me, fail because of my own defensiveness to sense my own feelings, then this kind of failure seems to result. It has made it seem to me that the most basic learning for anyone who hopes to establish any kind of helping relationship is that it is safe to be transparently real. If in a given relationship I am reasonably congruent, if no feelings relevant to the relationship are hidden either to me or the other person, then I can be almost sure that the relationship will be a helpful one.

One way of putting this which may seem strange to you is that if I can form a helping relationship to myself—if I can be sensitively aware of and acceptant toward my own feelings—then the likelihood is great that I can form a helping relationship toward another.

Now, acceptantly to be what I am, in this sense, and to permit this to show through to the other person, is the most difficult task I know and one I never fully achieve. But to realize that this *is* my task has been most rewarding because it has helped me to find what has gone wrong with interpersonal relationships which have become snarled and to put them on a constructive track again. It has meant that if I am to facilitate the personal growth of others in relation to me, then I must grow, and while this is often painful it is also enriching.

3. A third question is: Can I let myself experience positive attitudes toward this other person—attitudes of warmth, caring, liking, interest, respect? It is not easy. I find in myself, and feel that I often see in others, a certain amount of fear of these feelings. We are afraid that if we let ourselves freely experience these positive feelings toward another we may be trapped by them. They may lead to demands of us or we may be disappointed in our trust, and these outcomes we fear. So as a reaction we tend to build up distance between ourselves and others—aloofness, a "professional" attitude, an impersonal relationship.

I feel quite strongly that one of the important reasons for the professionalization of every field is that it helps to keep this distance. In the clinical areas we develop elaborate diagnostic formulations, seeing the person as an object. In teaching and in administration we develop all kinds of evaluative procedures, so that again the person is perceived as an object. In these ways, I believe, we can keep ourselves from experiencing the caring which would exist if we recognize the relationship as one between two persons. It is a real achievement when we can learn, even in certain relationships or at certain times in those relationships, that it is safe to care, that it is safe to relate to the other as a person for whom we have positive feelings.

4. Another question the importance of which I have learned in my own experience is: Can I be strong enough as a person to be separate from the other? Can I be a sturdy respecter of my own feelings, my own needs, as well as his? Can I own and, if need be, express my own feelings as something belonging to me and separate from his feelings? Am I strong enough in my own separateness that I will not

be downcast by his depression, frightened by his fear, nor engulfed by his dependency? Is my inner self hardy enough to realize that I am not destroyed by his anger, taken over by his need for dependence, nor enslaved by his love, but that I exist separate from him with feelings and rights of my own? When I can freely feel this strength of being a separate person, then I find that I can let myself go much more deeply in understanding and accepting him because I am not fearful of losing myself.

5. The next question is closely related. Am I secure enough within myself to permit him his separateness? Can I permit him to be what he is—honest or deceitful, infantile or adult, despairing or over-confident? Can I give him the freedom to be? Or do I feel that he should follow my advice, or remain somewhat dependent on me, or mold himself after me? In this connection I think of the interesting small study by Farson (6) which found that the less well adjusted and less competent counselor tends to induce conformity to himself, to have clients who model themselves after him. On the other hand, the better adjusted and more competent counselor can interact with a client through many interviews without interfering with the freedom of the client to develop a personality quite separate from that of his therapist. I should prefer to be in this latter class, whether as parent or supervisor or counselor.

6. Another question I ask myself is: Can I let myself enter fully into the world of his feelings and personal meanings and see these as he does? Can I step into his private world so completely that I lose all desire to evaluate or judge it? Can I enter it so sensitively that I can move about in it freely, without tramping on meanings which are precious to him? Can I sense it so accurately that I can catch not only the meanings of his experience which are obvious to him, but those meanings which are only implicit, which he sees only dimly or as confusion? Can I extend this understanding without limit? I think of the client who said, "Whenever

I find someone who understands a *part* of me at the time, then it never fails that a point is reached where I know they're *not* understanding me again. . . . What I've looked for so hard is for someone to understand."

For myself I find it easier to feel this kind of understanding, and to communicate it, to individual clients than to students in a class or staff members in a group in which I am involved. There is a strong temptation to set students "straight," or to point out to a staff member the errors in his thinking. Yet when I can permit myself to understand in these situations, it is mutually rewarding. And with clients in therapy, I am often impressed with the fact that even a minimal amount of empathic understanding—a bumbling and faulty attempt to catch the confused complexity of the client's meaning—is helpful, though there is no doubt that it is most helpful when I can see and formulate clearly the meanings in his experiencing which for him have been unclear and tangled.

7. Still another issue is whether I can be acceptant of each facet of this other person which he presents to me. Can I receive him as he is? Can I communicate this attitude? Or can I only receive him conditionally, acceptant of some aspects of his feelings and silently or openly disapproving of other aspects? It has been my experience that when my attitude is conditional, then he cannot change or grow in those respects in which I cannot fully receive him. And when—afterward and sometimes too late—I try to discover why I have been unable to accept him in every respect, I usually discover that it is because I have been frightened or threatened in myself by some aspect of his feelings. If I am to be more helpful, then I must myself grow and accept myself in these respects.

8. A very practical issue is raised by the question: Can I act with sufficient sensitivity in the relationship that my behavior will not be perceived as a threat? The work we are beginning to do in studying the physiological concomitants of psychotherapy confirms the research by Dittes in indicating how easily individuals are threatened at a physiological level. The psychogalvanic reflex—the measure of skin conductance—takes a sharp dip when the therapist responds with some word which is just a little stronger than the client's feelings. And to a phrase such as "My, you *do* look upset," the needle swings almost off the paper. My desire to avoid even such minor threats is not due to a hypersensitivity about my client. It is simply due to the conviction based on experience that if I can free him as completely as possible from external threat, then he can begin to experience and to deal with the internal feelings and conflicts which he finds threatening within himself.

9. A specific aspect of the preceding question but an important one is: Can I free him from the threat of external evaluation? In almost every phase of our lives—at home, at school, at work—we find ourselves under the rewards or punishments of external judgments. "That's good"; "that's naughty." "That's worth an A"; "that's a failure." "That's good counseling"; "that's poor counseling." Such judgments are a part of our lives from infancy to old age. I believe they have a certain social usefulness to institutions and organizations such as schools and professions. Like everyone else I find myself all too often making such evaluations. But, in my experience, they do not make for personal growth and hence I do not believe that they are a part of a helping relationship. Curiously enough a positive evaluation is as threatening in the long run as a negative one, since to inform someone that he is good implies that you also have the right to tell him he is bad. So I have come to feel that the more I can keep a relationship free of judgment and evaluation, the more this will permit the other person to reach the point where he recognizes that the locus of evaluation, the center of responsibility lies within himself. The meaning and value of his experience is in the last analysis something which is up to him, and no amount of external

judgment can alter this. So I should like to work toward a relationship in which I am not, even in my own feelings, evaluating him. This I believe can set him free to be a self-responsible person.

10. One last question: Can I meet this other individual as a person who is in process of *becoming*, or will I be bound by his past and by my past? If, in my encounter with him, I am dealing with him as an immature child, an ignorant student, a neurotic personality, or a psychopath, each of these concepts of mine limits what he can be in the relationship. Martin Buber, the existentialist philosopher of the University of Jerusalem, has a phrase, "confirming the other," which has had meaning for me. He says "Confirming means . . . accepting the whole potentiality of the other . . . I can recognize in him, know in him, the person he has been . . . *created* to become . . . I confirm him in myself, and then in him, in relation to this potentiality that . . . can now be developed, can evolve" (3). If I accept the other person as something fixed, already diagnosed and classified, already shaped by his past, then I am doing my part to confirm this limited hypothesis. If I accept him as a process of becoming, then I am doing what I can to confirm or make real his potentialities.

It is at this point that I see Verplanck, Lindsley, and Skinner, working in operant conditioning, coming together with Buber, the philosopher or mystic. At least they come together in principle, in an odd way. If I see a relationship as only an opportunity to reinforce certain types of words or opinions in the other, then I tend to confirm him as an object—a basically mechanical manipulable object. And if I see this as his potentiality, he tends to act in ways which support this hypothesis. If, on the other hand, I see a relationship as an opportunity to "reinforce" *all* that he is, the person that he is with all his existent potentialities, then he tends to act in ways which support *this* hypothesis. I have then—to use Buber's term—confirmed him as a living person, capable of creative inner development. Personally I prefer this second type of hypothesis.

CONCLUSION

In the early portion of this paper I reviewed some of the contributions which research is making to our knowledge *about* relationships. Endeavoring to keep that knowledge in mind I then took up the kind of questions which arise from an inner and subjective point of view as I enter, as a person, into relationships. If I could, in myself, answer all the questions I have raised in the affirmative, then I believe that any relationships in which I was involved would be helping relationships, would involve growth. But I cannot give a positive answer to most of these questions. I can only work in the direction of a positive answer.

This has raised in my mind the strong suspicion that the optimal helping relationship is the kind of relationship created by a person who is psychologically mature. Or to put it another way, the degree to which I can create relationships which facilitate the growth of others as separate persons is a measure of the growth I have achieved in myself. In some respects this is a disturbing thought, but it is also a promising or challenging one. It would indicate that if I am interested in creating helping relationships I have a fascinating lifetime job ahead of me, stretching and developing my potentialities in the direction of growth.

I am left with the uncomfortable thought that what I have been working out for myself in this paper may have little relationship to your interests and your work. If so, I regret it. But I am at least partially comforted by the fact that all of us who are working in the field of human relationships and trying to understand the basic orderliness of that field are engaged in the most crucial enterprise in today's world. If we are thoughtfully trying to understand our tasks as administrators, teachers, educational counselors, vocational counselors, therapists, then we are working on the problem which will determine the future of this planet. For it is not upon the physical sciences that the future will depend. It is upon us who are trying to understand and deal with the interactions between human beings—who are trying to create helping relationships. So I hope that the questions I ask of myself will be of some use to you in gaining understanding and perspective as you endeavor, in your way, to facilitate growth in your relationships.

REFERENCES

1. Baldwin, A. L., Kalhorn, J., and Breese, F. H. Patterns of parent behavior. *Psychol. Monogr.*, 1945, *58*, No. 268, 1–75.

2. Betz, B. J., & Whitehorn, J. C. The relationship of the therapist to the outcome of therapy in schizophrenia. *Psychiat. Research Reports #5. Research techniques in schizophrenia.* Washington, D.C.: American Psychiatric Association, 1956, 89–117.

3. Buber, M., & Rogers, C. Transcription of a dialogue held April 18, 1957, Ann Arbor, Mich. Unpublished manuscript.

4. Dittes, J. E. Galvanic skin response as a measure of patient's reaction to therapist's permissiveness. *J. Abnorm. & Soc. Psychol.*, 1957, *55*, 295–303.

5. Ends, E. J., and Page, C. W. A study of three types of group psychotherapy with hospitalized male inebriates. *Quar. J. Stud. Alchol.*, 1957, *18*, 263–277.

6. Farson, R. E. Introjection in the psychotherapeutic relationship. Unpublished doctoral dissertation, University of Chicago, 1955.

7. Fiedler, F. E. Quantitative studies on the role of therapists' feelings toward their patients. In Mower, O. H. (Ed.), *Psychotherapy: Theory and research.* New York: Ronald Press, 1953, Chap. 12.

8. Greenspoon, J. The reinforcing effect of two spoken sounds on the frequency of two responses. *Amer. J. Psychol.*, 1955, *68*, 409–416.

9. Halkides, G. An experimental study of four conditions necessary for therapeutic change. Unpublished doctoral dissertation, University of Chicago, 1958.

10. Harlow, H. F. The nature of love. *Amer. Psychol.*, 1958, *13*, 673–685.

11. Heine, R. W. A comparison of patients' reports on psychotherapeutic experience with psychoanalytic, nondirective, and Adlerian therapists. Unpublished doctoral dissertation, University of Chicago, 1950.

12. Lindsley, O. R. Operant conditioning methods applied to research in chronic schizophrenia. *Psychiat. Research Reports #5. Research techniques in schizophrenia.* Washington, D.C.: American Psychiatric Association, 1956, 118–153.

13. Page, C. W., & Ends, E. J. A review and synthesis of the literature suggesting a psychotherapeutic technique based on two-factor learning theory. Unpublished manuscript, loaned to the writer.

14. Rogers, C. R. The necessary and sufficient conditions of psychotherapeutic personality change. *J. Consult. Psychol.*, 1957, *21*, 95–103.

15. Quinn, R. D. Psychotherapists' expressions as an index to the quality of early therapeutic relationships. Unpublished doctoral dissertation, University of Chicago, 1950.

16. Seeman, J. Counselor judgments of therapeutic process and outcome. In Rogers, C. R., and Dymond, R. F. (Eds.), *Psychotherapy and personality change.* Chicago: University of Chicago Press, 1954, Chap. 7.

17. Verplanck, W. S. The control of the content of conversation: Reinforcement of statements of opinion. *J. Abnorm. Soc. & Psychol.*, 1955, *51*, 668–676.

18. Whitehorn, J. C., and Betz, B. J. A study of psychotherapeutic relationships between physicians and schizophrenic patients. *Amer. J. Psychiat.*, 1954, *111*, 321–331.

Chapter 16

Conceptual Framework for the Nursing Process

Throughout this book we have been working toward a complete understanding of the nursing process. Beginning in the early chapters with the most basic parts, we have been moving—step by step—toward a whole, integrated process. At the same time, we have been progressing toward understanding.

Parts I through V presented the phases of the nursing process: assessing, analyzing, planning, implementing, and evaluating. In addition, each method involved in each phase of the nursing process was detailed using a case example. The purpose for following the nursing process from step to step is to provide quality, individualized care—to assist the client to fullest health potential.

However, methods do not stand alone, and methods do not create a process nor do they create understanding of the process. Other variables affecting the nursing process—skills and quality systems—were also discussed. Thus, the seeds of the nursing process sown in earlier chapters have been cultivated, step by step and part by part, to yield a whole workable process.

Now, in this chapter we arrive at a more complete picture. Our discussion turns to the conceptual framework that holds all the parts of the nursing process together. This chapter presents the concepts guiding the nursing process, as well as a definition and statement of the purpose of the nursing process. In the final chapter of this book, one final element—humanism—will be added to the nursing process to color it in the human tones of the present and the future.

The conceptual framework upon which the nursing process is based employs General System Theory. The systems approach was first presented in the Introduction to this book, and parts of it have been discussed as it related to a particular method or phase. In the next section, however, we will combine the pieces already presented into a whole, workable theory that relates to nursing, health care, and all human life.

GENERAL SYSTEM THEORY

The systems framework provides a construct for studying people within an environment—and, indeed, as builders of their environment. General System Theory mandates analysis of all the parts of a system, the relationships between these parts, and the purposes, reasons, and tasks of the system. Simply stated, system approaches include purpose, content, and process (Yura & Walsh, 1983).

General System Theory is a model developed by von Bertalanffy (1969, 1975) that can be used to study designated phenomena, regardless of the properties contained within the event. Putt (1978) applied some of the tenets of General System Theory in nursing. The following assumptions of General System Theory were identified by von Bertalanffy (1969, 1975):

1. *A system is more than a sum of its parts.* More explicitly, the system develops a character of its own, subsumed by collective goals of the parts.

2. It is *ever changing*, since one change in any part affects the whole.

3. *Boundaries* are implicit in each system and are defined by its purpose. Closed systems end when a quantity needed for fulfillment is obtained. This phenomenon is not pertinent in human systems, as they are considered *open* and *dynamic*.

4. All systems must be *goal directed*, otherwise they fall apart. Goals of the individual parts of the system may not be directly in line with the group goal; however, these should not be in conflict. Even though the goal is often quite difficult to specify succinctly, it provides the core of a system's functioning.

The universe is perhaps our absolute outer system; all that goes on within the world falls into subsystems. It becomes necessary, however, to realize that one system is always related to or a part of a larger whole. Logical, systematic pursuits of a problem require that boundaries be designated. Figure 16–1 provides one example of the nursing profession's boundaries and how the profession can be portrayed as a hierarchical subsystem.

The most direct way to identify a system is to state its purpose (Banathy, 1968). This becomes paramount when studying a problem methodically, because the boundaries of any system must be circumscribed by the relevant parts of the environment as they pertain to the purpose. This answers the question: "What is the goal of a system, and what are the important components for this purpose within the relevant environment?" The purpose and goal of health-care systems, of course, is client care. It follows that each system is unique, developed from specified segments in a time and place. Therefore, what may be important in the care of one client in a certain place will probably not be totally appropriate for another. The systems framework facilitates delivery of individualized nursing care, since only those areas and people relevant in a client's care are included in the system, with purposes broadly *and* specifically

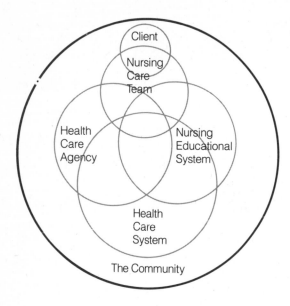

Figure 16–1

The System of Nursing Viewed from
an Overall Health-Care Perspective

stated. A hallmark of a systems approach is that importance is placed on diagnosing the needs of each unique system.

With a systems approach, the client becomes the focus of the purpose—care—but all of the facets of the system, in essence, receive care. A hypothetical example can be observed in Figure 16–2.

As can be seen in the figure, the client is, of course, the major segment of the system. Since the client is seen as being largely influenced by many other people and environmental factors, however, all relevant aspects then become part of the system. Each person or aspect is considered to have a relationship with and in the client's care; each must be assessed and included in the care-plan development, implementation, and evaluation. The size of the piece of the pie allotted to each facet of the system reflects the relative importance of the factor in the client's world.

NURSING THEORY

Nursing theorists have extensively applied systems approaches in their study of nursing practice, and this application is helpful in stressing the concept of individualized care in the nursing profession. Several theories are discussed.

Rogers's Theoretical Basis of Nursing

Rogers (1970, p. 3) discussed the concern of nursing as being "man in his entirety, his wholeness. Nursing's body of scientific knowledge seeks to describe, explain, and predict about human beings."

The assumptions described in General System Theory by von Bertalanffy (1969, 1975) relate directly to the following assumptions of the theoretic model developed by Rogers (1970):

1. Each person is a unique, unified whole being whose characteristics are different from or greater than the sum of his or her parts.

2. Matter and energy constantly exchange in persons and their environment(s). The system of a person's being is, therefore, dynamic.

3. The process of life is developmental within the space-time continuum. It is irreversible and linear in direction.

4. There is pattern and organization reflected in the whole entity of each person. It is primarily through this assumption that the study of human behavior is possible.

5. Each person's uniqueness is characterized by abstraction and behaviors that use language, emotion, feelings, and fantasy.

Rogers's (1970) belief about nursing implied a deep respect for the individuality of each person. This reflects study of the relationship between persons and their environment, with the goal of facilitating effective nursing-care outcomes. Disease is not the dominant focus; the unified

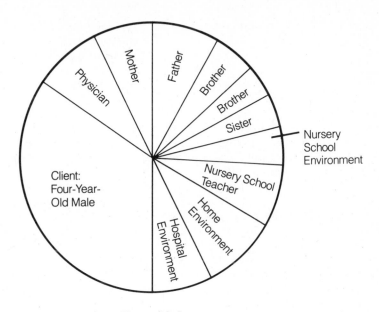

Figure 16–2

An Example of a Client's System

person and human functioning take priority. The well-being of society, the suprasystem of persons, must also be a focal point.

Roy's Adaptation Model

Developed subsequently to Rogers's model, Roy's model (1980) primarily used the systems approach in patient care. Similarities between the two theories become obvious as one looks at the assumptions presented by Roy (1980, pp. 180–182):

1. "The person is a bio-psycho-social being." Study of a human being must reflect all of these facets.

2. "The person is in constant interaction with a changing environment." Therefore, the dynamic aspect of being is portrayed.

3. Biologic, psychologic, and sociologic facets are used by people in coping with their ever changing world.

4. A person's life experience involves both health and illness. Moreover, illness is not idiosyncratic in living.

5. Adaptation to the environment is requisite in living.

6. The stimuli available in the particular environment guide the process of adaptation for an individual.

7. Positive adaptive responses result from stimuli that are within the individual's repertoire of response patterns.

8. The four basic adaptive modes of human beings are physiologic needs, self-concept, role function, and interdependent relations.

These adaptive modes guide the nursing process. The ultimate concern of nursing is the total person—supporting and promoting adaptation of the individual within the context of the person's own health-illness pattern, environmental process, and stimuli available for use

(Randell, Tedrow, & Landingham, 1982; Roy, 1980).

Other Nursing Models
Employing the Systems Approach

Hall's (1964) philosophy of nursing thoroughly supported a systems approach and the technical/professional position of the American Nurses' Association (1965). She described nursing practice as moving from simple to complex.

The simple/complex dichotomy is illustrated in the following example. A client in an ambulatory-care situation has a foot injury. She states that she is cold, and a blanket is offered by the nurse. This simple function of nursing is different from caring for a post-operative client who is in a recovery room following abdominal surgery. Should the recovering post-operative client complain of a chill, many complex factors must be considered as possible causes of the chill. These include low blood pressure, internal bleeding, reactions to transfusions, and so forth. Thus, it is the professional nurse's responsibility to do much more than simply offer the client a blanket.

The simple functions of nursing practice require consideration of very few factors prior to a discrimination or nursing judgment; as one moves outward into the complex realm, however, more and more items, facts, knowledge, and experience from the circumscribed system must be considered. Hall's (1964) belief in pro-fessional nursing is grounded on the idea that human beings are complex; professional nursing requires a broad range of knowledge and experience and a process by which complex decisions can be made with and for clients. Her concept of nursing practice compares easily with Reiter's (1966) and involves three essential components, seen in Table 16-1.

It becomes evident that the system developed for providing care must be concerned with biologic, psychologic, and sociologic facets of the individual. Figure 16-3 portrays the relationship among these facets of a person. The overlapping circles illustrate the autonomy of each human aspect, as well as the inter/intrarelationship of all three.

Other less-researched models of professional nursing practice that are also based on General System Theory are the following: Neuman's Health Care Systems Model (1980), the Johnson Behavioral System Model (Grubbs, 1980; Johnson, 1968), King's theory for nursing (1981), and Parse's theory of nursing (1981).

SUMMARY

Chapter 16 discussed the conceptual framework of the nursing process, specifying the systems approach as important and describing nursing theories that employ this approach. The nursing process has been defined, including a discussion of its goals.

Table **16-1**   Comparison of Lydia Hall's and Frances Reiter's Models of Nursing Care

Lydia Hall (1964)*		Frances Reiter (1966)
"The Person"	Social Sciences Therapeutic Use of Self	"The Core"
"The Body"	Biologic and Natural Sciences Bodily Care	"The Care"
"The Disease"	Pathology and Therapeutic Sciences	"The Cure"

*SOURCE: "Nursing: What is it?", by L. Hall, *The Canadian Nurse,* 1964, Vol. 60, No. 2. Reproduced with permission.

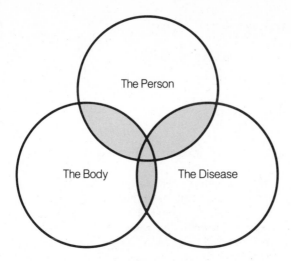

Figure 16-3

Schematic Diagram of Lydia Hall's Model of Nursing Care (SOURCE: "Nursing: What is it?", L. Hall, *The Canadian Nurse*, 1964, Vol. 60, No. 2. Reproduced with permission.)

REFERENCES

American Nurses' Association's First Position on Education for Nursing. (1965). *American Journal of Nursing, 65*, 106–111.

Banathy, B. (1968). *Instructional systems.* Palo Alto, CA: Fearon.

Carrieri, V., & Sitzman, J. (1971). Components of the nursing process. *Nursing Clinics of North America, 6*, 115–124.

Finch, J. (1969). Systems analysis: A logical approach to professional nursing care. *Nursing Forum, 8*, 176–190.

Grubbs, J. (1980). The Johnson behavioral systems model. In J. Riehl & C. Roy, *Conceptual models for nursing practice* (2nd ed.). New York: Appleton-Century-Crofts.

Hall, L. (1964). Nursing: What is it? *The Canadian Nurse, 60*, 150–154.

Johnson, D. (1968). *One conceptual model of nursing.* Unpublished paper presented at Vanderbilt University, Nashville, TN, April 25.

King, I. (1981). *A theory for nursing: Systems, concepts, process.* New York: Wiley.

Neuman, B. (1980). The Betty Neuman healthcare systems model: A total person approach to patient problems. In J. Riehl & C. Roy, *Conceptual models for nursing practice* (2nd ed.). New York: Appleton-Century-Crofts.

Parse, R. (1981). *Man-living-health: A theory of nursing.* New York: Wiley.

Putt, A. (1978). *General systems theory applied to nursing.* Boston: Little, Brown.

Randell, B., Tedrow, M., & Landingham, J. (1982). *Adaptation nursing: The Roy conceptual model applied.* St. Louis: Mosby.

Reiter, F. (1966). The nurse-clinician. *American Journal of Nursing, 66*, 274–280.

Rogers, M. (1970). *An introduction to the theoretical basis of nursing.* Philadelphia: F. A. Davis.

Roy, Sr. C. (1980). The Roy adaptation model. In J. Riehl & C. Roy, *Conceptual models for nursing practice* (2nd ed.). New York: Appleton-Century-Crofts.

von Bertalanffy, L. (1969). *General system theory.* New York: George Braziller.

von Bertalanffy, L. (1975). *Perspectives on general system theory: Scientific-philosophical studies.* New York: George Braziller.

Yura, H., & Walsh, M. (1983). *The nursing process: Assessing, planning, implementing, evaluating* (4th ed.). Norwalk, CT: Appleton-Century-Crofts.

SELECTED READINGS

Two selected readings follow, one studying the systems approach in professional nursing care, the other designating the components of the nursing process exemplified by a case analysis. Both are intended to amplify and reinforce the presentation already made by this author.

Systems Analysis: A Logical Approach to Professional Nursing Care

Joyce Finch, R.N., M.S.

Every day nurses are called upon to make choices among possible nursing actions: Is the anxiety of a pre-operative patient within tolerable limits or does he need assistance? Is a newly diagnosed diabetic patient ready to learn about insulin administration yet? Because of nursing error the narcotic order has "run out" but the patient is in pain. What is to be done? For the care given to be truly professional, the nurse's decisions should be based on a prediction of the probable consequences of the alternative actions. Too often, however, the nurse's action is an automatic response to the situation or the result of a hunch, rather than one that is based on a rational, replicable judgment. A body of knowledge is, of course, the raw material for making sound judgments, but knowledge is of little value unless nurses know how to use it. Therefore, as nurses develop a nursing science, they should concurrently develop strategies for applying their knowledge in the care of patients.

Systems analysis is one possible resource for the development of a tool for decision-making. The faculty of the College of Nursing at Arizona State University has begun developing and testing a systems analysis approach to nursing care in connection with a major curriculum revision.

The curriculum-planning group identified two critical variables which would affect its decisions. First, the faculty's philosophical com-

mitment required that the curriculum provide opportunities for the nursing student to learn to give patient-centered care. Second, the increase in knowledge relevant to nursing has been so rapid that to include all such knowledge in the curriculum is an impossibility. Therefore, the consensus was that the student should be provided with sufficient knowledge and skill to begin a professional career and with the competence needed to process the knowledge required for responsible decision-making.

The curriculum-planning group therefore sought an approach which would enable students to learn to focus on the patient rather than on the problem and which would enable graduates of the program to continue functioning at a high level in the future. A study of the reports of Howland and McDowell[1-3] on the use of systems engineering in hospital design and operation prompted the group to investigate the possibilities of systems analysis as an approach to the study of nursing.

In its simplest form a system is an entity "consisting of parts in interaction."[4] Systems analysis utilizes techniques that allow long-range planning and at the same time provides the means to update and maintain the current program. Techniques for evaluation of effectiveness are based upon the ongoing functioning of the program so that it can be altered to accommodate changing conditions and requirements. An example of a program that includes these techniques is SABRE, American Airlines' seat reservation system developed by the International Business Machines Corporation.[5] SABRE's long-range objective is continuous seat

Reprinted with permission of Nursing Publications, Inc., 194-B Kinderkamack Road, Park Ridge, New Jersey, from Nursing Forum, 1969, Vol. 8, No. 2, pp. 176–190.

inventory since American Airlines must be in minute-to-minute control of reservations in order to keep seats filled at the minimum occupancy that marks the difference between profit and loss. In seconds a central computer console handles requests for reservations from interchanges along American's route and also keeps track of all related operations such as those having to do with meals, connecting reservations, and baggage. The specifications contain more than a million instructions which fill five thick volumes.

Systems analysis is based upon probability theory and concepts. Probability recognizes a random element of chance in events. Outcomes are uncertain since alternative approaches may occur. This uncertainty was expressed colloquially by President Johnson when he said, "I'll see you, God willin' and if the creeks don't rise." To predict the consequences of a decision, it is necessary to determine the relative likelihood of occurrence of each of the possible outcomes of that decision. "Mathematically, probability represents a proportion or relative frequency that specifies the degree of assurance that an event will occur."[6]

Systems analysis is particularly applicable to the study of complex problems. It involves an organization of data that is achieved by breaking a whole into its component parts in such a way that the relationships of these parts may be studied and manipulated. Example: Health care involves not only physicians, nurses, hospitals, machines, and techniques but also such diverse elements as the standard of living, the tax base, transportation, the support of mass communications, and even opinions of the neighbors. Knowledge of the availability and value of health services may be outweighed by the relative difficulty of procuring these services; planning for health care, if it is to be successful, will have to include these less obvious variables. The logical relationship of such complex networks is called "organized complexity."[7]

A general systems theory is evolving "which can discuss the relationships of the empirical world."[8] This development has been stimulated by the rapid accumulation of knowledge and the resulting proliferation of specialization, which has necessitated the creation of a theoretical framework that enables one specialist to communicate with other specialists.

Systems can be closed or open. A closed system is one in which there is neither input nor output of information, materials, or energy from or to the environment. An open system is characterized by an exchange of energy in the form of information with the environment.[9] One way in which this exchange is accomplished is by feedback control mechanisms, whereby a part of the output of the system is fed back to the input in order to affect future outputs. Example: A measurement of the response of a patient to nursing intervention is fed back into the system and thus influences the plan for continuing care. Feedback control mechanisms are present in those systems that are self-regulating, that is, goal-directed.

Open systems are governed by the principle of equifinality, which states, "The same final state may be reached from different initial conditions and in different ways."[10] Example: It is possible for a person to become an effective contributing member of his community in a number of ways. He may learn a trade or he may become a professional person. He may become a member of a charitable organization or he may be an active member of his political party. The best possible decision will be in part dependent on the person's understanding of the available approaches.

Systems tend to maintain a state of equilibrium. Cannon, who outlined a systems approach to the study of physiology, identified internal self-regulating mechanisms which operate to maintain the physiological equilibrium, or homeostasis, of the organism.[11] A consideration of only those mechanisms that regulate fluid balance will lead one to see that systems analysis is an extremely useful method of studying both multivariable causation and multiple alternatives to action.

The goal of equilibrium implies that systems, like other organisms, suffer from wear and tear of their own activities. The over-all goal of systems analysis is to intervene in this process of disorganization, or entropy.[12] Constraints, or those relationships which reduce alternatives, are useful in this intervention.[13] Example: A person who has had the choice of four routes to the office finds that the highway department has closed one route for repairs and the police department has closed a second route for an official parade, thus reducing the possible choices by one half.

Cybernetics and decision theory have contributed to systems theory. Cybernetics, the science of communication and control, assumes that a system is goal-directed and asks the question: What does it do? When a set of possibilities is identified the focus is redirected to the regulating mechanism operant in the particular instance.[14] Example: Roses have the capacity to bloom or refrain from blooming. What prevents them from blooming at certain times, and what prompts them to bloom at times? Florists apply an understanding of the relationships between light, temperature, humidity, and water so that we may have roses any day of the year.

Decision theory supplies a framework for identifying criteria to be used in "analyzing rational choices, within human organizations, based upon examination of a given situation and its possible outcomes."[15] Goodenough describes the need for decision theory when he states:

> . . . there is frequently more than one course of action that will gratify a want. Which is most effective depends on how it affects conditions pertaining to other wants that one happens to have at the same time. For this reason we must qualify our definition of a need. In any situation the need is for a course of action that will be of maximum efficacy in relation to the gratification of all of one's wants. That is to say, for each want there is need for that one among the several possible means of gratifying it which will at the same time either maximally provide the grati-

fication of other wants or minimally interfere with their continued gratification.[16]

Goodenough then describes how this process increases in complexity when the number of people is increased and the number of wants is multiplied.

General systems theory makes possible the development of models that are abstractions of the real world. The model identifies essential variables that can be manipulated for optimal problem solution and in this way provides an opportunity to stimulate events that would not be feasible in an actual setting. The manned space program is an excellent example of development by simulation. Even if volunteers were foolhardy enough to offer their services, public opinion in an open society would not support the human wastage or the economic burden of trial-and-error testing of space vehicles. Models make it possible to compare the actual state with the ideal state; the consequences of the possible manipulations can then be predicted before a decision is reached. The process of selection of the best possible solution is called a "trade-off."

The simplest models are purely descriptive of the events occurring within a system. Analytical models explore alternatives that provide a logical basis for decision-making. The most sophisticated models are mathematical models developed for the purpose of predicting future outcomes.

The curriculum-planning group was intrigued by the possibilities of a systems approach to nursing care and decided to try to develop a nursing care system. In this undertaking the group has had the benefit of consultation from Dr. A. Alan B. Pritsker of the College of Engineering at Arizona State University.[17,18]

The outcome of the planning group's work was a descriptive model of professional nursing care which is based on the assumption that all nursing care is carried out through the nurse-patient relationship. The components of a nurse–patient relationship were identified as:

(1) a patient who is in a state of disequilibrium that can be resolved by nursing care; (2) a nurse who is prepared to assist in the resolution of this state of disruption; and (3) the termination of the relationship when equilibrium is restored. As a group has become more knowledgeable in the use of systems it has, with Dr. Pritsker's assistance, worked gradually toward the development of an analytical model. *Figures 1 and 2* represent the current level of development of our system of professional nursing care.

The operational features of the model are as follows:

- The patient is defined as an individual or a group of individuals and is seen as entering the system with expectations of benefiting from nursing care.

- The model is conceptualized as an open system so that the nurse who seldom operates independently of other health personnel may exchange information with other systems of health care.

- It is assumed that anyone can be trained to make observations and carry out nursing action; the professional nurse takes responsibility for assessment and decision analysis. Figure 1.

- The professional nurse makes two types of assessments. Operational assessments define the expectations of measurements related to the functional performance of the individual. Comparative assessments discriminate between measurements of an individual's current status and pre-set limits which have been established prior to the measurement.

- Strategic goals are defined as being concerned with over-all objectives of nursing care. Tactical goals are defined as being concerned with "what will help the patient feel better today."

- The patient exits from the system when the possible benefits have been derived; the nurse continues to work with the patient

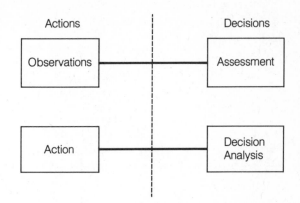

Figure 1

Professional Nursing Care System

as long as movement toward the desired state is feasible.

When the components of the professional nursing care model (Figure 1) are visualized it becomes clear that a subsystem can be developed within each component (Figure 2). The next steps will probably be directed toward the further development and refinement of the subsystems. The ultimate objective is a mathematical model that can be used to predict outcomes accurately as well as to describe and analyze problems. Since such a model can be programed for computers, simulated nursing problems can be worked out before the nursing student goes into an actual nurse–patient setting. The problem is to define clearly what the nurse is expected to achieve; the actual programing is then relatively simple.

The strategies dictated by the professional nursing care model constitute a basic feature of the revised curriculum. Learning experiences have been organized in two patterns. The students are given assignments concerned with general systems theory concurrent with assignments concerned with components of the nursing care system. Some of the students master the basic concepts of systems before proceeding with the components of the nursing care model.

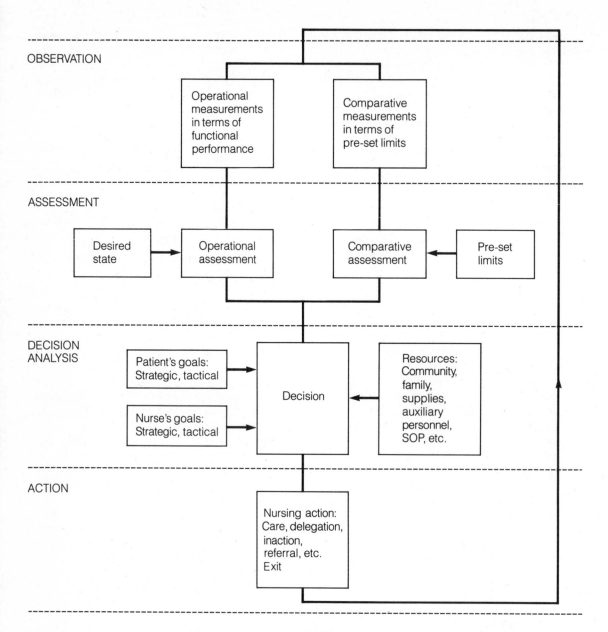

OBSERVATION

| Operational measurements in terms of functional performance | Comparative measurements in terms of pre-set limits |

ASSESSMENT

| Desired state | → | Operational assessment | Comparative assessment | ← | Pre-set limits |

DECISION ANALYSIS

| Patient's goals: Strategic, tactical | → | Decision | ← | Resources: Community, family, supplies, auxiliary personnel, SOP, etc. |

| Nurse's goals: Strategic, tactical | → |

ACTION

Nursing action: Care, delegation, inaction, referral, etc. Exit

Figure 2

System of Professional Nursing Care

Others work in reverse order. The student is thus allowed a degree of freedom in the selection of a learning method best suited to individual accomplishment. At succeeding levels of learning, students are given assignments in systems analysis of increasing complexity.

Final evaluation of the professional nursing care model will depend on a comprehensive evaluation of all curriculum revisions. In the meantime, current observations indicate a favorable reaction to this tool for decision-making from students and faculty alike.

The planning group has identified a number of positive values in the professional nursing care system:

- Primary focus upon the patient is maintained throughout the process.

- The plan of nursing can be altered to accommodate the changing condition and requirements of the patient, since continuous evaluation of patient responses to nursing intervention through feedback control is an integral part of the process.

- When problems in decision-making occur, the feedback control mechanism facilitates location of the point of departure from the process.

- The vocabulary of systems analysis transfers readily across the disciplinary lines. This increases the probability of accurate interpretation of the nursing care process by others.

After a year of experience with the revised curriculum, our junior students have learned to use the vocabulary of systems with confidence and are able to describe their activities meaningfully to others. They have acquired skill in looking critically at their own performance to determine where they need to focus their attention: they may need further data; their observations may have been inadequate or inaccurate; their knowledge of normal and pathological states may be faulty or inadequate; or they may have to reconsider their assessment

in regard to personal bias or in relation to the ordering of the data. The ability to withhold judgment until needed data are accumulated and ordered is acquired more slowly, but learning is enhanced as students recognize their maturation in this area. Example: A student became concerned about the quality of nursing care that she had given in a single three-hour experience with an elderly lady with a handicapping chest condition. She reported, "I didn't have an opportunity to see the patient before I took care of her. I knew her diagnosis and I had studied the pathological aspects and nursing care the night before I saw her, but I didn't know anything about her as an individual. After I had taken care of her I knew she felt better, for she was no longer in respiratory distress but was relaxed and comfortable. But I still did not know what it all meant to her." In a discussion about her reaction to this situation the student was able to recognize that she was attempting to make long-range goals operational in a situation in which only short-term goals were feasible. In a subsequent discussion the student said that as she had reflected upon the nurse–patient interaction she had learned much more about the patient than she had believed possible in such a short interval.

Nurses who would have confidence in their ability to evaluate their environment would appear to have a higher probability of success in acquiring knowledge and skills requisite to rational decision-making than do those who lack this self-confidence. Example: To test the effectiveness of the curriculum with respect to the integration of public health nursing content in the other courses, the NLN Achievement Test in this area was given to the junior students, who had not yet had the course in public health nursing. One student reported, "It wasn't too bad. Of course I didn't know a lot of the answers, but I discovered that many questions were asking for either observation or assessment and I could do that."

On the negative side, the precision of observation and communication dictated by the systems approach can be extremely frustrating if the necessity for sharpening skills is identified when the means of doing so are not clear. This problem has been a recurrent one in those situations in which the content was subjective and difficult to measure. The dynamic nature of the system has also caused problems to instructors and students who have been conditioned to traditional problem-solving methods. One student expressed the feelings of many when she said, "Just once I'd like to go to bed knowing that tomorrow I can get up without something still waiting to be finished." Upon reflection, the planning group has concluded that this ongoingness is one of the elements of the nursing program that is most representative of the real world.

Although the professional nursing care system model was developed as a learning tool for students, expectations are that further development will lead to a tool for the accurate measurement of nursing care in any setting. Through the use of this tool, the nurse will be able to predict the consequences of her behavior in the nurse–patient relationship and thus to make decisions in the best interests of the patient.

The use of systems analysis also has potential for facilitating the development of a science of nursing. Basically the problem in such development is to identify what is unknown about nursing care rather than what is known. Systems seem to hold promise of the ability to identify gaps in nursing knowledge which have so far eluded professional nurses.

In all efforts to develop and use systems in nursing, we must not lose sight of the fact that systems analysis is only a tool. Wiener has cautioned against the dehumanizing characteristics of systems; it is possible for the system to become more important than the persons involved.[19] The nurse's commitment will continue to be that aspect of good nursing care that cannot be programed into any system.

REFERENCES

1. Howland, Daniel, "Approaches to the Systems Problem," *Nursing Research*, Vol. 12, No. 3, Summer 1963, pp. 172–174.

2. Howland, Daniel, "A Hospital Systems Model," *Nursing Research*, Vol. 12, No. 4, Fall 1963, pp. 232–236.

3. Howland, Daniel and Wanda McDowell, "The Measurement of Patient Care: A Conceptual Framework," *Nursing Research*, Vol. 13, No. 1, Winter 1964, pp. 4–7.

4. von Bertalanffy, Ludwig, *General System Theory*, New York: George Braziller, Inc., 1968, p. 19.

5. Burck, Gilbert, *The Computer Age and Its Potential for Management*, New York: Harper & Row Publishers, Inc., 1965, pp. 31–34.

6. Armore, Sidney J., *Introduction to Statistical Analysis and Inference for Psychology and Education*, New York: John Wiley & Sons, 1966, pp. 187–197.

7. Rapoport, Anatol and William J. Horvath, "Thoughts on Organization Theory," *Modern Systems Research for the Behavioral Scientist*, Walter Buckley, Editor, Chicago: Aldine Publishing Co., 1968, pp. 71–75.

8. Boulding, Kenneth E., "General Systems Theory—The Skeleton of Science," *Modern Systems Research for the Behavioral Scientist*, Walter Buckley, Editor, Chicago: Aldine Publishing Co., 1968, pp. 3–10.

9. Hall, A. D. and R. E. Fagan, "Definition of System," *Modern Systems Research for the Behavioral Scientist*, Walter Buckley, Editor, Chicago: Aldine Publishing Co., 1968, pp. 81–92.

10. von Bertalanffy, *op. cit.*, p. 40.

11. Cannon, Walter B., *The Wisdom of the Body*, New York: W. W. Norton & Co., Inc. 1932.

12. Wiener, Norbert, *The Human Use of Human Beings: Cybernetics and Society*, New York: Doubleday & Company, 1950, p. 12.

13. Ashby, W. Ross, *An Introduction to Cybernetics*, New York: John Wiley & Sons, Inc., 1956, p. 127.

14. *Ibid.*, pp. 1–6.

15. von Bertalanffy, Ludwig, "General System Theory—A Critical Review," *Modern Systems Research for the Behavioral Scientist*, Walter Buckley, Editor, Chicago: Aldine Publishing Co., 1968, pp. 11–30.

16. Goodenough, Ward Hunt, *Cooperation in Change*, New York: John Wiley & Sons, Inc., 1963, p. 55.

17. Pritsker, A. A. B., GERT: Graphical Evaluation and Review Techniques, Santa Monica, The Rand Corporation, 1966.

18. Pritsker, A. A. B., The Formulation of Automatic Checkout Techniques, Battelle Memorial Institute, Technical Documentary Report #ASD-TDR-62-291, 1962.

19. Wiener, *op. cit.*, pp. 187–193.

Components of the Nursing Process

Virginia Kohlman Carrieri, M.S.
Judith Sitzman, M.S.

Nursing care is a continuous process. It must have coordination of parts without interruption or cessation. It must be set in motion and progress toward the integration of the whole individual or his highest achievable level of wellness. To achieve these goals patient care must be deliberate, systematic, and individualized through the use of the nursing process.

Many theoretical frameworks could be used to examine process as a concept. Parker defines process as "that intellectual scheme whereby relationships are put together." According to Parker, this encompasses the procedures of analysis, synthesis, and reduction to practice. Analysis involves the accumulation of, the classification of, and the distinction between differences in data. Synthesis includes establishing relationships between data, deriving trends, performing deductive and inductive analysis, and creating operational devices. Reduction to practice involves operational devices used on particular occasions in specific settings and testing for the effectiveness and validity of the operational devices.[1]

These concepts and additional resources have been used by various workers to outline the unique elements of the nursing process.[3,4,5] These elements have often been identified as: observation, inference, validation, assessment, action, and evaluation.

This model of the nursing process was

Reprinted with permission from *Nursing Clinics of North America*, 1971, Vol. 6, No. 1, pp. 115–124.

deliberately utilized by the present authors while caring for patients undergoing cardiac valve replacements. The process was initiated when data regarding a patient were obtained through interaction with the patient, from other health team members, or from patient records. Relationships with these patients usually began one week prior to surgery and were maintained until discharge.

OBSERVATION

The first step of the process, observation, is defined for this investigation as a deliberate search for relevant data about a patient with concurrent assignment of meaning to these data in light of the nurse's frame of reference.

It is realized that all observations are influenced by the nurse's previous experiences; however, what makes her observations scientific is the deliberateness and special care with which she makes reliable observations. The nurse is aware that observation is constantly subject to error and can be influenced by all past theoretical and experiential knowledge.

Kaplan contrasts scientific observation with casual everyday observations: "Observation is purposive behavior, directed toward ends that lie beyond the act of observation itself: the aim is to secure materials that will play a part in other phases of inquiry, like the formation and validation of hypotheses."[2]

Observation demanded the building of a trust relationship with the patient so that he felt free to verbalize all of his concerns. This relationship facilitated the collection of a wider range of observations about the physical and psychosocial status of the patient. Only through accumulation of significant information is the nurse able to progress beyond the first step of the process toward an accurate diagnosis and plan of care.

The authors utilized a nursing history form and a nursing diagnosis as the format for instituting the process, recording their findings, and retrieving information about the patient. All observations were categorized and coded using the following nursing history form unique to this report.

NURSING HISTORY FORM

Character of Information

1. Personal data, i.e., age, religion, marital status, etc.
2. Socio-economic and cultural influences
3. Concept or perception of self
4. Physiologic status
5. Adaptation to illness
   a. Current illness and life pattern of illness
   b. Hospital setting or health team
6. Understanding of treatments and procedures during hospitalization
7. Specific fears, i.e., fear of death, procedures, etc.

Source of Information

A. Observation or communication with the patient
B. Review of medical record
C. Communication with health team
D. Communication with significant others

Examples of selected observations and appropriate coding regarding one cardiac surgical patient are listed herewith:

Coding	Observations
(1B)	White male, 37, Protestant, divorced 3 years ago
(1B)	3 children with wife, many unskilled jobs
(4B)	Aortic stenosis, penicillin allergy, only sx "SOB"
(6A)	"All I know is they cut you open and sew you back together again"
(5aA)	"I came here for heart surgery, but they've had their fingers in everything I have"
(5bA)	"They're not going to throw something in my face and make me sign it"
(5aA)	"I've been having too much fun for the last 4 years to lie in bed for surgery"

(5A)   Moving constantly in bed

(1A)   Smoking frequently

(4A)   Skin color gray-white

These are examples of the significant information obtained during one interaction with a patient which had relevance for deliberate planning of nursing care, since they are clues about the patient as an individual. These are only a few of the many observations obtained during each interview with cardiac patients during the investigation of this interpersonal process.

INFERENCE

After coding all observations, the nurse initiated the second step in the process, that of inference. Inference is defined for purposes of this report as an interpretation of patient verbalization and behavior based on the nurse's prior theoretical knowledge of the type of problem with which the patient is confronted. The nurse infers, usually without sufficient data, that a certain type of problem exists for the patient. An awareness on the nurse's part that she is using the inference process, with its reliance on intuition as well as theoretical knowledge, in making decisions about the nature of her patient's problems should be a caution to her that she may, in fact, be functioning without sufficient data, and thus lead her to seek additional information before acting on the problem as she first perceives it.

The following are exemplary observations and inferences taken from a lengthy list of patterns of observations received each day throughout one patient's hospitalization.

Observations

Preop. Day #2
    "The only thing I hated was that tube down my nose—scared me to death"

Postop. Day #1
    "Froze all night, all I could think of was let me die warm"

    Rapid, shallow breathing. Rate 32/min. Flushed skin, restless.

Postop. Day #4
    "I thought I was going to die or faint, all I could see was my open chest on that pissy floor"

    "Now that I've gotten over the operation, I'll probably die of pneumonia"

Inferences

Fear of suctioning
Fear of nasogastric tube

Hypothermia mattress may be too high
Fear of death

Atelectasis, consolidation, drug reaction

Fear of death
Fear of pain
Fear of body mutilation

"My heart went all to pieces, guess I'm coming all unglued" } Fear of death
Fear of pain
Fear of body mutilation

Postop. Day #7

"Why don't they give me pain medication before the machine?"

"Now I know what pain is, it couldn't be worse" } Pain

"All I can do is say, buddy, I'm here . . . sometimes I don't think they know it's you"

Hostility toward staff
Impersonalization by staff

"I came here for heart surgery but they've had their fingers in everything I have"

Mistrust and resentment of staff

Postop. Day #8

"My heart beats faster and makes more noise than it did before surgery"

"I'm worse than before, weak as a cat, I'd rather give them their valve back and take mine; it was better" } Postoperative expectations of self not being met

VALIDATION

After the nurse formulated inferences as to the possibility of existing patient problems, she entered the third step of the nursing process, validation. Validation is defined as the corroboration of the patient's definition with that of the nurse's, and, when a discrepancy between the two occurs, attaining mutual agreement.

Agreement regarding definition of the problem can be achieved by various methods. If possible, verbal exploration of the situation with the patient should confirm the nurse's definition of the problem or necessitate its reformulation. The following exchange illustrates this method.

Patient discussing previous surgery: "The only thing I hated was that tube down my nose . . . scared me to death"

Based on the nurse's knowledge of the patient's previous appendectomy she inferred that he feared the nasogastric tube.

Nurse validating: "You're scared to death of which tube? The one put down your nose to make you cough or the tube which was inserted through your nose into your stomach for drainage?"

Patient response: "The one in my stomach that they put cold water down"

Thus, the patient confirmed the fact that in this case the nurse's definition and his own were the same. Further "hunches" explored by the authors were those based on their significance in terms of identification with patient problems.

If the problem cannot be confirmed verbally with the patient, the nurse has at her command alternate methods of identifying potential patient problems. Using all of her senses, available diagnostic tools, and/or actions on behalf of the patient, she indirectly validates her inferences.

For example, the authors observed that on the first postoperative day the patient had rapid, shallow respirations (32/min.), was restless, and had flushed skin. The following inferences were made: fever, atelectasis, consolidation, or possible drug reaction.

Nurse Validating

1. Felt skin for temperature and took temperature

2. Observed chest expansion, percussed chest, and used stethoscope to listen for quality and distribution of breath sounds

3. Observed amount and character of sputum

4. Examined chest films with M.D.

5. Checked laboratory reports for lowered arterial PO_2

Through several sources the authors were able to confirm their inference that the patient had developed right lower lobe atelectasis.

ASSESSMENT

Validation of patient problems allows the nurse to direct her attention toward assessment, the fourth component of the nursing process. The authors used assessment and the concept of nursing diagnosis interchangeably. Both of these steps were defined as relating knowledge to patient problems and determining central problems, which led to the development of alternative mitigating actions.

Peplau has summarized some of the steps involved in the process of assessment. Thought processes might include: sorting and classifying, comparing, applying concepts and relationships, and summarizing or synthesizing data.[6] Review of the literature also indicates many suggestions for categories to be used in assessing data or making a nursing diagnosis.[3,7,8]

However, the authors chose to code daily patient observations using the categories described above in the nursing history form. Inferences were made from these observations and were subsequently recorded. Based on frequency and importance, only certain validated inferences were recognized as central problems, and functioned as the assessment or nursing diagnosis. Just as the physician's diagnosis may change, the nurse's diagnosis also may vary from day to day or minute to minute. As the nurse's understanding and knowledge of the patient increases and as the patient presents new problems, the diagnosis should be revised accordingly.

A deliberative approach to diagnosis leads the nurse to decision making and priority-setting in the assessment of patient needs. The process enables formulation of nursing actions with a greater probability of success because more valid and comprehensive data are received.

The authors have included below one example of a preoperative nursing assessment or diagnosis. This assessment was formed by collecting many observations and inferences, similar to those shown above, during several interactions with the patient, family, or health team. Those validated inferences that demonstrated a pattern of frequency and importance were then established as the nursing diagnosis from which a plan of care was formulated.

ACTION

Nursing action, the next step in the process, is defined as the testing of alternatives and the carrying out of those considered the most suitable. The appropriate alternative actions chosen by the authors are listed below with the nursing diagnosis to illustrate these two steps in the process.

Nursing Diagnosis

1. Decreased energy with dypsnea on exertion.

2. Possible reaction to antibiotics and other medications.

3. Apparent anxiety and need for tension release.

4. Need for knowledge of procedures as they relate to self.

5. Possible low self-esteem and low masculine self-image.

6. Possible denial of illness leading to self-destruction.

7. Fear of losing body intactness and of death.

8. Unstable social environment.

Alternative Nursing Actions

1. Help patient to understand physical limitations prior to surgery in order to conserve energy; attempt to decrease environmental stressors.

2. Alert staff about possible drug reactions; observe for these reactions.

3. Assist patient to cope with illness by listening, focusing on what concerns him, and involving him in simple ward activities.

4. Investigate the patient's perception of the medical and nursing treatments in relation to himself; after investigation focus teaching on actual danger threats perceived by patient.

5a. Collect further data to validate low male identity.

5b. Allow patient to control his environment whenever possible.

5c. Involve patient in decision-making.

6a. Collect data to validate diagnosis of denial of illness and self-destructive behavior.

6b. Assist patient to develop a more realistic perception of postoperative self by focusing on realistic outcome of surgery.

6c. Help patient to gain understanding of rationale for M.D. order to stop smoking.

7a. Recognize nurse's behavior which may interfere with patient's ability to verbalize feelings about death.

7b. Listen for clues indicating patient's desire to express feelings about death.

8a. Collect more data to validate patient's life style and pattern of illness.

8b. Seek consultation from social worker and chaplain.

Nursing actions or interventions are in part dependent upon the nurse's theory of nursing. Such actions should encompass all activities from counseling and teaching to physical care and delegated medical therapy. Another important facet with which the nurse must concern herself is the priority of intervention. Although many factors beyond the scope of this report are significant, the patient's priority of needs primarily determines the type, level, and speed of intervention. Certainly, in particular patient situations, the nurse may need to act or intervene immediately after rapidly moving through the first steps of the process.

EVALUATION

The final step of these operational processes is that of evaluation. Evaluation is defined as a continuous process through which appraisal of the effectiveness of the previous steps in meeting the patient's needs is provided. Observation of patient behavior, communication with the patient, his family, and health team members, and diagnostic measurements were used to evaluate each step in the process and the total process. Because patient and nursing goals had been clearly defined, the authors were better able to determine the degree to which these goals had been achieved.

The following patient situations are presented to illustrate the process of evaluation. Previous steps in the process have been included in an attempt to describe more clearly the flow and developing nursing process for the reader.

Patient Situation I

Postop. Day #2

Observations:
Flushed skin color, elevated temp., restless
Rapid, shallow respirations, rate 32/min.
Greater expansion of left chest than right
Region of right lower lobe dull to percussion with diminished breath sounds
Decreased sputum in last 24 hours

Inferences:
Possible atelectasis or drug reaction

Validated Inference:
Chest film and M.D. physical examination confirmed right lower lobe atelectasis

Nursing Assessment/Diagnosis:
Right Lower Lobe Atelectasis

Nursing Actions:
1. Frequent change of position
2. Support incision during frequent deep breathing and coughing, clapping and vibrating, reemphasize need for all procedures
3. Contact physical therapist for chest therapy
4. Administer IPPB with bronchodilator as ordered
5. Observe for changes in expansion, rate, and breath sounds
6. Observe laboratory reports of blood gases for possible changes in acid-base balance, hypoxia
7. Force fluids

Postop. Day #5

Nurse Evaluation:
Chest film confirmed cessation of atelectatic process
Blood gases within normal limits

Patient Situation II

Postop. Days #8, 9

Observations:
"All I can do is say, buddy, I'm here . . . sometimes I don't think they know it's you."
"They're not going to throw something in my face and make me sign it again."
"That doctor is like a bull in a china shop."

Inference:
Impersonalization of patient by staff

Validated Inference:
Patient was asked his impressions of the health team, to which he replied, "They treat you like a guinea pig around here, sometimes I don't think they know it's you."

Nursing Assessment/Diagnosis:
Impersonalization by staff

Nursing Actions:
Discuss ways of personalizing care with nursing and medical staff.
1. Patient decision-making whenever possible
2. Possibility of one staff member caring for patient
3. Explain rationale for procedures before acting
4. Allow patient to express hostility

Postop. Day #13

Nurse Evaluation:
1. Patient's decreased frequency of negative comments about staff
2. Also increased positive clues, such as:
"Dr. B. didn't yank out those stitches so hard today."
"Oh, I know that, Miss J. told me all about that pill this morning."

CONCLUSIONS

The authors formulated the following conclusions while putting this process into operation. The daily recording of all observations, inferences, diagnoses, actions, and evaluations in horizontal sequence within one notebook assisted the authors and the staff to see definite patterns of patient behavior and subsequent nursing actions for this group of patients. This method of recording and coding data also was practical, time-conserving, easy to use, and could actually be implemented in the patient setting.

It is apparent that this process requires the use of both theory and expert clinical practice in order that valid nursing actions can be derived and evaluated for effectiveness.

Continuity of care was necessarily increased as nurses gained an understanding of the process through discussions and care conferences. With increased knowledge of the process and recording designs they assisted the authors in establishing nursing histories, diagnoses, alternative actions, and evaluations. With such assistance a wider range of patient problems was identified and a unified plan of care achieved. Care plans were transferred with patients as they moved from preoperative to postoperative settings. These plans were easily communicated to other health team members and community agencies.

A trust relationship with the patient was the cornerstone of this process. The accumulation of data would have been impossible if the authors had not conveyed interest and concern, and used all their abilities to form relationships that became therapeutic catalysts.

One of the most important findings was that patients evaluated this process favorably. They expressed opinions that knowledge of procedures and potential danger threats, exposure to the intensive care unit preoperatively, and identification with one nurse throughout their hospitalization helped them to understand and anticipate events during hospitalization. Anxiety appeared to be reduced, and postoperative expectations seemed more realistic.

In conclusion, a more scientific approach to the nursing process has enabled the investigators to identify a wider range of patient problems, to apply theoretical knowledge toward the solution of identified patient needs, and to define a rationale for nursing action which has a higher probability of success. It is the authors' opinion that the use of this nursing process would help to increase understanding of individual patient problems and give insight into patterns of behavior to be used for future prediction.

REFERENCES

1. Parker, C. J., and Rubin, L. J.: *Process as Content: Curriculum Design and the Application of Knowledge.* Chicago, Rand McNally & Co., 1966.

2. Kaplan, Abraham: *The Conduct of Inquiry: Methodology for Behavioral Science.* San Francisco, Chandler Publishing Co., 1964, p. 127.

3. Lewis, L., Carozza, V., Carroll, M., Darragh, R., Patrick, M., and Schadt, E.: *Defining Clinical Content Graduate Nursing Programs: Medical-Surgical Nursing.* Colorado, Western Interstate Commission for Higher Education, 1967.

4. Wiedenbach, Ernestine: *Clinical Nursing—A Helping Art.* New York, Springer Publishing Co., 1964.

5. Orlando, Ida Jean: *The Dynamic Nurse– Patient Relationship.* New York, G. P. Putnam's Sons, 1961.

6. Peplau, Hildegard E.: *Process and Concept Learning.* In Burd, Shirley, and Marshall, Margaret A., Eds.: *Some Clinical Approaches to Psychiatric Nursing.* New York, The Macmillan Co., 1963, pp. 333–336.

7. McCain, R. Faye: Nursing by assessment—not intuition. *Am. J. Nursing,* 65: 82–84, April, 1965.

8. Little, Dolores E., and Carnevali, Doris L.: *Nursing Care Planning.* Philadelphia, J. B. Lippincott Co., 1969.

Chapter 17

The Humanistic Approach in Learning and in Nursing Practice

Part VI has studied nursing as a helping profession, discussing the dimensions of helping according to researchers in counseling psychology. General System Theory, the theoretic framework encompassing the nursing process, was also discussed in Chapter 16, and models of nursing care developed by various theorists focusing on the systems approach were presented.

Chapter 17 is devoted to an added dimension, the humanistic approach to the nursing process—that is, the humanistic approach both in practicing and in learning the process. The conceptual framework for humanistic education begins the chapter, followed by a theoretic model that is the foundation of all the concepts presented in each chapter of this book.

THE CONCEPTUAL FRAMEWORK

It is important to remember that the nursing process involves a constant state of learning, whether in learning nursing techniques, or in learning about a particular client in order to provide care. The conceptual framework for humanistic education focuses primarily on attitudinal development and then on behavioral manifestations in practice. Attitudes are of great importance because they pervade all aspects of self: thoughts, feelings, values, experiences, desires, behaviors, and even the body. The learner's belief systems become the core of the educational process (Combs, 1972). Attitudes are then developed, and consonant behaviors follow. Rogers (1967a) synthesized from research findings (Aspy, 1965; Barrett-Lennard, 1962; Emmerling, 1961; Schmuck, 1963, 1966) that having attitudinal development as the primary focus in a learning process effectively facilitates deeper learning with self-understanding and is a characteristic of practitioners who are regarded as effective. Recognizing the significance of research findings, it becomes necessary to explore attitudinal development.

Attitudes as Determinants of Behavior

A general characteristic of an attitude is its tendency to cause one to evaluate an object in a certain way (Katz & Stotland, 1959). This definition was elucidated earlier by Campbell (1947) when he described a social attitude as a syndrome of response consistency toward social objects. Perceptual sets (see Chapter 2) formulated in past experience are another dimension added by Asch (1948, 1952). Yet, all of these definitions include an essential similarity: an attitude is a mental posture toward an object or person that leads to behavior.

Attitudinal Structure.   Social psychologists break down attitudes into three highly correlated aspects: affective, cognitive, and behavioral (Katz & Stotland, 1959). Lott (1973) viewed the *affective* facet as relating to dichotomous feelings of good/bad, like/dislike, approach/avoidance, and so forth. He stated that many theorists see the affective aspect of attitudes as providing the motivational energy for behavior.

The *cognitive* dimension is useful in determining the information and beliefs held about an object or person (Katz & Stotland, 1959) and was seen by Osgood (1962) and Osgood, Suci, and Tannenbaum (1967) as having evaluative dimensions. This implies that there is no neutrality in cognition and thereby couples the cognitive and affective aspects.

The third aspect of attitudinal structure is termed *behavioral*, or action, and consists of a predisposed response to a certain stimulus (Lott, 1973). The strength of the predisposed response directly relates to what is elicited behaviorally (Lott, 1973). It can be concluded at this point that attitudes have a positive relationship with behavior.

Hersey and Blanchard (1982) simplified attitudinal structure by saying that behavior is a function of motives and goals. Motives are defined as needs, wants, desires, and conscious and unconscious beliefs within an individual; goals are external factors influencing the individual and, among others, include incentives, responsibilities, anticipated results, or behavioral outcomes. Both combine to yield behavior (Hersey & Blanchard, 1982).

Since it becomes evident that attitudes are responsible for behavior as well as for behavioral intent, the development of a positive attitude toward nursing care becomes paramount, and this positive attitude must be integrated with knowledge and experience. If clear understanding and positive attitudes are not developed, the negative ramifications will extend throughout a lifelong nursing career: it is the seed from which all grows. Moreover, since negative experiences require extra effort to be first neutralized and then relearned (Carkhuff, 1969c) it becomes paramount that initial contact with the nursing process must be positive and firmly based in individual belief systems. This will provide the opportunity to truly learn and know, to integrate the foundations of nursing practice with personal meaning and individual experience.

The Existential Base

Attitudes have been described as being composed of an individual's beliefs, values, response sets, and perceptions about an object, person, or process. These, together with motives, lead to behavior. For a nurse's behavior to be based on positive attitudes paralleled with an awareness of what must be accomplished in helping, education must focus on both dimensions. The awareness of requirements for helping is usually developed in educational systems and practice experience in nursing. The high correlation of attitudes to behavior mandates that attitudes be equally studied. Attitudinal development involves primary focus on internal processes of the learner: it involves *knowing* rather than *knowing about*, and includes understanding self.

The conceptual model used by the author for facilitating knowing in a learner is existentially based. One knows only because one experiences and is so aware—uniquely. This concept is crystallized in the words of Axline (1976, p. 20): "Even though we do not have the wisdom to enumerate the reasons for the behavior of another person, we can grant that every individual does have his private world of meaning, conceived out of the integrity and dignity of his personality."

Weisman (1965) said that all persons regard themselves as unique, significant entities. When every human being is seen as a unique entity, it is possible to visualize the differences in people's thoughts, interpretations, and beliefs. Pain/pleasure, harmony/dissonance, and beauty/ugliness then become real as one explores one's own feelings and thoughts regarding an object, person, or process. Indeed, thoughts and feelings are valid and cannot be excused as prejudice or preference—thoughts and feelings are reality, but valuable only to the individual (Weisman, 1965).

Existentialism is the philosophy that provides the foundation for a humanistic approach to learning and to using the nursing process. Existentialism describes an attitude and an approach to human beings. It is concerned with human longing and man's search for importance within self. Beck (1963) viewed the existential philosophy as that which emphasizes the view of reality that is most meaningful to a person— the person's own existence and being. Camus (1946, 1956, 1959, 1947/1972) wrote extensively on being, pointing out three corollaries

(1959). The first is that we can understand another human being only as we see what that human is moving toward, what that person is becoming; we can understand ourselves only as we project our potentialities into action. The second aspect of *being*, according to Camus (1959), is that it is not an inherent given. In other words, being does not unfold automatically as the flower from a seed; it can be forfeited or sloughed off. Self-consciousness is an element inseparable from the human being; humans are the particular beings who must become aware of themselves if they are to become themselves. The third distinctive aspect described by Camus (1959) is that humans are the beings who know that at some future moment they will not be; in effect, the person is in relation with nonbeing, or death. If one is to grasp what it means to exist, one must confront the fact that at any moment one may cease to exist and that death will inescapably arrive at some moment in the future. With this awareness of nonbeing, however, existence takes on vitality and immediacy, and the individual experiences a heightened consciousness of self, the world, and others at the same time.

Harper (1974) stated that, in existential therapy, emphasis is placed on the importance of the individual's goals and values, with attention directed toward understanding an individual's personal world and carousel of values. Existentialists analyze the meaning structure of each person's unique world of values by consciously attempting to strip themselves of preconceived notions about the nature and values of Man.

Existentialism Applied to Nursing.   It has been shown that attitudes relate positively to behavior; therefore, *one's beliefs about the nursing process will affect practice.* Referring back to the question of how to develop positive attitudes in nurses, and integrating the described conceptual framework, the following conclusions can be synthesized: A nurse must be aware of personal experience in relation to the nursing process, recognize this as true and valid, and respond to clients in concert with the individual reality of both self and client. The objective is to have motives and goals in harmony with elicited behavior.

The conceptual framework discussed the underlying philosophy of humanistic education: individuality and self-knowledge as the basis of learning. This has been portrayed by La Monica and Parisi-Carew (1975) in the PELLEM Pentagram (Figure 17-1).

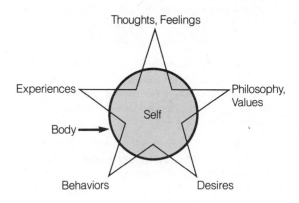

Figure 17-1

The PELLEM Pentagram (SOURCE: La Monica and Parisi-Carew, 1975.)

The PELLEM Pentagram

The PELLEM Pentagram (named for its originators, Elaine L. La Monica and Eunice M. Parisi-Carew) is a model of self, comprised of five interrelated, yet separate, composite parts:

1. Thoughts, Feelings
2. Philosophy, Values
3. Desires
4. Behaviors
5. Experiences

It is symbolized by a five-pointed star as shown in Figure 17-1. Each point represents one aspect of self. These aspects merge in the center to form the total self. The body is represented by the line of a circle running through each point. It is symbolized in this way because of the interrelating effect of the body on how and what one experiences, feels and thinks, and how one behaves.

The points of the model represent what is thought by theorists to be operating within a person's total experience. An individual's body is the vehicle for self-expression and, therefore, crosses all facets of the Pentagram; it is one's language. Self, signified by the center of the model, is the blending of all.

Absent from the model is the influence of psychic powers and mystical phenomena that may play a part. To date, their influence is undetermined and indeed looked upon by many "concrete scientists" as superstitions or at best unknowns. These energies are neither denied nor claimed as fact.

The self is studied holistically. It is the interplay of all parts that produces the unique phenomenon of the individual, just as it is all the components acting in unison that provides the reasons for experience at any given moment. To deny the importance of any one of these parts is to deny an important aspect of our being.

This model provides a simple way to view the complexities of a person. It stems from a personal and professional struggle to know, understand, and be self-directive. In analyzing why people are perceived in a certain way with particular feelings, the areas of the PELLEM Pentagram should be explored. When these are studied, problem areas and actions seem to fall into place. A feeling of more fully knowing oneself can lead to self-acceptance concurrent with self-worth even though the life process usually prohibits such a level of truth. This ideologic level of truth exists, however, only if the knowing process occurs in an atmosphere of complete safety and trust.

Use of the model in learning the nursing process becomes important because the process is the professional guideline for *all* nursing practice. The nurse who is aware of the complex nature of self is also likely to be aware of the complexities of the client, thus leading to care based on the whole person.

Actualizing the humanistic approach becomes the next step. Humanism refers to anything that involves thought and human ideals. Therefore, humanism refers to the process of learning as well as to learning's affective part in particular. Equally important in dealing with the whole person are the cognitive and psychomotor aspects of learning. In this book, the theory of the nursing process has been provided, as well as guidelines for using the humanistic approach in learning the psychomotor skills necessary to implement the process; this book also provides guidelines for exploring and developing affective attitudes. The dynamic, personal learning experience necessary in learning and using the nursing process is achieved by human-relations education.

The Human-Relations Educational Mode in Attitudinal Development

Looking at the history of the human-relations model, Matarazzo (1965) reviewed counseling and psychotherapeutic processes and concluded that the group helping process was a self-taught art with few guiding principles. There were controversies between practitioners who concentrated upon the individual helpee within the group, those who fixed upon interpersonal relationships within the group, and others who gave chief attention to the interaction between the group and the individual, with no definite conclusions being reached. Out of the traditional model of group psychotherapy, there developed a number of experiential types. For example: growth groups (Gazda, Asbury, Balzer, Childers, Desselle, & Walters, 1973, 1977; Lubin & Lubin, 1967), encounter and marathon groups (Bach, 1966; Moustakas, 1972; Murphy, 1969; Stoller, 1967), the self-directed groups (Berzon & Soloman, 1966; Rogers, 1967b), sensitivity and "T" groups (Benne, 1969; Brad-

ford, Gibb, & Benne, 1964; Schein & Bennis, 1965), and humanistic-experiential ones (Berne, 1978; Perls, 1969; Schutz, 1967). The human-relations training model, which grew out of the T-group model, was developed at Bethel by the organization called the National Training Laboratories. The model has been documented as being effective (Appley & Winder, 1973).

There are several underlying assumptions about the nature of the learning process distinguishing T-groups and human-relations training from other models of learning. All of these assumptions are directly applicable to the nursing process. According to Seashore (1970, pp. 15–16),[1] these assumptions are:

1. *Learning Responsibility.* Each participant is responsible for his own learning. What a person learns depends upon his own style, readiness, and the relationships he develops with other members of the group.

2. *Staff Role.* The staff person's role is to facilitate the examination and understanding of the experiences in the group. He helps participants to focus on the way the group is working, the style of an individual's participation, or the issues that are facing the group.

3. *Experience and Conceptualization.* Most learning is a combination of experience and conceptualization. A major T-group aim is to provide a setting in which individuals are encouraged to examine their experiences together in enough detail so that valid generalizations can be drawn.

4. *Authentic Relationships and Learning.* A person is most free to learn when he establishes authentic relationships with other people and thereby increases his sense of self-esteem and decreases his defensiveness. In authentic relationships persons can be open, honest, and

---

[1]From *The Reading Book for Human Relations Training,* by C. Seashore, pp. 9–10. Copyright © 1979 by NTL Institute. Reprinted by permission.

direct with one another so that they are communicating what they are actually feeling rather than masking their feelings.

5. *Skill Acquisition and Values.* The development of new skills in working with people is maximized as a person examines the basic values underlying his behavior, as he acquires appropriate concepts and theory, and as he is able to practice new behavior and obtain feedback on the degree to which his behavior produces the intended impact.

The intent of the group-dynamics laboratory is to accomplish one or more of the following changes in attitude or behavior on the part of the trainees (Stogdill, 1974, p. 182):

1. Greater sensitivity to follower needs and desires;

2. Greater openness and sharing of information;

3. Greater sharing of decision-making responsibilities with followers;

4. More intimate, friendly, and equalitarian interaction with followers; and

5. Less structuring, personal dominance, and pushing for productive output.

The goals and outcomes of human-relations training are classified according to potential learning involving individuals, groups, and organizations (Seashore, 1970). The metagoals of the laboratory method involve inquiry, collaboration, rational conflict resolution, and the freedom to exercise choice. These processes are shared by the staff and the participants (Appley & Winder, 1973). These researchers further stated that, in a relatively safe world, members can test and learn trust, risk-taking, openness, and interdependence. Studies by Gibb (1971), Harrison and Lubin (1965), and Miles (1965) have all found the T-group method an effective one for increasing interpersonal communication.

Blumberg (1971, pp. 7–8) asserted that, in order for training goals in laboratory education to be realized, certain conditions in the laboratory must be met:[2]

1. *Presentation of Self.* Until the individual has an opportunity to reveal the way he sees things and does things, he has little basis for improvement and change.

2. *Feedback.* Individuals do not learn from their experiences. They learn from bringing out the essential patterns of purposes, motives, and behavior in a situation where they can receive back clear and accurate information about the relevancy and effectiveness of their behavior. They need a feedback system which continuously operates so that they can change and correct what is inappropriate.

3. *Atmosphere.* An atmosphere of trust and nondefensiveness is necessary for people both to be willing to expose their behavior and purposes, and to accept feedback.

4. *Cognitive Map.* Knowledge from research, theory, and experience is important to enable the individual both to understand his experiences and to generalize from them. But normally, information is most effective when it follows experience and feedback.

5. *Experimentation.* Unless there is opportunity to try out new patterns of thought and behavior, they never become a part of the individual. Without experimental efforts, relevant change is difficult to make.

6. *Practice.* Equally important is the need to practice new approaches so that the individual gains security in being different.

7. *Application.* Unless learning and change can be applied to back-home situations, they are not likely to be effective or lasting. Attention needs to be given to helping individuals plan application.

---

[2]From *Sensitivity Training: Processes, Problems, and Applications,* by A. Blumberg. Copyright © 1971 by Syracuse University Publications in Continuing Education. Reprinted by permission.

8. *Relearning How to Learn.* Because much of our academic experience has led us to believe that we learn from listening to authorities, there is frequently need to learn from presentation–feedback–experimentation.

Carkhuff, Collingwood, and Renz (1969) investigated the effects of didactic training upon trainee levels of discrimination and communication. Their results indicated that exclusively didactic training yielded significant improvement in discrimination but very little generalization of learning in communication skills.

Carkhuff and Truax (1965) evaluated the effects of an integrated didactic and experiential approach to training. They found that these two combined were basic to the training program, along with having a trainer who was a role model in offering high levels of empathy, respect, concreteness, and genuineness.

Carkhuff (1969e), Carkhuff and Banks (1970), and Carkhuff and Bierman (1970) discovered that, to effect differences in communication, training must employ a behavioristic, interpersonal approach preceding practice in communication. Several studies confirmed the need and success of providing experiential, interpersonal, and intrapersonal group training for helping professionals (Berenson, Carkhuff, & Myrus, 1966; Foulds, 1969; Martin & Carkhuff, 1968; Vitalo, 1971). With conclusions based on research and experience, Carkhuff (1969d, p. 130) offered several propositions that led him to prefer the group training mode:

1.. *Proposition I.* "The core of functioning or dysfunctioning (health or psychopathology) is interpersonal."

2. *Proposition II.* "The core of the helping process (learning or relearning) is interpersonal."

3. *Proposition III.* "Group processes are the preferred mode of working with difficulties in interpersonal functioning." Group processes can obviously insure the greatest amount of learning for the greatest number of people at one time.

4. *Proposition IV.* "Systematic group training in interpersonal functioning is the preferred mode of working with difficulties in interpersonal functioning."

Carkhuff (1969d) made use of all sources of learning: experiential, didactic, and role modeling. He stressed that the key in all group helping processes is the level of functioning of the leader (Carkhuff, 1969a, 1969b). The use of high-functioning leaders results in an atmosphere whereby trainees/helpees can move toward higher levels of functioning; it also provides multiple potential helpers/trainers for individual group members (Carkhuff, 1969d).

The advantages of human-relations-modeled group processes that include all sources of learning under the direction of a high-functioning leader are numerous. They apply in both training and helping. Each helpee has the following opportunities, according to Carkhuff (1969d, p. 181):

1. to act out his characteristic behaviors;

2. to observe the characteristic behaviors of others;

3. to communicate directly with another person other than the helper;

4. to dispense with unsuccessful defenses and express himself freely in the context of a facilitative group atmosphere;

5. to share in the helper's clarification and interpretation of the behavior of another;

6. to try out new behaviors directly with others;

7. to have the experience of helping as well as being helped;

8. to be valued by more than one person;

9. to focus upon the generalities of experience within the group; and

10. to obtain a definition of social reality.

Advantages of group over individual processes for the trainer/helper are also significant.

According to Carkhuff (1969d, p. 181), the helper has the following opportunities:

1. observe directly the behaviors of the individual helpees;

2. facilitate communication between individual helpees;

3. create a facilitative group atmosphere within which each group member may come to serve as a helper;

4. focus directly upon the generalities in the group experience; and

5. utilize his resources in such a way as to get a maximum return in human benefits for a minimum of investment of time and energy on the part of the helper.

It is important, however, to note the limitations of group processes for the helper/trainer and helpee/trainee. Group processes may be more difficult for the helper to control, since there are more individuals and interactions to which the helper must attend. An effective leader can minimize these conditions, however, and handle group crises just as the leader would handle a crisis in individual treatment. If necessary, individual treatment can be offered concurrently with group processes (Carkhuff, 1969d).

Several conclusions can be reached regarding the preference for the human-relations model in training and treatment. This model is goal and action directed and provides a work-oriented structure through which experiential and therapeutic processes can take place. It emphasizes practice in the behavior one wishes to effect and leaves the trainee/helpee with tangible and usable skills. Longer retention of these skills is promoted, since they are learned as a result of direct teaching, shaping, and modeling. Group members can be systematically selected, and there is a built-in means for assessing the effectiveness of the program because the very nature of systematic training involves steps that lead to measurable outcomes (Carkhuff, 1969d). Stated Carkhuff (1969d, p.

184): "In summary, what can be accomplished individually can be accomplished in groups—and more! What can be accomplished in groups can be accomplished in systematic training—and more!"

APPLICATION OF HUMANISTIC LEARNING TO NURSING PRACTICE

Throughout this book it has been stressed that learning occurs continually. Therefore, the elements of humanistic learning are easily applied to nursing practice.

Humanistic learning emphasizes the individuality of the student. The student, of course, can be the actual student nurse, or, in the case of giving client care, the caregiver may be the student, learning about the client as data are collected, processed, compiled into a care plan, and evaluated. Indeed, all members of the health-care system learn as care is given. Williamson (1981) called this model of nursing "mutual interaction." Humanistic education emphasizes long-term changes in behavior through attitudinal development. Therefore, both caregivers and care-receivers experience learning throughout the nursing process as behaviors are studied and changed to coincide with good health. Members of the health-care system learn from each other and with each other; they are interdependent.

By integrating content with knowledge and experience and, of course, feelings, the caregiver and care-receiver can work together to achieve an individualized, quality care plan that will help the client toward the all-important goal: the client's fullest health potential.

In addition, the humanistic approach emphasizes change. Therefore, in nursing practice the nurse becomes aware of change in personal perceptions, change in both client and health-team attitudes, change in the client's conditions, and change in personal experience. Each of these aspects builds on the nurse's experiential foundation; the nurse can only grow.

Humanism emphasizes the interrelationship of persons, the environment, and the inner self. In giving care, therefore, all concerning the client—and all concerning the nurse—is taken into consideration. The result is humanistic care of the whole person; the nursing process achieves its ultimate goal.

SUMMARY

The humanistic approach used throughout this book and conceptualized in this chapter is a combination of many facets of learning theory. Content material, outside experiences related to actual practice, and direct nursing care are elements of the humanistic approach to learning and applying the nursing process as presented in this book. The continuous bond between elements of humanistic learning is that the learning is intended to focus on the individuality of the student. In other words, the designs are built so that the student can take a new body of knowledge; use background, expectations, and experience; and work through an exercise related to the content needing to be learned. Sharing with fellow students enables one to be aware of a broader range of perceptions, all adding to self-learning. Through this personalization of content, one brings outside experiences into one's life, adding significance. This significance is necessary if learning is to bring long-term change in behavior, since this type of change will greatly help in ensuring that students continue to strive toward carrying the high ideals learned in academic environments into their service institutions. Humanistic psychologists have documented that people learn more fully when the learning involves themselves (Combs & Syngg, 1959; Jourard, 1971; Rogers, 1961). Ultimately, then, through humanistic learning of the nursing process, a behavior pattern is established in which the nurse later applies a humanistic approach to exploring client care, giving client care, and, indeed, learning about the individual client.

REFERENCES

Alschuler, A. (1970). Humanistic education. *Educational Technology Magazine, 10* (5), 58–61.

Appley, D., & Winder, A. (1973). *T-groups and therapy groups in a changing society.* San Francisco: Jossey-Bass.

Asch, S. (1948). The doctrine of suggestions, prestige, and imitations in social psychology. *Psychological Review, 55,* 250–276.

Asch, S. (1952). *Social psychology.* Englewood Cliffs, NJ: Prentice-Hall.

Aspy, D. (1965). *A study of three facilitative conditions and their relationship to the achievement of third grade students.* Unpublished doctoral dissertation, University of Kentucky.

Axline, V. (1976). *Dibs: In search of self.* New York: Ballantine.

Bach, G. (1966). The marathon group: I. Intensive practice of intimate interaction. *Psychological Reports, 18,* 995–1002.

Barrett-Lennard, G. (1962). Dimensions of therapist response as causal factors in therapeutic change. *Psychological Monographs, 76* (No. 562).

Beck, C. (1963). *Philosophical foundations of guidance.* Englewood Cliffs, NJ: Prentice-Hall.

Benne, K. (1969, January). *The self, the group or the task: Differences among growth groups.* Paper presented at "The growth groups: Encounter, marathon, sensitivity and 'T'," Ninth Annual Conference, Personality Theory and Counseling Practice, University of Florida, Gainesville.

Berenson, G., Carkhuff, R., & Myrus, P. (1966). The interpersonal functioning and training of college students. *Journal of Consulting Psychology, 13,* 441–446.

Berne, E. (1978). *Games people play: The psychology of human relationships.* New York: Ballantine.

Berzon, B., & Soloman, L. (1966). Research frontiers: The self-directed therapeutic group. *Journal of Counseling Psychology, 13,* 491–497.

Blumberg, A. (1971). *Sensitivity training: Processes, problems, and applications.* Syracuse, NY: Syracuse University Publications in Continuing Education.

Bradford, P., Gibb, J., & Benne, K. (Eds.) (1964). *T-group theory and laboratory method: An innovation in re-education.* New York: Wiley.

Campbell, D. (1947). *The generality of social attitudes.* Unpublished doctoral dissertation, University of California, Berkeley.

Camus, A. (1946). *The stranger.* New York: Knopf.

Camus, A. (1956). *The rebel.* New York: Knopf.

Camus, A. (1959). *The myth of Sisyphus.* New York: Random House.

Camus, A. (1972). *The plague.* New York: Random House. (Originally published 1947).

Carkhuff, R. (1969a, January). *Critical perspectives on group processes.* Paper presented at "The growth groups: Encounter, marathon, sensitivity and 'T'," Ninth Annual Conference, Personality Theory and Counseling Practice, University of Florida, Gainesville.

Carkhuff, R. (1969b). Critical variables in effective counselor training. *Journal of Counseling Psychology, 16,* 238–245.

Carkhuff, R. (1969c). *Helping and human relations: A primer for lay and professional helpers* (Vol. 1). New York: Human Resource Development Press.

Carkhuff, R. (1969d). *Helping and human relations: A primer for lay and professional helpers* (Vol. 2). New York: Human Resource Development Press.

Carkhuff, R. (1969e). The prediction of the effects of didactic training in discrimination. *Journal of Clinical Psychology, 25,* 460–461.

Carkhuff, R., & Banks, G. (1970). Training as a preferred mode of facilitating relations between races and generations. *Journal of Counseling Psychology, 17,* 413–418.

Carkhuff, R., & Bierman, R. (1970). Training as a preferred mode of treatment of parents of emotionally disturbed children. *Journal of Counseling Psychology, 17,* 157–161.

Carkhuff, R., Collingwood, T., & Renz, L. (1969). The effects of didactic training upon trainee levels of discrimination and communication. *Journal of Clinical Psychology, 25,* 460–461.

Carkhuff, R., & Truax, C. (1965). Training in counseling and psychotherapy: An evaluation of an integrated didactic and experiential approach. *Journal of Consulting Psychology, 29,* 333–336.

Combs, A. (1972). *Educational accountability: Beyond behavioral objectives.* Washington, D.C.: Association for Supervision and Curriculum Development.

Combs, A. (1973). The human side of learning. *The National Elementary Principal, 52* (4), 38–42.

Combs, A., & Syngg, D. (1959). *Individual behavior.* New York: Harper and Row.

Emmerling, F. (1961). *A study of the relationships between personality characteristics of classroom teachers and pupil perceptions.* Unpublished doctoral dissertation, Auburn University, Auburn, Alabama.

Foulds, M. (1969). Self-actualization and the communication of facilitative conditions during counseling. *Journal of Counseling Psychology, 16,* 132–136.

Gazda, G., Asbury, F., Balzer, F., Childers, W., Desselle, R., & Walters, R. (1973). *Human relations development: A manual for educators.* Boston: Allyn and Bacon.

Gazda, G., Asbury, F., Balzer, F., Childers, W., Desselle, R., & Walters, R. (1977). *Human relations development: A manual for educators* (2nd ed.). Boston: Allyn and Bacon.

Gibb, J. (1971). The effects of human relations training. In A. Bergin & S. Garfield (Eds.), *Handbook of psychotherapy and behavior change.* New York: Wiley.

Harper, R. (1974). *Psychoanalysis and psychotherapy.* Englewood Cliffs, NJ: Prentice-Hall.

Harrison, R., & Lubin, B. (1965). Personal style, group composition and learning. *Journal of Applied Behavioral Science, 3,* 286–301.

Hersey, P., & Blanchard, K. (1982). *Management of organizational behavior: Utilizing human resources* (4th ed.). Englewood Cliffs, NJ: Prentice-Hall.

Jourard, S. (1971). *The transparent self* (2nd ed.). New York: Van Nostrand Reinhold.

Katz, D., & Stotland, E. (1959). A preliminary statement to a theory of attitude and structure change. In S. Koch (Ed.), *Psychology: A study of a science* (Vol. 3). New York: McGraw-Hill.

La Monica, E., & Parisi-Carew, E. (1975). The PELLEM Pentagram. Unpublished material. University of Massachusetts.

Lott, A. (1973). Social psychology. In B. Wolman (Ed.), *Handbook of general psychology*. Englewood Cliffs, NJ: Prentice-Hall.

Lubin, B., & Lubin, A. (1967). *Group psychotherapy: A bibliography of the literature from 1956 to 1964.* East Lansing: Michigan State University Press.

Martin, J., & Carkhuff, R. (1968). Changes in personality and interpersonal functioning in counselors in training. *Journal of Clinical Psychology, 24,* 109–110.

Matarazzo, J. (1965). Psychotherapeutic processes. *Annual Review of Psychology, 16,* 181–219.

Miles, M. (1965). Changes during and following laboratory training: A clinical experimental study. *Journal of Applied Behavioral Science, 1,* 215–242.

Moustakas, C. (1972). *The authentic teacher: Sensitivity and awareness in the classroom.* Cambridge, MA: Howard A. Doyle.

Murphy, M. (1969, January). *The growth center phenomenon.* Paper presented at "The growth groups: Encounter, marathon, sensitivity and 'T'," Ninth Annual Conference, Personality Theory and Counseling Practice, University of Florida, Gainesville.

Osgood, C. (1962). Studies on the generality of affective meaning systems. *American Psychologist, 17,* 10–28.

Osgood, C., Suci, G., & Tannenbaum, P. (1967). *The measurement of meaning.* Urbana: University of Illinois Press.

Perls, F. (1969). *Gestalt therapy verbatim.* Lafayette, CA: Real People Press.

Rogers, C. (1961). *On becoming a person.* Boston: Houghton-Mifflin.

Rogers, C. (1967a). The interpersonal relationship in the facilitation of learning. In R. Leeper (Ed.), *Humanizing education: The person in the process.* Washington, D.C.: Association for Supervision and Curriculum Development.

Rogers, C. (1967b). A plan for self-directed change in an educational system. *Educational Leadership, 24,* 717–731.

Schein, E., & Bennis, W. (Eds.). (1965). *Personal and organizational change through group methods: The laboratory approach.* New York: Wiley.

Schmuck, R. (1963). Some relationships of peer liking patterns in the classroom to pupil attitudes and achievement. *The School Review, 71,* 337–359.

Schmuck, R. (1966). Some aspects of classroom social climate. *Psychology in the Schools, 3,* 59–65.

Schutz, W. (1967). *Joy: Expanding human awareness.* New York: Grove Press.

Seashore, C. (1970). What is sensitivity training? In R. Golembiewski & A. Blumberg (Eds.), *Sensitivity training and the laboratory approach: Readings about concepts and applications.* Itasca, IL: F. E. Peacock.

Stogdill, R. (1974). *Handbook of leadership.* New York: Free Press.

Stoller, F. (1967). The long weekend. *Psychology Today, 1,* 28–33.

Vitalo, R. (1971). Teaching improved interpersonal functioning as a preferred mode of treatment. *Journal of Clinical Psychology, 27,* 166–171.

Weisman, A. (1965). *The existential core of psychoanalysis.* Boston: Little, Brown.

Williamson, J. (1981). Mutual interaction: A model of nursing practice. *Nursing Outlook, 29,* 104–107.

SELECTED READINGS

Two articles written by pioneers in the area of humanistic education are included for further reading. Both discuss humanistic learning philosophy as it was originally developed. Humanism as a philosophy has its roots in educational systems. The essence of these articles, among others, has been synthesized and applied in nursing practice. Practice implies education and the circularity of this process becomes evident. Each article is intended to provide a clearer understanding of the historical development of humanism and its application in our nursing profession.

The Human Side of Learning

Arthur W. Combs

Anyone who doesn't know that education is in deep trouble must have been hiding somewhere for the last fifteen years. Somehow we have lost touch with the times, so we find young people opting out, copping out, and dropping out of the system. The processes of education have become concerned with nonhuman questions, and the system is dehumanizing to the people in it. Earl Kelley once said, "We've got this marvelous school system with beautiful buildings and a magnificent curriculum and these great teachers and these marvelous administrators, and then, damn it all, the parents send us the wrong kids."

For a number of generations now, we have been dealing with learning from a false premise. Most of us are familiar with Pavlov's famous experiment conditioning a dog to respond to a bell. The principles he established then are the ones we still use to deal with the problems of learning in our schools today. But Pavlov's system depended on: 1) separating his dogs from all other dogs, which made the learning process an isolated event; 2) tying his dogs down so that they could only do precisely what he had in mind, a technique not very feasible for most elementary teachers; 3) completely removing the dogs from all other possible sources of stimuli, a hard thing to do in a classroom.

This point of view has taught us to deal with the problem of learning as a question of stimulus and response, to be understood in terms of input and output. Currently it finds its latest expression in behavioral objectives, performance based criteria for learning that systematically demand that you: Establish your objectives in behavioral terms; set up the machinery to accomplish them; and then test whether or not you have achieved them. Such an approach seems straightforward, businesslike, and logical; and that's what is wrong with it. I quote from Earl Kelley again, who once said, "Logic is often only a systematic way of arriving at the wrong answers!"

I'm not opposed to behavioral objectives. Nobody can be against accountability. The difficulty with the concept is that its fundamental premise is only partly right. The fact is that behavioral objectives are useful devices for dealing with the simplest, most primitive aspects of education, the things we already do quite well. Unfortunately, they do not serve so well when they are applied to other kinds of objectives, such as intelligent behavior requiring a creative approach to a problem. Behavioral objectives do not deal with the problem of holistic goals. They do not help us in dealing with the things that make us truly human—the questions of human beliefs, attitudes, feelings, understandings, and concerns—the things we call "affective." Nor do they deal with the problems of self-actualization, citizenship, responsibility, caring, and many other such humanistic goals of educators.

Using this approach, we are evaluating schools and circumstances on the basis of what we know how to test. As a result, we are finding that our educational objectives are being established by default because the things we know how to test are the simplest, smallest units of cognitive procedures, which don't really matter much anyway.

We are spending millions and millions of dollars on this very small aspect of dealing with the educational problem, while the problems of self-concept, human attitudes, feelings, beliefs, meanings, and intelligence are going unexplored.

Although I do not oppose behavioral objectives, I do believe that those who are forcing accountability techniques on us need also to be held accountable for what they are doing to American education.

Performance based criteria is the method of big business, a technique of management, and we are now in the process of applying these industrial techniques to education everywhere. We ought to know better. When industry developed the assembly line and other systematic techniques to increase efficiency, what happened? The workers felt dehumanized by the system and formed unions to fight it. And that is precisely what is happening with our young people today. They feel increasingly dehumanized by the system, so they are fighting it at every possible level. Applying industrial techniques to human problems just won't work. A systems approach, it should be understood, is only a method of making sure you accomplish your objectives. Applied to the wrong objectives, systems approaches only guarantee that your errors will be colossal.

The trouble with education today is not its lack of efficiency, but its lack of humanity. Learning is not a mechanical process, but a *human* process. The whole approach to learning through behavioral objectives concentrates our attention on the simplest, most primitive aspects of the educational endeavor, while it almost entirely overlooks the human values. I believe we can get along better with a person who can't read than with a bigot. We are doing very little to prevent the production of bigots but a very great deal to prevent the production of poor readers.

Learning is a human problem always consisting of two parts. First, we have to provide people with some new information or some new experience, and we know how to do that very well. We are experts at it. With the aid of our new electronic gadgets, we can do it faster and more furiously than ever before in history. Second, the student must discover the meaning of the information provided him. The dropout is not a dropout because we didn't give him information. We told him, but he never discovered what that information meant.

I would like to give an alternate definition to the S–R theory most of us cut our teeth on: Information will affect a person's behavior only in the degree to which he has discovered its personal meaning for him. For example, I read in this morning's paper that there has been an increase in the number of cases of pulmonic stenosis in the state of Florida in the past two years. I don't know what pulmonic stenosis is, so this information has no meaning for me. Later in the day I hear a friend talking about pulmonic stenosis, so I look it up and find that it's a disorder that produces a closing up of the pulmonary artery. It's a dangerous disorder, and it produces blue babies. Now I know what it is, but it still doesn't affect my behavior very much. Later in the day I received a letter from a mother of one of my students who says, "Dear Teacher, we have taken Sally to the clinic, where we learned that she has got pulmonic stenosis, and she's going to have to be operated on when she reaches adolescence. In the meantime, we would appreciate it if you would keep an eye out for her."

This information has more meaning to me now because it's happening to one of my students, and my behavior reflects that meaning. I protect the girl, and I talk to other people on the faculty: "Did you hear about Sally? Isn't it a shame? She's got pulmonic stenosis. Poor child, she's going to have to be operated on."

Let's go one step further. Suppose I have just learned that my daughter has pulmonic stenosis. Now this information affects my behavior tremendously, in every aspect of my daily life.

This explains why so much of what we do

in school has no effect on students. Sometimes we even discourage them from finding the personal meaning of a piece of information. We say, "Eddie, I'm not interested in what you think about that, what does the book say?" which is the same as telling him that school is a place where you learn about things that don't matter.

What do we need to do, then, if we're going to humanize the business of learning? We have to see the whole problem of learning differently. We have to give up our preoccupation with objectivity. In our research at the University of Florida, we find that objectivity correlates negatively with effectiveness in the helping professions we have so far explored.

Freud once said that no one ever does anything unless he would rather. In other words, no one ever does anything unless he thinks it is important. So the first thing we must do to humanize learning is to believe it is important.

Let me tell you another story by way of illustration. In the suburbs of Atlanta there was a young woman teaching first grade who had beautiful long blonde hair which she wore in a pony tail down to the middle of her back. For the first three days of the school year she wore her hair that way. Then, on Thursday she decided to do it up in a bun on top of her head. One of the little boys in her class looked into the room and didn't recognize his teacher. He was lost. The bell rang, school started, and he didn't know where he belonged. He was out in the hall crying. The supervisor asked him, "What's the trouble?" and he said, "I can't find my teacher." She said, "Well, what's your teacher's name? What room are you in?" He didn't know. So she said, "Well, come on, let's see if we can find her." They started down the hall together, the supervisor and the little boy, hand-in-hand, opening one door after another without much luck until they came to the room where this young woman was teaching. As they stood there in the doorway, the teacher turned and saw them and she said, "Why, Joey, it's good to see you. We've been wondering where you were. Come on in. We've missed you." And the

little boy pulled away from the supervisor and threw himself into the teacher's arms. She gave him a hug, patted him on the fanny, and he ran to his seat. She knew what was important. She thought little boys were important.

Suppose the teacher hadn't thought little boys were important. Suppose, for instance, she thought supervisors were important. Then she would have said, "Why good morning, Miss Smith. We're so glad you've come to see us, aren't we boys and girls?" And the little boy would have been ignored. Or the teacher might have thought the lesson was important, in which case she would have said, "Joey, for heaven's sake, where have you been? You're already two pages behind. Come in here and get to work." Or she might have thought that discipline was important, and said, "Joey, you know very well when you're late you must go to the office and get a permit. Now run and get it." But she didn't. She thought little boys were important. And so it is with each of us. We have to believe humanizing learning is important.

To humanize learning we must also recognize that people don't behave according to the facts of a situation, they behave in terms of their beliefs. In the last presidential election, those who thought that the Democrats would save us and the Republicans would ruin us voted for the Democrats. And those who thought the Republicans would save us and the Democrats would ruin us voted for the Republicans. Each of us behaved not in terms of "the facts," but in terms of our beliefs. A fact is only what we believe is so. Sensitivity to the beliefs of the people we work with is basic to effective behavior. In our research on the helping professions, we found the outstanding characteristic of effective helpers was that the good ones are always concerned with how things look from the point of view of the people they are working with.

Let me give another illustration of what I mean by being aware of the other person's point of view. A supervisor and a teacher were talking about a little boy: "I don't know what to do with him," the teacher said. "I know that he can do it;

I tell him, 'It's easy, Frank, you can do it' but he won't even try." The supervisor said, "Don't ever tell a child something is easy. Look at it from the child's point of view. If you tell him it's easy and he can't do it, he can only conclude that he must be stupid, and if he can do it, you have robbed it of all its thrill! Tell him it's hard, that you know it's hard, but you're pretty sure he can do it. Then if he can't do it, he hasn't lost face, and if he can do it, what a glory that is for him."

So much of what we do in teaching is not concerned with people. It is concerned with rules, regulations, order, and neatness. I visited a school some years ago, and as I sat in the principal's office one of the bus drivers came in with a little boy in one hand and a broken arm from one of the seats of the bus in the other hand. How did this principal behave? He became very angry. It was as if the little boy had broken the principal's arm. And, in a sense, the boy had, I suppose.

In contrast to that, I am reminded of a visit I made to a school in Michigan. As I walked down the hall with the principal, a teacher and a group of children came out of one of the rooms of this very old building. We walked into the room and saw that it was in complete havoc. The principal said, "It's a mess isn't it? And it can stay that way. That teacher has raised the reading level of her classes by two grades every year she's had them. If that's the way she wants to teach, it's all right with me!"

We walked along to the gymnasium and looked in. He said as we looked at the floor, "That's the third finish we've had on that floor this year. We use it in the evenings for family roller skating!" There is a man whose values are clear. He is more concerned with people than things.

There are hundreds of ways we dehumanize people in our schools, and we need to make a systematic attempt to get rid of them.

In *Crisis in the Classroom*, Charles Silberman says that he believes one of the major problems in American schools is "mindlessness." We do so many things without having the slightest idea of why we're doing them. One dehumanizing element is the grading system. Grades motivate very few people, nor are they good as an evaluative device. Everyone knows that no two teachers evaluate people in exactly the same terms. Yet we piously regard grades as though they all mean the same thing, under the same circumstances, to all people at all times.

I remember my son coming home from college and asking, "Dad, how can you, as an educator, put up with the grading system? Grading on the curve makes it to my advantage to destroy my friends. Dad, that's a hell of a way to teach young people to live." I'd never thought of it that way before.

Another thing we need to understand is the serious limitation of competition as a motivational system. Psychologists know three things about motivation:

1. The only people who are motivated by competition are those who think they can win. And that's not very many. Everyone else sits back and watches them beat their brains out.

2. People who do not feel they have a chance of winning and are forced to compete are not motivated. They are discouraged and disillusioned by the process, and we cannot afford a discouraged and disillusioned populace.

3. When competition becomes too important, morality breaks down, and any means becomes justified to achieve the ends—the basketball team begins to use its elbows and students begin to cheat on exams.

Grade level and grouping is another mindless obstacle to humanizing. All the research we have on grouping tells us that no one method of grouping is superior to any other. And yet we go right on, in the same old ways, insisting that we must have grade levels. As a result, we might have an eleven-year-old child in the sixth grade reading at the third-grade level. Every day of his life we feed him a diet of failure because we can't find a way to give a success experience to such a child.

If we want to humanize the processes of learning, we must make a systematic search for the things that destroy effective learning and remove them from the scene. If we're going to humanize the processes of learning, we must take the student in as a partner. Education wouldn't be irrelevant if students had a voice in decision making. One of my friends once said that the problem of American education today is that "all of us are busy providing students with answers to problems they don't have yet." And that's true. We decide what people need to know and then we teach it to them whether they need it or not. As a result some students discover that school is a place where you study things that don't matter and so they drop out. It's intelligent to drop out. If it isn't getting you anywhere, if it doesn't have any meaning, if it doesn't do something for you, then it's intelligent to drop out. But we seldom think of it that way. Most of us regard the dropout as though there is something wrong with him.

Part of making education relevant to the student is allowing him to develop responsibility for his own learning. But responsibility can only be learned from having responsibility, never from having it withheld. The teacher who says, "You be good kids while I'm out of the room" is an example of what I'm talking about. When she comes back the room is bedlam. "I'll never leave you alone again," she says. By this pronouncement she has robbed the children of any opportunity to learn how to behave responsibly on their own.

Not long ago, I arrived at a school just after the election for student body president, and the teachers were upset because the student who was elected president had run on a platform of no school on Friday, free lunches, free admissions to the football games, and a whole string of other impossible things. The teachers thought it was "a travesty on democracy" and suggested that the student body have another election. I said, "If you do that, how are these kids ever going to discover the terrible price you have to pay for electing a jackass to office?"

We know that what a person believes about himself is crucial to his growth and development. We also know that a person learns this self-concept from the way he is treated by significant people in his life. The student takes his self-concept with him wherever he goes. He takes it to Latin class, to arithmetic class, to gym class, and he takes it home with him. Wherever he goes, his self-concept goes, too. Everything that happens to him has an effect on his self-concept.

Are we influencing that self-concept in positive or negative ways? We need to ask ourselves these kinds of questions. How can a person feel liked unless somebody likes him? How can a person feel wanted unless somebody wants him? How can a person feel acceptable unless someone accepts him? How can a person feel he's a person with dignity and integrity unless somebody treats him so? And how can a person feel that he is capable unless he has some success? In the answers to those questions, we'll find the answers to the human side of learning.

Humanistic Education

Alfred S. Alschuler

In the Symposium, Alcibiades praised Socrates by saying, "He is exactly like the busts of (the god) Silenus which are set up in the statuaries' shops, holding pipes and flutes in their mouths; they open in the middle and have images of gods inside them. When I opened him (Socrates) and looked within at his serious purpose, I saw divine and golden images of such fascinating beauty that I was ready to do in a moment whatever Socrates commanded." Silenus was a minor Greek deity, a follower of Dionysus, disconcertedly homely, and nearly human. Usually he was seen drunk, sitting precariously on the back of an ass, yet he was renowned for the unsurpassed wisdom and knowledge of past and future that emerged, as with Socrates, in any dialogue. Silenus was a popular god, for he symbolized the universal desire to be discovered and valued for one's inner virtues. All of us want to be a Silenus and to have our Alcibiades. "His words are ridiculous when you first hear them," continues Alcibiades, "but he who opens the bust and sees what is within will find that they are the only words which have a meaning in them, and also the most divine, abounding in fair images of virtue and extending to the whole duty of a good and honorable man." As Humanistic Educators, we are Alcibiades for our students, opening them up, discovering their inner virtues and drawing forth (literally, "educating") the "good and honorable man."

Only a small number of events in a lifetime radically change the way a person lives—a deeply religious experience, getting married or divorced, having a child, the death of parents, involvement in a serious accident. These dramatic, singular events transform a person's outlook, relation to others and view of himself. By comparison, daily learning experiences in school are undramatic, regularized and designed to promote steady, small increments in external knowledge rather than rapid changes in motives, values and relationships. Obviously we do not want to create regular apocalyptic events that drastically change students' personal lives. However, the ultimate teaching goal of Humanistic Education is to develop effective strategies and humane technology for educating inner strengths as profoundly as these rare life-changing events.

UNIQUELY HUMAN LEARNING

Inchoate work in Humanistic Education exists. Scattered across the United States a handful of individuals working in isolated independence have created programmatic approaches to the discovery and enhancement of inner strengths. These Humanistic Education courses respond directly to previously unanswered student questions about setting goals, clarifying values, forming identify, increasing their sense of personal efficacy and having more satisfying relationships with others. The array of humanistic education courses include training in: achievement motivation, awareness and excitement, creative thinking, interpersonal sensitivity, affiliation motivation, joy, self reliance, self esteem, self assessment, self renewal, self actualization, self understanding, strength training, development of moral reasoning, value clarification, body awareness, meditative processes and other aspects of ideal adult functioning.* The variety of virtuous sounding titles testifies to the extent of developmental efforts underway, and also reflects the absence of a definitive description of ideal end states. In spite of this diversity, most of these courses share four general goals, in addition to their unique and specific emphases.

First, most courses attempt to develop a person's *imagination* by using procedures that encourage a constructive dialogue with one's fantasy life. In Synectics training, a creativity course, students are asked to "make the strange familiar" by fantasizing themselves inside a strange object, or to "make the familiar strange" by fantasizing about a common object. In other creativity courses, remote associations are encouraged in order to attain a new, useful and creative perspective on some problem. In other courses, students are taken on guided tours of day dreams and night dreams and on fantasy trips into their own body. In achievement motivation courses, students are encouraged to fantasize about doing things exceptionally well and are taught how to differentiate between achievement imagery and plain old task imagery. Later in the course, these achievement images are tied to reality through careful planning and projects. These procedures often bring previously ignored aspects of one's personality into awareness. Usually this is a joyful, enhancing experience in contrast to psychoanalytic dream analysis and free association, which are oriented to uncovering unconscious conflicts. The implication is that most adults don't make constructive use of their fantasy life and have forgotten how to enjoy fantasy in a childlike but healthy way.

Second, most courses try to develop better *communication skills* by using non-verbal exercises, such as silent theater improvisations, free expression dance movements, meditation, the exaggeration of spontaneous body movements and a wide variety of games. In sensitivity training and encounter groups, non-verbal exercises are used to increase channels of communication. Some personal feelings can be expressed more effectively in motions than in words. Other times, dance and theater improvisations are used because they increase one's expressive vocabulary and are simply joyful experiences. As with constructive fantasizing, proponents of these methods believe that this type of expression, communication and learning is underdeveloped in most people.

A third goal common to these courses is to develop and explore individuals' *emotional responses* to the world. In most courses, how people feel is considered more important than what they think about things. Without these emotional experiences, ranging from laughter and exhilaration to tears and fear, the teacher is likely to consider the course a failure. For example, if an adolescent is scaling a cliff in an Outward Bound course and does not feel any fear, he will not increase his self confidence through his accomplishment. In Achievement Motivation courses, strong group feelings are developed to help support the individual in whatever he chooses to do well. In all of these courses, there is a shared belief that affect increases meaningful learning and that the capacity for the full range of affective responses is a crucial human potentiality often underdeveloped in adults. As a

*Descriptions of a number of these courses along with a comprehensive bibliography are contained in *New Directions in Psychological Education*, A. S. Alschuler, *Educational Opportunities Forum*, whole issue, January, 1970, State Education Department, Albany, New York. The three most well developed sets of curriculum materials exist for: (1) *Teaching Achievement Motivation*, by A. S. Alschuler, D. Tabor, J. McIntyre, Education Ventures, Inc., Middletown, Connecticut, 1970; (2) "Urban Affairs and Communications," T. Borton and N. Newberg, specialists in Humanistic Education, Philadelphia Board of Education Building, Philadelphia, Pa.; (3) "Value Clarification," see *Values and Teaching*, L. Raths, M. Harmon, S. Simon, Columbus, Ohio: Charles Merrill Books, 1966.

result, a wide range of techniques to enhance affect have been created.*

A fourth goal emphasizes the importance of *living fully and intensely* "here and now." The emphasis takes many forms. In Gestalt awareness training, the goal is philosophically explicit. In most courses, it is subtle and implicit. Usually courses are held in retreat settings which cut people off from past obligations and future commitments for brief periods of time. The isolated resort settings dramatize the "here and now" opportunities. In general there is little emphasis on future "homework" or past personal history as an explanation for behavior. A vivid example is Synanon, a total environment program for drug addicts, which promotes "self actualization," and in the process cures addiction. Synanon requires the addict to kick drugs immediately upon entering the program. Other "bad" behavior which stands in the way of self actualization is pointed out as it occurs. Historical explanations for bad behavior are considered excuses and are not tolerated. In other Humanistic Education programs, the games, exercises, group process, etc., are model opportunities to explore, discover, and try out new behavior here and now. The assumption is that if a person can't change "here and now," where the conditions for growth are optimal, he is not likely to continue growing outside and after the course.

The existing procedures for developing new thinking, action and feelings in the "here and now" constitute humane methods for educating inner strengths. These methods make it possible to create, without trauma, the sequence of uniquely human learning that occurs during and after rare, dramatic, life-changing events.

In most of these naturally occurring events there is a strong focus of attention on what is

happening "here and now." Whether it is a mother's labor during birth, the taking of marriage vows, the shock of realizing your arm is broken, or the ecstasy of a religious vision, the intensity of that experience crowds out familiar reactions. One characteristic that sets these experiences apart is the simultaneous intensity of radically new thoughts, actions and feelings. Usually these experiences break established relationships, as when a parent dies. Often they disrupt habitual patterns of living, or dissolve longtime beliefs. Whether the experience is revelatory or traumatic in nature, it breaks basic continuities in a person's life. After the peak of the experience is passed, there is a period of some confusion and puzzlement, during which the person attempts to make sense out of what happened and to establish meaningful new continuities. This attempt takes many forms, from conversation with friends to meditation and prayer. Even if the experience is never fully understood, in time the consequences become clearer—how relationships are altered, what goals and values are different, and what new behaviors occur. After a while these changes seem more familiar and practiced. For example, new roles become less confusing. As the newness of being a parent wears off, the role becomes an integral part of a person's life, with its own rich set of relationships, behaviors and meanings. Similarly, in time, the traumatic loss of a loved one results in new relationships, behaviors and meanings that we internalize in our way of living.

This sequence of learning can be conceptualized as a six-step process and used as a guideline in planning Humanistic Education courses and sequencing existing humanistic procedures.

1. Focus attention on what is happening here and now by creating moderate novelty that is slightly different from what is expected.

2. Provide an intense, integrated experience of the desired new thoughts, actions and feelings.

---

*Human Relations Education: A Guidebook to Learning Activities, prepared by the Human Relations Project of Western New York, reprinted by the University of the State of New York, the State Education Department, Curriculum Development Center, Albany, New York, 1969.

3. Help the person make sense out of his experience by attempting to conceptualize what happened.

4. Relate the experience to the person's values, goals, behavior and relationships with others.

5. Stabilize the new thought, action and feelings through practice.

6. Internalize the changes.

This teaching strategy is not simply a heuristic device. A considerable amount of support for the validity of these guidelines exists in the theoretical and empirical research literature on personality change.*

This strategy indicates a number of ways that Humanistic Education differs from more traditional academic training. The most effective way to proceed through this learning sequence is to set aside a large block of time, often as long as a week or more, in a special location for a concentrated workshop. The untypical setting helps create moderate novelty, reduces distractions and helps focus attention on the new experiences. The concentrated time period is needed to allow the participants to follow new thoughts, to try out new behavior and to stick with their feelings to a natural conclusion. *Emotions*, in contrast to *thoughts*, tend to be non-reversible and difficult to stop quickly at the end of a 45-minute class period. This inhibits the expression of feelings, just as longer time periods encourage the expression of feelings. In this sense, Humanistic Education is experience based and inductive, in contrast to

academic learning—which tends to be more abstract, logical and deductive.

A less obvious difference is the integration and simultaneous development of thoughts, feelings, and actions. Learning achievement motivation, for example, involves developing a specific cognitive pattern of planning, a special type of excitement and a set of related action strategies. Most normal learning situations differ by rewarding expertise as a "thinker" in academic courses, or as a doer in physical courses like vocational education or athletics. This makes it especially difficult for teachers to be concerned in practice with educating the "whole child." However, there is some justification for the way schooling fragments human functioning into component parts. It does prepare students for adult lives in which separate role performances are played out in many directions. Just as students move from class to class during the day, adults move from role to role. We work in one place, have our intimate, loving relationships in another place, and usually travel to still other places for recreation. In each role adults are known for a narrow set of behaviors, just as students are known by their teachers as a math student, or typing student and rarely as a complex, many-sided individual. Experience-based learning integrates human functioning in the service of balanced maturation.

The art and technology of Humanistic Education, in large part, lies in the creation of productive learning experiences. Only the outlines of this technology are clear at this time. Teachers must be insightful diagnosticians of children's experience, so that moderately novel situations can be created. These situations bridge the gap between where the child is and where he can be. Thus, teachers must know a wide range of Humanistic Education procedures and be knowledgeable about the goals of human development. This expertise allows them to help students conceptualize, relate and apply their new experiential knowledge. Few learning experiences require extensive hardware and materials. Most procedures involve the person in

---

*The most relevant summaries of this literature can be found in D. C. McClelland, "Toward a Theory of Motive Acquisition," *American Psychologist*, May, 1965; D. C. McClelland and D. G. Winter, *Motivating Economic Achievement*, Free Press, 1969; Campbell, J., Dunnette, M., "Effectiveness of T-Group Experience in Managerial Training and Development," *Psychological Bulletin*, August, 1968, pp. 73–104.

relation to his own body, feelings and imagination or in relation to his environment and other people. A comprehensive source book of humanistic methods would be useful, but ultimately each teacher must adapt and sequence these methods to create the course of learning, i.e., the curriculum. In this sense, curriculum innovation is constant, and Humanistic Educators need to become adept at improvising sequences of learning that lead to internalization.

Compared to typical school goals, Humanistic Education courses aim for long-term internalization, not short-term gains in mastery. More precisely, these courses attempt to increase "operant" behavior as well as respondent behavior. Operant behavior is voluntary, seemingly spontaneous and certainly not required by the situation. What a person does with his leisure time is an indication of his operant behavior. Respondent behavior requires external cues and incentives before it will occur, just as an examination question brings forth respondent knowledge that otherwise probably would not have been demonstrated. In practice, most school learning calls for respondent behavior: multiple choice and true-false questions, reading assigned chapters, solving a given set of mathematics problems correctly, or writing an essay to a prescribed theme. To be most meaningful to a student, Humanistic Education must result in operant, internalized behavior, since after the course is over there will not be anyone to follow him around defining the problems, presenting the alternatives, guiding the response and evaluating the results. Paradoxically, the most important thing to do in helping a person develop long-term operant behavior is to stop doing anything. Support must be gradually transferred from external sources to the person's own inner resources. The problem is to leave on time—not too soon, because guidance is needed in the early phases, and not too late because that retards essential self reliance. At the present time, staging perfectly timed exits is an art in need of becoming a technology.

HUMANIZING SCHOOLS

Educating the "good and honorable man" is a ubiquitous aim of schooling. The problem is not the legitimacy of humanistic goals for public education, but how to translate these goals fully into practice. Specifically, it is unethical to develop students' ability to relate more warmly and directly their achievement motivation, their capacity for creative thinking through Humanistic Education courses, and then send them back into normal classrooms where these processes are not functional. For example, many Humanistic Education courses teach people how to develop collaborative and trusting relationships. Only in schools are there so few structured opportunities for practicing team-work and cooperation. From the humanistic point of view, the way people learn is just as important as what they learn. Ideally, there should be at least as much variety in the teaching-learning process within a single school as exists outside and after school, where students are variously required, ordered, coached, coaxed, persuaded, led, followed, threatened, promised, lectured, questioned, joined, challenged and left alone. Compared to this handsome array of naturally occurring learning processes, the typical range within a school is embarrassingly narrow. As Humanistic Education courses are introduced in schools, corresponding new processes should be available in regular courses in order for students to *practice what they have learned.*

How students learn is determined in large part by the rules of the implicit learning game and the teacher's leadership style. Both rules and leadership styles can be modified easily, although these methods of changing the processes of learning generally are not used. One of the first errors made by teachers who decide to increase the number of alternative learning processes is to decrease the number of rules and amount of teacher leadership, because this seems to decrease authoritarianism while increasing the possibility of many types of student initiative and learning styles. The key to a systematic variation in learning processes, however, is not how many rules and directions, but *what kind.* For example, such highly rule-governed activities as baseball and square dancing are non-authoritarian, and stimulate specific human processes. A variety of desired learning processes can be aroused by changing the rules which govern the nature of the scoring system, the type of obstacles to success and how decisions about strategy and tactics are made.* Implementing a variety of "learning games" requires of teachers great flexibility and repertoire of personal styles; they must have actualized many of the "divine and golden images" within themselves.

Just as it is unethical to develop inner strengths in students and put them into classrooms with a narrow range of legitimate learning styles, so too is it unethical to expect this flexibility within teachers or among a school faculty in a school that does not encourage, support and reward this variety. Ultimately, the administrative style, rules and rewards in a whole school must implement a pluralistic philosophy of education. The task of humanizing schools is, of necessity, multi-leveled and holistic.

The technology of planned change in schools is just now emerging. As recently as 1965 there was only one book devoted exclusively to the problem. Since then, the Office of Education and the National Training Laboratories have sponsored a large-scale investigation of how to increase innovation in teaching, learning and human relations at all levels in school systems—The Cooperative Project for Educational Development (COPED). The results of COPED suggest a four-phased strategy

for maximizing the likelihood of effectively introducing Humanistic Education in a school.†

1. *Selection.* The top administrator and other key decision makers should be committed in principle to innovation in advance of specific training programs. Representatives from all groups within the school should be eligible for the special training programs.

2. *Diagnosis.* Organizational strengths and weaknesses need to be assessed. This can be done most effectively through interviews with potential participants prior to the major change efforts. Information is obtained on such factors as the reward system, rules, communication patterns, current school issues and individual goals. Often it helps if these data are shared with the school system in a "diagnostic workshop." The purpose of this collaborative meeting is to further clarify the problem and place priorities on the goals of change.

3. *Introductory Training.* A training program is designed to meet the defined needs. This workshop introduces the members of the school to relevant aspects of Humanistic Education. The workshop follows the six-step sequence described earlier. During the final phase, the school is encouraged to select an ongoing "change management team" with representatives from all groups in the school.

4. *Follow Through.* After the initial training the aim is to build into the school system a permanent team of self-sufficient change management experts and well-trained Humanistic Educators. The "change management team" coordinates this development, and conscientiously supports the introduction of Humanistic Education. These changes can be accomplished through internal task forces, additional specialized training or a variety of organizational

---

*For a complete explication of this position see "The Effects of Classroom Structure on Motivation and Performance," A. S. Alschuler, *Educational Technology*, August, 1969, and "Motivation in the Classroom," Chapter 3 in *Teaching Achievement Motivation*, A. Alschuler, D. Tabor, J. McIntyre, Education Ventures, Inc., Middletown, Connecticut, 1970.

†Based on a private conversation with Dr. Dale G. Lake, Director of COPED and editor of the *COPED, Final Report*, April, 1970, ERIC Files, U.S. Office of Education, Division of Research.

development services from outside consultants. To start the "follow through," the team is encouraged to implement a high visibility project likely to succeed.

This strategy for change differs markedly from traditional approaches through graduate school teacher education and curriculum reform. It more closely resembles the creation of a Research and Development group within a corporation. This comparison highlights the fact that businesses often spend as much as 10–15% of their budget on R & D activities whereas the typical corresponding allocation by schools is less than 1%. The absence of this strong coordinating group in schools vitiates the effectiveness of "new curricula" and restricts the influence of well-trained new teachers. The creation of an effective change management team coordinates and internalizes curriculum innovation within the school.

Although the existence of this coordinating group does facilitate changes in the character of schooling, it does not guarantee perfect guidance towards ultimate human goals. For instance, some teachers make humanistic methods ends in themselves. The use of game simulations and role playing, ipso facto, is considered good. Creativity training courses are endorsed whether or not the problems to be solved are meaningful. Courses in Theater Improvisation are introduced to develop non-verbal behavior independent of significant personal relationships and goals. As a result, these courses and methods often fail precisely in what they are trying to accomplish. Strengthening imagination simply becomes bizarre fantasizing; a narrow focus on feelings leads to misunderstanding; exclusive attention to non-verbal communication stimulates anti-intellectual distrust of rational, goal-directed behavior.

Major advances in Humanistic Education are not likely to come simply from the proliferation of methods, training, teacher-curriculum-developers or the creation of self-renewing schools, although each of these tasks is worthy. We need guiding visions of the "good and honorable man" and utopian models for the places where we live. Human abilities are strengthened, integrated, balanced and given meaning only in the pursuit of these goals. The essentially heuristic value of these unattainable ideals is conveyed in the word "Utopia," a pun made by Thomas More on "Eutopia" (good place) and "Outopia" (no place). In the last century, over 200 utopian communities were started—and none has survived. The longest-lived utopian communities are those which face the question of life and death daily (kibbutzim, Synanon) or which surround a single charismatic leader (Ashrams with their gurus) or those which share an ultimate faith (Amish, Oneida). In the United States, most of us no longer face daily life–death issues. We are surrounded by anti-heroes, who command our sympathy by their stand against those public figures who would be our gurus. Ultimate faith is being replaced by immediate action concerns against visible injustice and for personal pleasure. This is reflected in our schools, where pluralistic demands for innovation often mask the loss of an ultimate sense of mission.

The consequences of this value crisis are to leave key ethical questions unanswered for all types of education: What kind of teaching and subject matter is in the best interests of students? Who is to decide? How? How do you know when a teacher is competent? How do you know when teaching is effective, ineffective, or negative? Choices about what new curricula to develop, how to train teachers, what kinds of learning outcomes to assess and how best to humanize schooling depend on answers to these ethical questions. Obviously, there is no single set of definitive conclusions; but, instead, there is the opportunity for all educators to engage in a uniquely human search for values. The continuing attempt to discover "divine and golden images" and to draw forth the "good and honorable man" is the mission of Humanistic Education.

Epilogue

The Golden Helping Rule

Whenever you feel unable to respond to a client;
Whenever you do not know what to say;
Whenever you want to help but do not know
        what would be helpful . . .

Place yourself in the client's world;
Be in that time and space;
Ask yourself the questions asked you;
Feel what you think the client feels. . . .

Then say what you would like to hear;
Do what you would like to have done.

                    Elaine Lynne La Monica

Humanistic Exercises*

Nursing: A Helping Profession

Exercise 16   Getting Acquainted and
Ice-Breaking

Exercise 17   Getting Acquainted and
Ice-Breaking

Exercise 18   Thoughts and Feelings

Exercise 19   Thoughts and Feelings

Exercise 20   Philosophy and Values

Exercise 21   Philosophy and Values

Exercise 22   Desires and Goals:
What I Want in Nursing

Exercise 23   Behaviors

Exercise 24   Behaviors

Exercise 25   Experiences

Exercise 26   Experiences

Exercise 27   Body Expression

Exercise 28   Body Expression

Exercise 29   Self: My Nursing Shield

---

*Jointly created and designed by Elaine L. La Monica and
Eunice M. Parisi-Carew. These exercises follow the
aspects of the PELLEM Pentagram, discussed in Chapter
17.

Exercise 16

Getting Acquainted and Ice-Breaking

Purposes	1. To introduce the participants to each other.
	2. To begin formation of the group.
	3. To establish an atmosphere conducive to humanistic learning.
Facility	Large room.
Materials	None.
Time Required	One hour.
Group Size	Unlimited groups of two.
Design	1. Pair group members, including self.
	2. Request that pair members share information about themselves with each other—thoughts, experiences, backgrounds, goals, hobbies, and so forth (20 minutes).
	3. Form large group.
	4. Ask each member of each pair to introduce the other to the rest of the class.
	5. Provide an overview of the course to the entire class.
Variations	1. Have members wear name tags on which they have only drawn a picture. Instruct them to mill around and find a partner. Then proceed with design.
	2. Use adjectives in the variation above instead of a picture.

Exercise 17

Getting Acquainted and Ice-Breaking

Purposes	1. To facilitate development of positive group-member relationships. 2. To create an atmosphere of openness and sharing. 3. To encourage self-expression.
Facility	Large room (with tables or carpeted floor) to accommodate class size and extra space for working.
Materials	Construction paper Scissors Magazines Paste Crayons Assorted media
Time Required	One hour.
Group Size	Unlimited groups of six.
Design	1. Using the materials provided, ask each individual to develop a collage that represents a self-portrait (20 minutes). 2. In groups of six, have everyone share their collages, telling what each item means, how their feelings, beliefs, and so forth are represented in the design (20 minutes). 3. Discuss the experience in the total group.
Variations	1. This exercise can be done with any media available or just with crayons and paper. 2. A second collage can be done on a self-portrait as a nurse, comparing the two in a group discussion.

Exercise 18

Thoughts and Feelings

Purposes
1. To identify feelings aroused in the course of one's work.
2. To form a composite of feelings that gives an indication of the emotional climate and attitudes one faces in the nursing profession.

Facility
A room large enough for groups of five to talk without disturbing one another.

Materials
Crayons—assorted colors for each participant
Paper—36" × 24".

Time Required
45 minutes.

Group Size
Unlimited groups of five—preferably at least ten participants in all.

Design
CONCEPT LIST

helping	life	client
death	doctor	hospital
baccalaureate degree	nursing history	NLN
professionalism	dedication	ANA
nurse	associate degree	education
uniform	community	discharge
Florence Nightingale	sacrifice	client

1. Each participant has assorted colored crayons and papers. Participants are told that the purpose of the exercise is to identify the feelings that are constantly flowing within them at work.
2. Twelve (or more) concepts are going to be read aloud slowly, with a pause between each word. The participant is to identify the major feeling he or she has when thinking of that word. Then the person is to choose a color and draw with it. All word "responses" are done on a single paper, forming a collage.
3. Upon completion, the participants are given some time to reflect upon their product, its major characteristics, meaning, and use of colors.
4. Request that individuals share their collages in five-person groups.

5. Have each person speak out to the large group the one or two words that best represent their emotional state while they are at work in a clinical agency.

6. Discuss the experience.

Variations

1. Mill around, holding collages in view. Find one or two others whose collages strike you in a particular way. Discuss your collages together.

2. Mill around, holding collages in view. Find the one or two persons whose collages are most dissimilar to yours. Share the differences and their meaning.

Exercise 19

Thoughts and Feelings

Purpose
: To identify the thoughts and feelings generated by particular nursing situations.

Facility
: A room large enough for groups of five to converse without disturbing others or being disturbed.

Materials
: Paper, pencils/pens.

Time Required
: 45 minutes or longer.

Group Size
: Unlimited groups of five.

Stories
:
1. It is 8 P.M. in the Emergency Room. The telephone call a few minutes ago said the ambulance is on its way. There has been an automobile accident: one dead and two injured. The ambulance arrives. I meet it at the door. I feel _____

_____

_____ .

I think _____

_____

_____ .

I do _____

_____

_____ .

2. I have been working in Room 310 for three hours with no break. The light in 311 goes on. I walk in _____

_____

_____ .

3. Ms. R., age 25, is scheduled to leave at 11 A.M. today. She has recovered from a panhysterectomy. It is my task to discharge her. I enter the room _____

_____

_____ .

4. It is noon. All clients are having lunch. I am waiting to go to the cafeteria. The loud speaker comes on: "Code Blue, cardiac intensive care." I feel _____

_____

_____ .

I think _____

_____

_____ .

I do _____

_____

_____ .

Design

1. The participants are informed of the goal of the exercise and are instructed as to the nature of the experience. They are told to complete a story using the first person—"I"—approach. Focus should be on what they think, feel, and would do in response to the situation. This assists in realizing the differences and interrelatedness of the three experiences.

2. Read one or two situations to the participants, allowing them ten minutes to finish a story.

3. Divide into groups of five to share the stories, with all the drama the participants desire.

4. After sharing, have them discuss in small groups the similarities and differences in thoughts and feelings among persons and how the feelings could affect their behavior during each situation.

5. The process can be repeated with each story if desired.

6. Discuss the experience.

Variations

1. The facilitator writes a nursing-focused story, leaving out all adjectives and descriptive words. These are to be filled in by the participants and discussed.

2. Within small groups, a couple of volunteers each write situations from their own experiences similar to the examples given. The other participants finish the stories as they would respond personally. These are then shared and compared with the writer's experience.

3. Give the participants all four situations, of which they are to choose one to finish. In the sharing, ask them to explain why they chose that particular one.

Discussion

Thoughts and feelings may have an impact on how you behave, as well as your relationship to self, other staff members, and clients.

Exercise 20

Philosophy and Values

Purposes	1. To identify what nursing means to each participant.
	2. To identify any generalization among nurses as to what values underlie the profession.
Facility	A room large enough for groups of five to converse undisturbed.
Materials	None.
Time Required	One hour.
Group Size	Unlimited groups of five. A minimum of ten is preferable for the entire group.
Design	1. Each participant is to lie on the floor and relax, breathing deeply.
	2. The facilitator asks the participants to think back to when they first felt like nurses.
	a. When was it?
	b. What did it feel like?
	c. What did it mean to feel like a nurse?
	Time should be provided to have participants be able to appreciate the experience fully.
	3. After individually responding to the questions above, groups of five or the total group should form to devise a consensual list as to what the underlying values are.
	4. Participants should compare their own lists to the consensual one and think about some of the following questions.
	a. How similar or different is it?
	b. Does this say anything about me? If so, what does it say?
	c. When is the last time I felt like a nurse?
	d. Do I feel like a nurse all the time? When do I and when don't I?
	e. Do we as a group have a value system or philosophy of nursing? Does it match what is written in nursing history and literature?
Variations	Ask participants whether the feelings of being a nurse have changed since the first time they thought of themselves as nurses. Have the participants trace the development of these feelings.

Discussion   What happens if we as nurses do not experience what we value? What kind of effect does this have on us? How much room is there for diverse value systems? What are the parameters? Discuss the importance of philosophy and values as a framework and pathway in nursing. It is our philosophy and values that dictate how we work, why we work, and how comfortable and satisfied we are in our journey.

Exercise 21

Philosophy and Values

Purposes	1. To identify the values underlying self as a nurse.
	2. To compare values and philosophies with other nurses.
Facility	A room large enough for groups of eight to converse without disturbance.
Materials	Paper, pencils.
Time Required	45 minutes.
Group Size	Unlimited groups of eight.

Sentence
Completions

1. I am a nurse because _____

_____ .

2. As a nurse I should be _____

_____ .

3. As a nurse I should not _____

_____ .

4. The most important thing for me to remember as a nurse is _____

_____

_____ .

5. I am different from other nurses in that _____

_____

_____ .

6. The one thing all nurses have in common is _____

_____

_____ .

7. The thing I like most about nursing is _____

   _____

   _____ .

8. Some nurses make me angry because _____

   _____

   _____ .

Design

1. Give instructions for participants to complete the eight sentences above. Read them to the group, allowing time for participants to respond thoughtfully.
2. Once these have been completed, the participants should form groups of eight to discuss their responses and identify the similarities and differences between them. After discussion the group is then asked to make generalized statements about nurses and themselves as nurses.
3. Discuss the experience.

Variations

Choose one or two people whom you would expect to have answers very different from yours. Discuss responses, where they came from, and why you expected them to be different.

Discussion

Explore the effect of values on the everyday operation of nursing. Stress the importance of values as a personal framework within which a person functions and a generalized direction or path for the profession. How do great similarities or great discrepancies in values among nurses affect the individual nurse or the "nursing profession"?

Exercise 22

Desires and Goals: What I Want in Nursing

Purposes	1. To discuss the facets of nursing practice that prevent it from being personally fulfilling.
	2. To begin to explore the areas of nursing practice that one may wish to change.
Facility	Large, comfortable room.
Materials	Paper, pen, or pencil.
Time Required	One hour.
Group Size	Groups of six; maximum number of total group, eighteen.

Sentence Completions

1. If there is one thing I would change about myself as a nurse, it would be

   _____

   _____ .

2. If there is one thing I would change about my profession, it would be

   _____

   _____ .

3. In five years I would like to be _____

   _____

   _____ .

4. Nursing is more than _____

   _____ ,

   it is _____

   _____ .

5. An aspect of nursing that is missing for me is _____

   _____

   _____ .

6. In nursing school, the experience is/was _____

   _____

   _____ .

7. Now, nursing is _____

   _____ and I feel _____

   _____ about this.

Design
1. Have participants complete the statements individually.
2. In groups of six, ask members to share their completions one by one. Advise them to react to each other's statements and note significant and/or dissimilar/similar thoughts. Look at how the thoughts evolved and why they are important.
3. Discuss small-group activities.
4. Ask the small groups to come together and form a total group. Have each small group report their significant and similar feelings.
5. Discuss the similarities and differences within the group.
6. Request that individuals think about what they have learned from others in the experience.

Variations
Ask members of the group to add any sentence completions that seem appropriate.

Discussion
To isolate problem areas, one has to discriminate perceived reality from the ideal. This exercise begins to uncover the discrepancy.

Exercise 23
Behaviors

Purposes

1. To find out how others perceive your behavior.
2. To learn possible alternative ways of behaving.

Facility

Room with ample size to sit in dyads without being cramped.

Materials

None.

Time Required

30 minutes.

Group Size

Unlimited dyads.

Design

1. Explain the purpose of this exercise and the importance of feedback from someone who knows you.
2. The participants are asked to form dyads with the person who best knows them.
3. The first person describes to the other how he/she thinks he/she is generally viewed by others. Next, the first person is asked to focus on his/her behavior in situations he/she has a problem handling, then in situations that he/she feels he/she handles well.
4. The partner confirms or denies these self-perceptions. The partner may share the effects of the other's behavior on self. Alternative suggestions for ways of behaving can then be developed by the first person and checked with the partner.
5. The roles are now reversed and the design repeated.
6. Discuss the experience.

Variations

1. Members may meet in larger groups to get a number of perceptions. This is a bit riskier but may give a more valid picture of the person.
2. In dyads, each participant takes a few moments to think not only of self but of the partner. Then the person describes the situations that he/she feels the partner has the most trouble with and the situations that the partner handles well. The partner compares these perceptions with his/her own. These are shared and the discussion reversed.

Discussion

Feedback can be a helping process. Without feedback from others on the effect of one's behavior, one's self-perception may not be accurate. One must work toward an accurate view of how one is affecting others to be successful in reaching one's own ends. In support of these statements people may be encouraged to discuss times when they have been misunderstood.

Exercise 24

Behaviors

Purposes	1. To receive feedback from others in the profession.
	2. To learn some behavioral alternatives to situations.
Facility	A room large enough to allow for milling around of participants. As little furniture as possible is ideal.
Materials	Roles for various participants—if desired. Costumes may be devised.
Time Required	1½ hours.
Group Size	Approximately twenty.

Role-Play Situations

1. A head nurse's or team-conference meeting concerning a client or a particular problem.
   a. Ms. Rudcliff in Room 313 will not take her medicine and is very uncooperative.
   b. The team is in "bad" shape. Colleagues do not help one another. There is no overt hostility; it's just that no one seems to care. This attitude has had an effect on the client. The atmosphere is gloomy. Something has to be done.
2. The same person should star in all three of the following scenes to determine the behavioral differences among situations if they should occur.
   a. Two nurses talking about a client in the client's room.
   b. Two nurses talking about a client while standing in the hall.
   c. Two nurses talking about a client in the parking lot after work.
3. A nurse feeding four clients dinner.

   Client A—impatient, irritable

   Client B—seems lonely, wants to talk

   Client C—extremely concerned about her condition

   Client D—apathetic, does not seem to care about anything, including dinner
4. A student nurse with the instructor and a client. The student is being evaluated by the instructor.

| Design | 1. A participant who wishes to receive feedback is selected to star in a role-play situation. The participant is asked to choose one of the four situations, either the one the person feels most identified with or the one the person feels most distant from. Two stars may be required. |

Design

1. A participant who wishes to receive feedback is selected to star in a role-play situation. The participant is asked to choose one of the four situations, either the one the person feels most identified with or the one the person feels most distant from. Two stars may be required.

2. The supporting cast (all group members) is given a minute to think about the role each person will play. They may portray any attitude or role they desire.

3. The supporting cast's job is to observe the behavior of the star(s) and provide feedback as to its effect, both to the other role players and themselves in their role. If appropriate, more effective ways of behaving can be suggested.

4. The sequence is repeated with new actors or actresses or subsequent stories.

5. Discuss the experience.

Variations

1. Each participant dons a sign bearing key words that describe the person as a practicing nurse. Examples might be: operating room, ICU, staff nurse, supervisor, or student. These signs are to include the position held and area of nursing in which identified. The participants mill around and group with others bearing the same or similar sign. This group makes up a short role-play typifying a situation in which they are likely to be involved. The audience observes, giving feedback to each role player on the effect of the person's behavior on other role players and on the person.

2. Suggestions of more effective ways of behaving may be offered. Feedback may be provided for all role players instead of just the star.

Discussion

Emphasize the importance of knowing how you affect others on the job. Intent may not always match behavior. Stress also the value of developing a trusting support system where honest reactions are a norm.

Exercise 25

Experiences

Purpose
To begin to get in touch with the experiences one has had that have affected the choice of nursing as a profession.

Facility
Large room, preferably with a carpet; if room is not carpeted, participants can be asked to bring their own blankets or towels.

Materials
None.

Time Required
45 minutes to one hour.

Group Size
Groups of three; maximum number of groups depends on size of room.

Design

1. Each participant is asked to lie down on the floor and take several slow, deep breaths.

2. Speaking quietly and slowly, tell participants to gradually turn off everything in their personal worlds and concentrate only on the air they are breathing, their bodies, and the floor on which they rest.

3. After a few minutes of quiet, ask the participants to look back into their history and ponder the following questions. State each in a slow, subdued voice to maintain the mood of oneness with the time, place, and thoughtfulness. Allow time between questions.

4. Questions:

    a. Who was the most impressive nurse you remember in your life?

    b. How old were you when you first met this nurse?

    c. What was the nurse like physically?

    d. What was the nurse like as a person?

    e. What was there about the nurse that impressed you?

    f. Why was the nurse so important in your life?

5. After allowing about fifteen minutes of reminiscence, ask the members to get up and form triads. Instruct them to share their thoughts with the other two members of their groups. You may place these questions on a blackboard or piece of newsprint for easier recall.

6. Following the sharing in triads, ask each group of three to identify any particularly significant or similarly shared experiences.

7. Move into one large group to share and discuss significant or similar factors.

8. Discuss the experience.

Discussion   It is important to become aware of the sets and expectations that nurses have had in their past experiences to enable them to formulate their real goals and rationale in the present framework. The identification and modeling processes are influential in our sociologic development.

Exercise 26
Experiences

Purpose   To look at past experiences that most affected one's practice in nursing.

Facility   Large, comfortable room where people can sit in small groups.

Materials   Drawing paper or newsprint.
                       Crayons or felt-tipped pens.

Time Required   One hour.

Group Size   Unlimited groups of six.

Design   1. Having six participants sit in a circle, instruct them to draw a picture of
                          the most critical experiences they have had in their nursing practice.
                       2. When members are finished, have them share their picture with others
                          in the group. In sharing, have them explain the incident and how they
                          pictured it, discuss why it was critical, and look at how it currently
                          affects them. Other members of the group may react to the incidents.
                       3. Discuss the experience in small groups.

Discussion   Looking at important points in one's career is useful in raising conscious-
                       ness on who a nurse is in the here and now. Discovering incidents that are
                       critical in one's experience may help one formulate reasons for present
                       behavior.

Exercise 27
Body Expression

Purpose	To explore changes in body language when one plays a professional role.
Facility	Large room.
Materials	None.
Time Required	One hour.
Group Size	Unlimited groups of twelve.
Design	1. In the middle of a large circle have participants individually or in pairs act out one of the following scenes:

      a. Strolling on the beach with someone of the opposite sex.

      b. Chatting in the hall with a friend.

      c. Introducing one good friend to another good friend.

    Then have them act out one of the next scenes:

      d. A nurse in a client's room when the client is of the opposite sex.

      e. A nurse speaking with the head nurse.

      f. A nurse on a break in the lounge.

  2. Ask the observers to give feedback to the role players. They should be concerned with the following:

      a. How did the role player use his/her body in the scenes? Were there any differences between the two scenes? What were they?

      b. What changes occurred in the physical being of the role player between scenes? In which did the person appear more comfortable?

  3. Ask the role player to discuss feelings in the two scenes and respond to the feedback.

  4. Discuss the experience.

Discussion	When one gets into a role, one may change. Being aware of the kind of change that may occur is an important consciousness-raising activity.

Exercise 28

Body Expression

Purpose	To develop an image of one's physical self-concept and how one relates through it in nursing practice.
Facility	Large comfortable room.
Materials	Drawing paper or newsprint. Crayons.
Time Required	45 minutes to one hour.
Group Size	Unlimited groups of six.

Design

1. Using paper and crayons, have individuals draw and color a uniform that they feel would best suit their body.
2. In groups of six, have them describe their uniform, the reason for the colors, and their bodies in it. Have them think about and share thoughts related to the following questions:
   a. How does it differ from the uniform I wear?
   b. Why is it me?
   c. What does my body feel like in it?
   d. Why does it most suit me?
   e. Why does it least suit me?
3. Discuss the experience.

Variations

1. Have people draw as described and then draw another picture of what they actually wear while nursing. Compare and share the pictures and what each person feels like in each picture.
2. Ask members to draw the ideal nurse's uniform. Ask what it represents in terms of physical self-image. Share these sketches in small groups.

Discussion

It is important to look at the feelings, values, and the emphasis that one places on a uniform. Clothing is an extension of one's self-concept. Learning and awareness may be derived from exploring the similarities and/or differences between nursing and personal values.

Exercise 29
Self: My Nursing Shield

Purposes

1. To look at the thoughts, feelings, and experiences that developed one's desire to become a nurse.
2. To become aware of one's personal values or philosophy of nursing.
3. To explore one's desires and beliefs in ideal nursing practice.
4. To probe into ways one actually practices while in a nursing position.

Facility

Large room, preferably with small tables.

Materials

Construction paper.
Felt-tipped pens or crayons.

Time Required

One hour.

Group Size

Groups of four; maximum twenty-four.

Design

1. In groups of four, have participants draw a large shield on paper and divide it into six parts as shown.

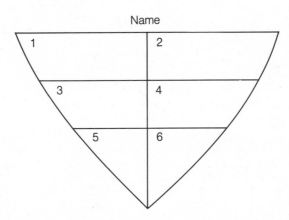

2. Have them place their names at the top of the shield. Explain that this is their personal nursing shield and symbolizes various aspects of themselves as nurses.

3. Request that the areas in the shield be numbered from one to six.
4. Ask participants to draw in the designated area pictures or symbols that answer the following six questions:
   a. What or who was significant to me in developing a desire to become a nurse?
   b. Describe the "best" nurse I knew/know.
   c. What do I believe is the essence of nursing to be?
   d. What signifies my personal practice in nursing?
   e. How do I experience my body at work?
   f. In five years, if all were ideal, how would I be as a nurse?
5. After completing the shield, ask the groups of four to discuss their shields with each other. Suggest that they explore the symbols, reasons, thoughts, and feelings that went into each picture.
6. Discuss the experience.

Variations

The questions to be answered and pictured in the shield can be changed according to the needs of the group.

Discussion

It is necessary for a person to explore globally the various feelings and experiences that formulated what the person is professionally today. From this point, the person can begin to conceptualize the ideal versus reality.

SELECTED BIBLIOGRAPHY ON
EXPERIENTIAL LEARNING

The following are suggested as sources of further humanistic exercises.

Benne, K., Bradford, L., & Gibb, J. (Eds.). (1975). *The laboratory method of changing and learning.* Palo Alto, CA: Science and Behavior Books.

Brill, N. (1976). *Teamwork: Working together in human services.* Philadelphia: Lippincott.

Corey, G., & Corey, M. (1977). *Groups: Process and practice.* Monterey, CA: Brooks/Cole.

Crosbie, P. (1975). *Interaction in small groups.* New York: Macmillan.

Dyer, W. (1972). *Modern theory and method in group training.* New York: Van Nostrand Reinhold.

Egan, G. (1970). *Encounter: Group processes for interpersonal growth.* Monterey, CA: Brooks/Cole.

Egan, G. (1973). *Face to face: The small-group experience and interpersonal growth.* Monterey, CA: Brooks/Cole.

Ellenson, A. (1973). *Human relations.* Englewood Cliffs, NJ: Prentice-Hall.

Finch, F., Jones, H., & Litterer, J. (1976). *Managing for organizational effectiveness: An experiential approach.* New York: McGraw-Hill.

Gazda, G., Asbury, F., Balzer, F., Childers, W., Desselle, R., & Walters, R. (1973). *Human relations development.* Boston: Allyn and Bacon.

Gazda, G., Asbury, F., Balzer, F., Childers, W., Desselle, R., & Walters, R. (1977). *Human relations development* (2nd ed.). Boston: Allyn and Bacon.

Golembiewski, R., & Blumberg, A. (Eds.). (1970). *Sensitivity training and the laboratory approach: Readings about concepts and applications.* Itasca, IL: F. E. Peacock.

Golembiewski, R., & Blumberg, A. (Eds.). (1973). *Sensitivity training and the laboratory approch: Readings about concepts and applications* (2nd ed.). Itasca, IL: F. E. Peacock.

Golembiewski, R., & Blumberg, A. (Eds.). (1977). *Sensitivity training and the laboratory approach: Readings about concepts and applications* (3rd ed.). Itasca, IL: F. E. Peacock.

Goodstein, L., & Pfeiffer, J. (Eds.). (1983). *The 1983 annual for facilitators, trainers, and consultants.* San Diego: University Associates.

Grove, T. (1976). *Experiences in interpersonal communication.* Englewood Cliffs, NJ: Prentice-Hall.

Harvard Business Review—On human relations. (1979). New York: Harper and Row.

Howe, L. (1977). *Taking charge of your life.* Niles, IL: Argus Communications.

Johnson, D. (1981). *Reaching out: Interpersonal effectiveness and self-actualization* (2nd ed.). Englewood Cliffs, NJ: Prentice-Hall.

Johnson, D., & Johnson, F. (1975). *Joining together: Group theory and group skills.* Englewood Cliffs, NJ: Prentice-Hall.

Jones, J., & Pfeiffer, J. (Eds.). (1975). *The 1975 annual handbook for group facilitators.* La Jolla, CA: University Associates.

Jones, J., & Pfeiffer, J. (Eds.). (1977). *The 1977 annual handbook for group facilitators.* La Jolla, CA: University Associates.

Jones, J., & Pfeiffer, J. (Eds.). (1979). *The 1979 annual handbook for group facilitators.* La Jolla, CA: University Associates.

Jones, J., & Pfeiffer, J. (Eds.). (1981). *The 1981 annual handbook for group facilitators.* La Jolla, CA: University Associates.

Kemp, C. (1970). *Foundations in group counseling.* New York: McGraw-Hill.

Kolb, D., Rubin, I., & McIntyre, J. (1974). *Organizational psychology: An experiential approach* (2nd ed.). Englewood Cliffs, NJ: Prentice-Hall.

Krupar, K. (1973). *Communication games.* New York: Free Press.

Lieberman, M., Yalom, I., & Miles, M. (1973). *Encounter groups: First facts.* New York: Basic Books.

Lifton, W. (1972). *Groups: Facilitating individual growth and societal change.* New York: Wiley.

Luft, J. (1970). *Group processes: An introduction to group dynamics* (2nd ed.). Palo Alto, CA: National Press Books.

Maier, N., Solem, A., & Maier, A. (1975). *The role-play technique: A handbook for management and leadership practice.* La Jolla, CA: University Associates.

Morris, K., & Cinnamon, K. (1974). *A handbook of verbal group exercises.* Kansas City, MO: Applied Skills Press.

Morris, K., & Cinnamon, K. (1975). *A handbook of non-verbal group exercises.* Kansas City, MO: Applied Skills Press.

Napier, R., & Gershenfeld, M. (1981). *Groups: Theory and experience* (2nd ed.). Boston: Houghton-Mifflin.

O'Banion, T., & O'Connell, A. (1970). *The shared journey: An introduction to encounter.* Englewood Cliffs, NJ: Prentice-Hall.

Pfeiffer, J., & Goodstein, L. (Eds.). (1982). *The 1982 annual for facilitators, trainers, and consultants.* San Diego: University Associates.

Pfeiffer, J., Heslin, R., & Jones, J. (1976). *Instrumentation in human relations training* (2nd ed.). La Jolla, CA: University Associates.

Pfeiffer, J., & Jones, J. (Eds.) (1974–1981). *A handbook of structured experiences for human rela-tions training* (8 vols.). La Jolla, CA: University Associates.

Pfeiffer, J., & Jones, J. (Eds.). (1976). *The 1976 annual handbook for group facilitators.* La Jolla, CA: University Associates.

Pfeiffer, J., & Jones, J. (Eds.) (1978). *The 1978 annual handbook for group facilitators.* La Jolla, CA: University Associates.

Pfeiffer, J., & Jones, J. (1979). *Reference guide to handbooks and annuals* (3rd ed.). La Jolla, CA: University Associates.

Pfeiffer, J., & Jones, J. (Eds.) (1980). *The 1980 annual handbook for group facilitators.* San Diego: University Associates.

Saulnier, L., & Simard, T. (1973). *Personal growth and interpersonal relations.* Englewood Cliffs, NJ: Prentice-Hall.

Schein, E., & Bennis, W. (1965). *Personal and organizational change through group methods: The laboratory approach.* New York: Wiley.

Vaughn, J., & Deep, S. (1975). *Instructor's manual to accompany program of exercises for management and organizational behavior.* Beverly Hills: Glencoe Press.

Vaughn, J., & Deep, S. (1975). *Program of exercises for management and organizational behavior.* Beverly Hills: Glencoe Press.

Appendix

Key to Abbreviations

A.A.	Alcoholics Anonymous	IV	intravenous
AC	before meals	lb(s)	pound(s)
ANA	American Nurses' Association	L & W	living and well
BID	twice per day	mg	milligram
BP	blood pressure	MI	myocardial infarction
BRP	bathroom privileges	min	minute
BS	blood sugar	MS	morphine sulfate
BUN	blood urea nitrogen	NLN	National League for Nursing
CBC	complete blood count	O^2	oxygen
CCU	coronary-care unit	OOB	out of bed
c̄	with	PC	after meals
cc	cubic centimeters of fluid	PO	given orally
c/o	complains of	PRN	according to necessity
ECG	electrocardiogram	Pt	patient
FBS	fasting blood sugar	PVC	premature ventricular contraction
GI	gastrointestinal		
h	hour	Q	every
HS	hour of sleep	QD	every day
ICU	intensive-care unit	Q 2h	every two hours
I & O	intake and output	QH	every hour

403

QHS	every night	tbl	tablespoon
QID	four times per day	TPR	temperature, pulse, and respiration
S/A	sugar and acetone		
SC	subcutaneously	U-100	units of insulin—100
S. Car.	South Carolina	VDRL	venereal disease research laboratory—test for syphilis
STT	particular waves on an ECG		

Name Index

Subject Index